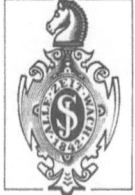

T. Nakashima M. Kojiro

Hepatocellular Carcinoma

An Atlas of Its Pathology

Foreword by H. Popper

With 368 Figures, Mostly in Color

Springer Japan KK

TOSHIRO NAKASHIMA, M.D.
Professor Emeritus, Kurume University School of Medicine
Chief, Research Institute, Kurume Koga Hospital, Kurume, 830 Japan

MASAMICHI KOJIRO, M.D.
Professor and Chief, The First Department of Pathology,
Kurume University School of Medicine, Kurume, 830 Japan

ISBN 978-4-431-68336-0   ISBN 978-4-431-68334-6 (eBook)
DOI 10.1007/978-4-431-68334-6

© Springer Japan 1987
Originally published by Springer-Verlag Tokyo in 1987
Softcover reprint of the hardcover 1st edition 1987

Typesetting: Asco Trade Typesetting Ltd., Hong Kong

Foreword

Hepatocellular carcinoma is one of the most common fatal malignancies of mankind. Up to a few decades ago it was looked upon as a cancer which aroused mainly academic concern but relatively little clinical interest, because its therapy and prognosis had a most unfavorable outlook. Indeed, it was mostly recognized only at autopsy. Recently this pessimism has radically changed and is disappearing to a rapidly accelerating degree. Many of the scientific contributions at this change in outlook are the result of research in the Far East, first, Japan and then gradually extending to its neighbors. The introduction of experimental hepatocarcinogens by Yoshida more than 50 years ago may have been one of the first important steps. Hepatocellular carcinoma shows a characteristic geographical distribution. With the highest incidence in China, Taiwan, Southeast Asia and sub-Saharan Africa, followed by southern and eastern Europe, while generally the incidence is rather low in western and northern Europe and North and South America.

But this uneven distribution explains only in part the great role of Japanese contributions to hepatocellular carcinoma research, of which this volume represents an excellent example. Many epidemiologic, morphologic, clinical, molecular biologic, and comparative pathologic observations have strongly suggested, if not already proven, the relation between hepatocellular carcinoma and persistent hepatitis B virus infection. This causative relation has raised the possibility of eventual prevention of hepatocellular carcinoma by hepatitis B vaccination, supplemented in the newborn by hyperimmune gamma-globulin. Thus, this one of the most common malignancies may be the first to be eliminated by a vaccine, at least in the bulk of the cases. This heightened interest in the tumor is augmented by the possibility of therapy even after onset of the carcinoma. These Endeavors in this direction have been favored by recent devices for early detection as screening with tumor markers, e.g., alpha-fetoprotein, imaging techniques, and liver biopsy. Indeed, the existence of the small (minute) hepatocellular carcinoma has been recognized. Removal in what has been called the subclinical stage, again mainly supported by Far Eastern investigations, seems to provide frequent 5-year survival by so-called secondary prevention. In addition, in the symptomatic stage, operative and, to a lesser degree, chemotherapeutic strategies appear to be becoming increasingly successful.

The key to diagnosis and prognosis in these therapeutic attempts is the gross and microscopic pathologic features of the hepatocellular carcinoma and of the surrounding liver. This volume is probably the most completely, attractively, and instructively illustrated atlas of hepatocellular carcinoma in existence. The senior author, who has just retired from his prestigious chair, and his successor and equally gifted colleague leave us this as a heritage of their endeavors in investigating, describing, and classifying hepatocellular carcinoma. They bring together here the results of their extensive investigations published in many journals. Thus, they provide the attending physician, surgeon, gastroenterologist, and radiologist with information invaluable in their attempts at management. The authors had the opportunity to collect, catalogue, and study with various techniques unusual material which has been worked up in an exemplary and meticulous fashion. The result is a most informative, luxuriously illustrated, and esthetically pleasing book. I hope that the reader will get as much pleasure as I did from studying the illustrations with their learned legends and useful introductions.

New York   HANS POPPER, M.D. Ph. D.

Preface

With the remarkable advances in diagnosis and therapy for hepato-cellular carcinoma and the discovery of a possible pathogenetic role of hepatitis B virus, the study of this malignancy is entering a new era. Parallel to this, development of the pathological study of hepatocel-lular carcinoma is expected.

At the time of the transition to this new era, we publish this book in which we present our accumulated pathomorphogical knowledge of hepatocellular carcinoma, based on the examination findings in 439 cases of hepatocellular carcinoma autopsied at our department during the past 20 years. We are indebted to the colleagues who assisted us during this time. We are also grateful to Professors Wataru Mori of Tokyo University, Kunio Okuda of Chiba University, Masahiko Okudaira of Kitazato University, and Nobu Hattori of Kanazawa University, Emeritus Professor Toru Miyaji of Osaka University, late Professor Robert L. Peters of the University of Southern California, Professors Teruyuki Nakashima and Minoru Morimatsu of the Second Department of Pathology of Kurume University, the physicians and surgeons of the Departments of Medicine and Surgery of Kurume University Hospital, colleagues in our department, and many other friends for their helpful comments and encouragement.

We also extend our appreciation to Mr. Kimitaka Inamasu and Mr. Kazuo Takashima for photomicrographs and Springer-Verlag Tokyo for their kind cooperation in publication.

Many of the studies in this book were supported by a grant-in-aid for cancer research from the Ministry of Health, a grant-in-aid for scientific research from the Ministry of Education, Science and Cul-ture, and the Sarah Cousins Fund.

We hope that this book will contribute to advances in the study of hepatocellular carcinoma.

Kurume, Japan   TOSHIRO NAKASHIMA

MASAMICHI KOJIRO

Contents

Chapter 4: Histological Growth Patterns of Hepatocellular Carcinoma

Chapter 5: Angioarchitecture of Hepatocellular Carcinoma

Chapter 6: Tumor Thrombus of the Hepatic and Portal Veins

Chapter 7: Intra-Atrial Tumor Invasion in Hepatocellular Carcinoma

Chapter 8: Tumor Growth in the Bile Ducts in Hepatocellular Carcinoma

Chapter 9: Extrahepatic Metastasis of Hepatocellular Carcinoma

Chapter 10: Hepatocellular Carcinoma and Liver Cirrhosis

Chapter 11: Hepatitis B Virus and Hepatocellular Carcinoma

Chapter 12: Hepatocellular Carcinoma and Multiple Cancer

Chapter 13: Histological Changes in Hepatocellular Carcinoma Associated with Transcatheter Arterial Embolization Therapy

Chapter 14: Tissue Culture of Hepatocellular Carcinoma Cells and Hetero-Transplantation to the Nude Mouse

Chapter 15: Metastatic Liver Cancers

Introduction

History of Studies on Hepatocellular Carcinoma

The description of liver cancer in the second century A.D. by the Greek physicians Galen and Aretaeus is cited as the oldest record of this tumor [1]. Morgagni [2] has been referred to as a pioneer of pathological anatomy; his work ushered in the dawn of medicine in a true sense, and he also left his mark on liver cancer research. The case of liver cancer he reported, however, was associated with tumors in the stomach and spleen, suggesting a metastatic origin [1]. Virchow [3], who has been called the father of modern pathology, gave a detailed description of the difference between primary liver cancer and metastatic liver cancer. Von Hanseman [4], who reviewed a total of 258 cases of malignant tumor in the liver at the Berlin Pathological Institute, demonstrated that in Europe the incidence of primary liver cancer was far lower than that of metastatic liver cancer. The gross classification of primary liver cancer was further developed by Hanot and Gilbert [5] in 1888 and Eggel [6] in 1901. In 1911, Yamagiwa [7] and Goldzieher and Bokay [8] classified primary liver cancer on the basis of histology. In particular, the classification by Yamagiwa, in which a hepatoma arising from a hepatocyte was differentiated from a cholangioma arising from bile duct epithelium, remained in use throughout the world until quite recently. Outstanding research in this field by Berman [1] and Edmondson and Steiner [9, 10], formed the basis for current investigation of primary liver cancer.

Pathogeographical Characteristics of Hepatocellular Carcinoma

It is a well-known fact that hepatocellular carcinoma (HCC) shows a characteristic geographical distribution. Berman [1] listed South Africa, India, Indonesia, the Philippines, China, and Japan as the countries with a high incidence. HCC is one of the commonest malignant tumors in Asia and South Africa, and in Japan its incidence follows that of gastric cancer, leukemia, and lung cancer. Miyaji [11], reviewing the Annual of Pathological Autopsy Cases in Japan from 1958 to 1973, reported that HCC composes 2.5% of all autopsy cases and is thus far more frequent in Japan than in the United States and Europe. In our department, 439 (8.0%) of 5449 adults autopsied had HCC.

Geographical differences are also noted in age and sex. In most of the areas with high incidence, including Japan, HCC is prevalent in the 6th and 7th decades of life. In South Africa, however, HCC is most frequent in the 4th decade (average age 33.4 years) and more than 50% of the victims are under 30 years old [12]. In the areas of high incidence, HCC is predominant in males, with a frequency several times higher than that in females. However, even in the areas with a low incidence of HCC, such as the United States and Europe, the male to female ratio is around 2.5 : 1.

Geographical differences in the morphological features of HCC are also noted. Okuda et al. [13] reported that the encapsulated type of HCC is more frequent in Japan than in South Africa and the United States. Furthermore, fibrolamellar-type HCC [14], found in a high proportion of young adults with a favorable prognosis, is extremely rare in Asian countries, including Japan, but not so uncommon in the United States.

With such clear geographical differences in HCC, it is predicted that various factors, such as pathogenesis, race, and environment, may be involved. These geographical differences may be clarified in the near future with the increasing exchange of data among researchers in different parts of the world.

Tumor Markers of Hepatocellular Carcinoma

Alpha-fetoprotein (AFP) was first demonstrated in calf serum by Pedersen [15] in 1944, and the appearance of AFP in HCC was first mentioned by Abelev et al. [16] in 1963. In 1964, Tatarinov [17] described the presence of AFP in the serum of a patient with HCC and examination of serum AFP became indispensable for the diagnosis of HCC. The more sensitive radioimmunoassay made it possible to detect minimal alterations of AFP levels, facilitating early diagnosis of HCC in patients with chronic hepatitis and liver cirrhosis, assessment of the effect of therapy, and detection of postoperative recurrence of HCC [18].

Hepatocellular Carcinoma and its Diagnosis by Means of Imaging Techniques

During the past 10 years, diagnostic imaging techniques for the detection of HCC, such as celiac angiography, computed tomography (CT), and ultrasonography (US), have advanced remarkably. These advances have facilitated early diagnosis of HCC, leading to an increase in the number of cases treated by curative surgery.

Hepatocellular Carcinoma and Hepatitis Virus

The close association of HCC with hepatitis virus, in particular hepatitis B virus (HBV), has been proven in South Africa, Japan, and Southeast Asia, where HBV infection is endemic [19–23]. Hepatitis B surface antigen (HBsAg) in serum is more frequently positive in patients with HCC than in controls, and the high incidence of HCC in healthy carriers of HBsAg has been reported from endemic areas [24–26]. In addition to the establishment of HCC cell lines continuously producing HBsAg [27–29], integration of HBV DNA into the hepatocyte DNA has been proven in patients with HCC, and it is presumed that following integration of HBV DNA into the hepatocyte DNA, cancerous changes of hepatocytes may occur after a long latent period. It has been surmised that DNA in liver cells predisposes to structural and functional change subsequent to the incorporation of viral DNA [30–34].

Chapter 1
Gross Features and Gross Classification of Hepatocellular Carcinoma

Hanot and Gilbert [5] first undertook a gross classification of primary liver cancer in 1888. They divided primary liver cancer into three types: (1) *cancer massif*, (2) *cancer nodulaire*, and (3) *cancer avec cirrhose*. This classification was modified in 1901 by Eggel [6], who painstakingly reviewed the records of 164 cases of primary liver cancer, including one of his own cases. His classification is still widely used.

Eggel's Classification

Nodular form. This type occurs as solitary or multiple (few to many) nodules, which vary in size and are sharply demarcated. These cancers accounted for 64.4% of Eggel's cases.

Massive form. Massive tumors involving the whole of the right or left lobe are included in this category. The tumor mass is not well demarcated and is frequently accompanied by small intrahepatic metastatic nodules. Eggel found this type in 23% of cases.

Diffuse form. Numerous small foci, about as large as the pseudolobules of a cirrhotic liver, are scattered throughout the liver. Each focus is surrounded by connective tissue. Grossly, this type is frequently difficult to distinguish from the pseudolobules of liver cirrhosis. This type accounted for 12.4% of Eggel's cases.

Steiner [35] made an epidemiological comparison between HCC in parts of Africa known to have a high incidence and HCC in the United States, and he found that the fundamental macroscopic and histological features of HCC did not vary with race and geographical region, except that the affected livers of Negroes in nine areas of Africa weighed between 3045 and 3891 g and were on average about 800 g heavier than those of Caucasians. He stated that this difference was statistically significant. Recent active cultural exchanges between Japan and other countries have brought us more information about HCC from both Western and African countries. As a result, it has become progressively evident that HCC varies strikingly in its gross features in different parts of the world. According to Okuda et al. [13], who compared the gross features of HCC in the United States, South Africa, and Japan in 1984, the most prominent difference is that the incidence of encapsulated HCC is high in Japan, but low in the other two countries.

Gross Classification of HCC by the Present Authors

Our classification was elaborated under consideration of the following three main factors [36].

Capsule. The incidence of encapsulated HCC, in which there is enclosure by a fibrous capsule, is higher in Japan than in the United States or South Africa [13, 37, 38]. In cases of encapsulated HCC, it is often possible to accomplish a cure by surgery if the diagnosis can be established early, before cancer infiltration extends beyond the capsule and the tumor thrombus of the portal vein is formed. The presence or absence of encapsulation is thus an important factor in the gross classification of HCC.

Liver cirrhosis. Although the incidence of HCC in association with liver cirrhosis varies between about 60% and 90% by report and area, it mostly falls between 70% and 80%. Underlying liver cirrhosis should be taken into consideration because the presence or absence of liver cirrhosis, and its prognosis, greatly influence the gross features of HCC.

Tumor thrombus of the portal vein. HCC invades the portal vein at an early stage, and the tumor thrombus of the portal vein is one of the factors which greatly determine the gross morphological features.

Infiltrative HCC

A typical morphological feature of the infiltrative type is seen in HCC without liver cirrhosis, in which the tumor-nontumor boundary is irregular and indistinct (Figs. 1.1–4). In cases with associated cirrhosis, none of the cancerous foci are clearly demarcated even if all the whole liver slices are examined, and foci varying in size fuse to form larger foci. Such findings suggest that HCC of this type spreads through the liver mainly via the tumor thrombus of the portal vein. At the tumor-nontumor boundary, the tumor extends out as if replacing the pseudolobules of liver cirrhosis (Figs. 1.5–8). Large infiltrative HCC corresponds to Eggel's massive form. This type accounts for 33% of our series.

Expansive HCC

Expansive HCC extends as if it were thrusting intact tissues aside. The foci are sharply demarcated and mostly nodular. Most of the cases associated with liver cirrhosis have a fibrous capsule. In the early stage, tumor infiltration over the capsule and portal vein tumor thrombus are absent or mild. The earlier the diagnosis is established, therefore, the greater the chance of a complete cure by surgery. Expansive HCC is subclassified into the single nodular and the multinodular types.

Single nodular HCC. This type of HCC is relatively clearly demarcated. In particular, those cases associated with liver cirrhosis have a distinct fibrous capsule and are also termed encapsulated HCC (Figs. 1.13, 14). The capsule is, however, frequently indistinct in cases without associated liver cirrhosis (Figs. 1.1–9). Daughter nodules, which also grow in an expansive fashion, are formed around this type of HCC

[39]. The tumor grows expansively by merging with daughter nodules, and the portal veins are occasionally involved (Figs. 1.1–20). This type accounts for 10% of our series.

Multinodular HCC. This type of HCC involves no fewer than two nodules of the expansive type, regardless of intrahepatic metastasis or multicentric origin. The foci are uniform in size and are greater than 2 cm in diameter, with or without liver cirrhosis (Figs. 1.17–24). In the case of the latter, there is a capsule of variable thickness which is apparently nodular (Figs. 1.1–20). This type accounts for 7.7% of our series.

Mixed infiltrative and expansive HCC

The primary foci of expansive HCC may be identified in association with infiltrative foci outside the capsule, intrahepatic metastasis, and/or an intrahepatic tumor whose spread is mediated by a tumor thrombus. This type of HCC, which accounts for 33% of our series, is divided into two subtypes depending on the number of expansive tumor nodules.

Mixed infiltrative and single nodular HCC. A solitary encapsulated HCC with a distinct fibrous capsule, a possible primary focus, is seen together with evidence indicating tumor infiltration beyond the capsule, apparent intrahepatic metastasis, and/or an intrahepatic tumor spreading through a tumor thrombus (Figs. 1.25–28).

Mixed infiltrative and multinodular HCC. Relatively long-standing encapsulated HCC with no fewer than two nodules is seen in association with distinct intrahepatic metastatic foci and/or a tumor spreading via a tumor thrombus of the portal vein (Figs. 1.29–32).

Diffuse HCC

Diffuse HCC (Figs. 1.33–40) occurs as multiple nodules, 0.5–1.0 cm in diameter, scattered throughout the liver, which do not fuse and are always associated with liver cirrhosis. The nodules proliferate as if they were replacing cirrhotic pseudolobules, and are therefore occasionally indistinguishable from such pseudolobules. An intrahepatic tumor spreading through a tumor thrombus of the portal vein plays an important role in forming this type of HCC; however, the diffuse type should be distinguished from the infiltrative type because of the lack of confluence. Diffuse HCC corresponds to *carcinoma avec cirrhose* in the classification by Hanot and Gilbert [5] and to the diffuse form in Eggel's classification [6]. The incidence of this type of HCC varies widely among reports: a figure of 12.4% was reported by Eggel's [6], 17% by Mori [40], 6.2% by Miyaji [41], and we found 5.4% in our series. The discrepancy may be attributed to differences in interpretation.

Special types
In addition to the four basic gross types of HCC described above, there are special
types, such as small liver cancer and pedunculated HCC.

Small liver cancer. Small liver cancer (Figs. 1.41–56) is defined as HCC in the form
of a solitary tumor less than 2 cm in maximum diameter. In the past, it was not of
such great interest because it was found only by chance in autopsy cases. Recent
progress in diagnostic imaging techniques, however, has facilitated detection, and
this has brought about the need for full pathomorphological information about
small liver cancer. In the absence of a widely accepted definition or terminology,
this type of HCC, which is mostly less than 3–5 cm in maximum diameter, was
variously defined and given different names, such as minute HCC and small liver
cancer. Thus, a good deal of confusion ensued from the lack of standardization
[42–45]. In Japan, a solitary HCC less than 2 cm in maximum diameter is defined
as "small liver cancer" in *General Rules for the Clinical and Pathological Study of
Primary Liver Cancer*, issued by the Liver Cancer Study Group of Japan in 1983
[46]. This definition, which is gaining progressively wider currency in Japan, was
employed in our classification.
    The morphological features of noncancerous areas of the liver in victims of small
liver cancer differ markedly between autopsy and surgical cases. In surgical cases,
small liver cancer was found in both noncirrhotic and cirrhotic livers, but liver
function was sufficiently preserved. On the other hand, many small liver cancers
seen in our autopsy cases were associated with advanced cirrhosis in which the
livers were highly atrophic and weighed between 500 and 800 g (Fig. 1.42). A small
liver cancer occurring in a highly atrophic liver may be considered latent carcinoma
rather than early cancer. In fact, some small HCCs remain unchanged in size for a
considerable time, and there have been many clinical reports on long survival
without specific treatment. While small liver cancer in surgical cases is usually
solitary, that found in our autopsy cases was solitary or multiple with about equal
frequency—13 solitary and 14 multiple. The multiple lesions comprised two, three,
or more small cancer nodules up to 2 cm in diameter. Of the multiple cases, those in
which the constituent foci are close together are believed to result from early
intrahepatic metastasis, while a multicentric origin cannot be excluded for those
foci located at some distance from each other (Fig. 1.42c, d).
    A common morphological feature of small liver cancers, seen in both surgical
and autopsy cases, is that they are mostly nodular. However, it is presumed that the
infiltrative type of small liver cancer may be as frequent as advanced HCC (about
30%). Such infrequency of infiltrative small liver cancer among surgical and autopsy cases may be explained by the difficulty of detecting infiltrative small liver cancer
with diagnostic imaging techniques and by the fact that most cases of infiltrative
HCC occur in noncirrhotic livers; few patients die of hepatic failure or other causes
while HCC is small.
    Of tumors greater than 2 cm in diameter found in association with liver cirrhosis,
approximately 70% had a fibrous capsule, but capsule formation was seldom found
in tumors smaller than 1 cm in diameter. Among 10 resected tumors less than 2 cm
in diameter at our institute, capsule formation was not found in all three tumors less
than 1.0 cm in diameter but was found in five tumors between 1.0 and 2.0 cm in
diameter. Thus, capsule formation in HCC seems to become apparent when tumors

increase to 1–2 cm in diameter. When tumors become as large as 3–5 cm in diameter, extracapsular tumor growth and tumor thrombus of the portal vein frequently become evident, leading to changes in morphology to the expansive type.

Some small liver cancers extend in an infiltrative fashion even in the early stage. We once encountered a case of infiltrative small liver cancer in which a remarkable tumor thrombus of the portal vein was grossly evident, although the tumor was only 2 cm in maximum diameter (Figs. 1.1–45)

Pedunculated HCC. Massive tumors proliferating extrahepatically with or without a peduncle are included in the category of pedunculated HCC (Figs. 1.57–64). Edmondson and Steiner [9] suggested that the cases which had been reported by Roux [47] and by Goldberg and Wallenstein [48] should be assigned to a new subclass in the gross classification of HCC. In Japan, since Kato et al. [49] first reported a case of pedunculated HCC, a number of cases of this type, including our cases, have been reported [50–57]. Recent advances in diagnostic imaging techniques have made the diagnosis of pedunculated HCC easier. Ninomiya et al. [54] stressed that celiac angiography was one of the most reliable diagnostic procedures. In addition to celiac angiography, CT scan is considered to be a reliable procedure. Pedunculated HCC is further divided into two subtypes—intrahepatic origin (type I) and extrahepatic origin (type II).

Pedunculated HCC type I. In this type of HCC (Figs. 1.57–59, 61–63), the tumors grow expansively to form a large hemispheric protrusion from the surface of the liver. A cancer of the expansive type which has arisen directly beneath the capsule of the liver extends outside the liver by growth. The addition of extracapsular daughter nodules is also responsible for the formation of prominent extrahepatic protrusions. The occurrence of this type is higher in HCC with expansive growth. Most cases of this type are of well-to moderately differentiated HCC exhibiting a trabecular or pseudoglandular pattern. In our 439 cases of HCC, 17 (3.8%) were type I pedunculated HCC. Horie et al. [53] found three cases (2.4%) of pedunculated HCC among 123 HCC cases.

There are, however, pedunculated tumors which exhibit marked degeneration and/or a sarcomatous appearance, and it is frequently difficult to distinguish these cases from those of HCC concomitant with sarcoma. We have experienced eight such cases (0.2%) in our 439 autopsy findings of HCC. Many of these cases were described as having undergone transformation into sarcomas, because most of these liver tumors and their metastatic foci presented sarcoma-like histological features, although the histological features of typical HCC were demonstrated in part of each tumor.

Pedunculated HCC type II. In cases reported by Miyoshi et al. [57], it was demonstrated by means of celiac angiography that a tumor mass was nourished by means of a branch of the right hepatic artery, although no connection between the liver and the tumor was grossly evident. HCC that develops outside the liver cannot be diagnosed as having arisen from an accessory hepatic lobe, as described by Cullen [58], unless the presence of such a lobe can be proven by the demonstration of liver cells in addition to cancer cells in the relevant area. If no liver cells are evident because they have been completely replaced by tumor cells, it is mere speculation to say that the HCC developed from an accessory hepatic lobe. We have encountered only one case of this type in which the fibrous connection between the extrahepatic tumor and the liver was preserved: The bile duct was found in the tumor tissue, and the presence of numerous intrahepatic metastatic foci suggested metastases through the portal vein. These findings supported the view that this HCC had arisen from an accessory hepatic lobe (Figs. 1.60, 64).

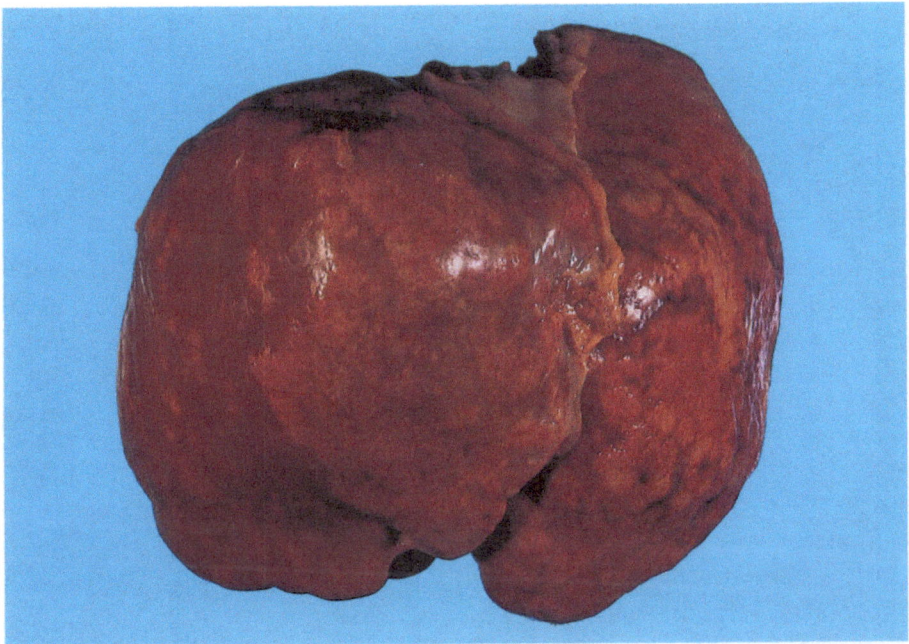

Fig. 1.1. Infiltrative HCC without associated liver cirrhosis. Macular tumor nodules recognizable in liver surface

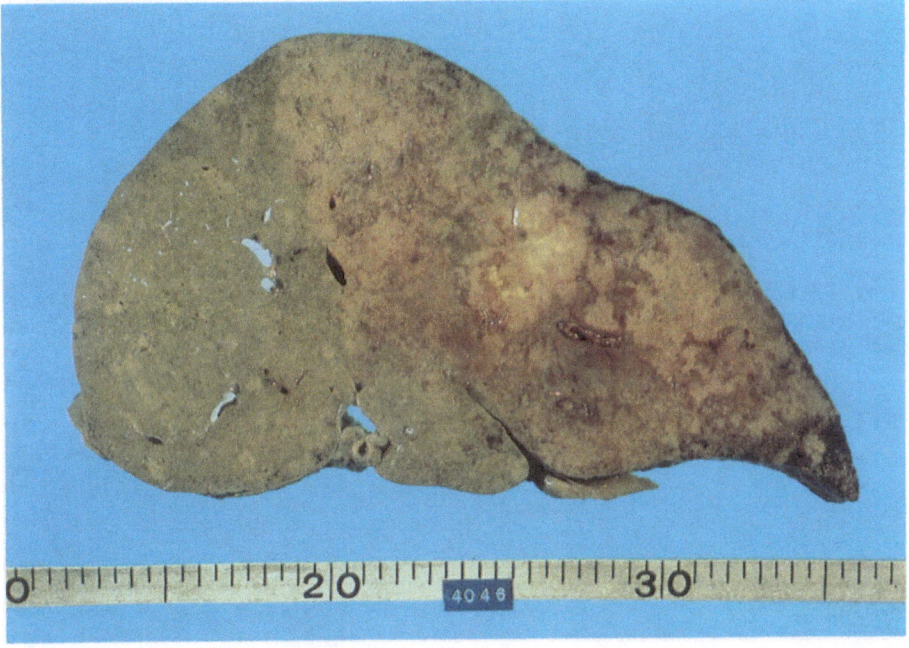

Fig. 1.2. Same case. The tumor is occupying the entire left lobe and proliferating in an infiltrative fashion. The tumor-nontumor boundary is not clear

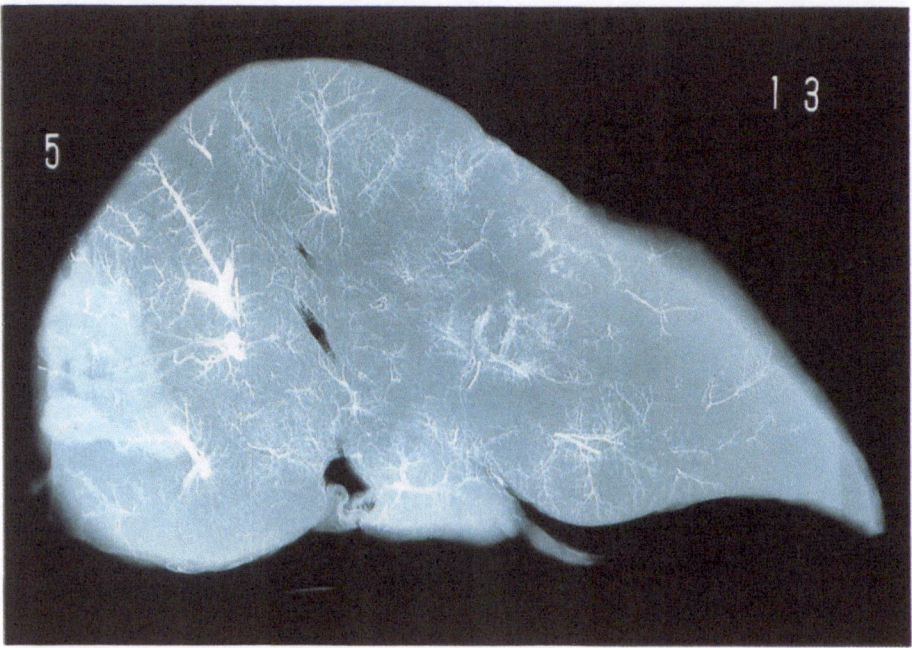

Fig. 1.3. Same case, soft X-ray finding. Tumor shadows are not clear. Contrast medium could not be injected into the portal vein because of obstruction by a massive tumor thrombus

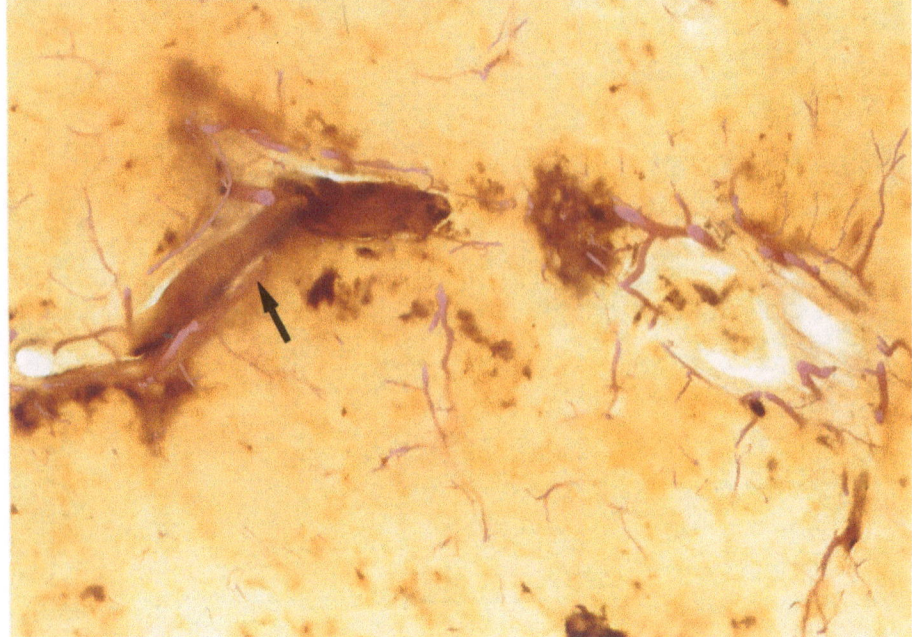

Fig. 1.4. Same case. Portal vein branch is filled with tumor thrombus (*arrow*). The arterial branches are markedly narrowed and interrupted in the cancerous tissue

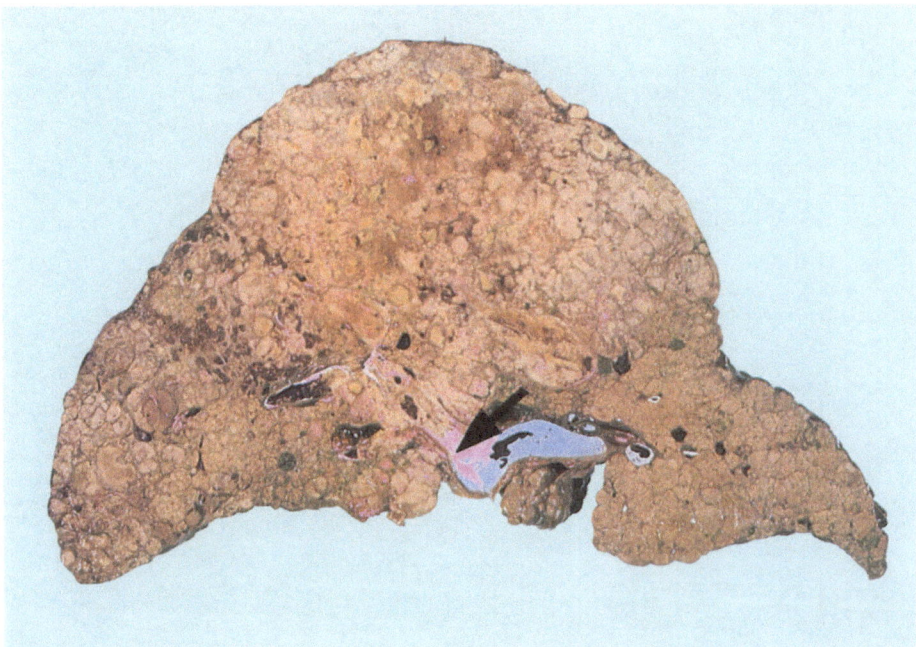

Fig. 1.5. Infiltrative HCC associated with liver cirrhosis. The tumors are proliferating as they replace the cirrhotic pseudolobules. Mixture of arterial blood (*red*) and portal vein blood (*blue*) through tumor thrombus is observed in the portal trunk (*arrow*)

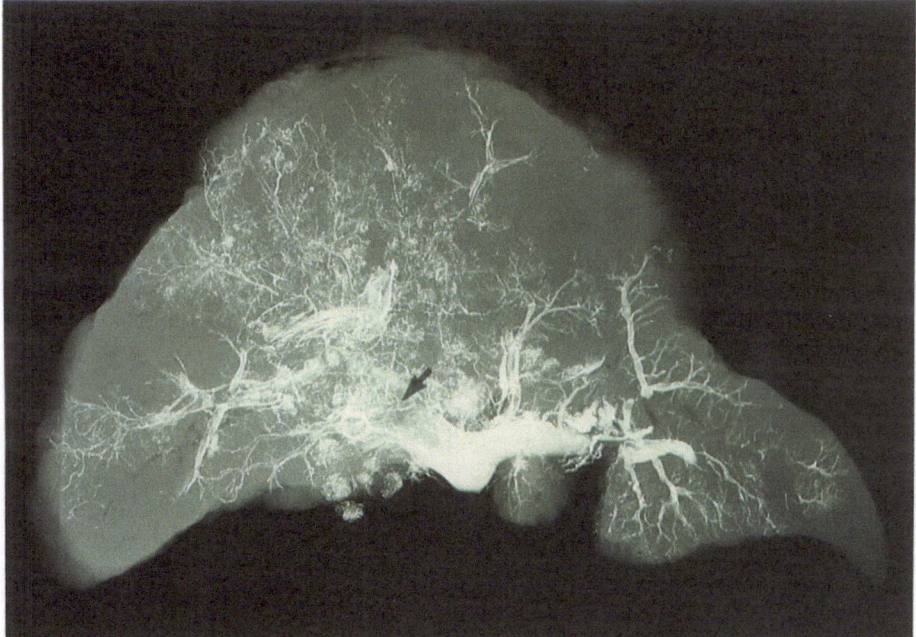

Fig. 1.6. Same case, soft X-ray finding. The confluent tumor is hypervascular. The periportal arterial branches are dilated and the portal vein branches are not demonstrated due to the massive tumor thrombus in the portal trunk (*arrow*)

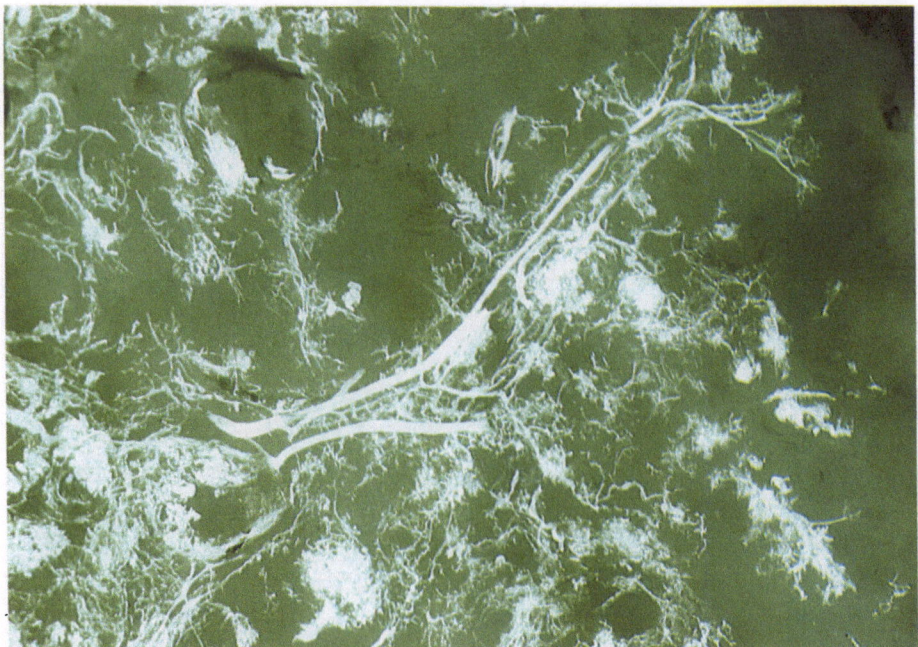

Fig. 1.7. Same case, soft X-ray finding. The periportal arterial branches are markedly dilated and intrahepatic metastatic foci around the portal vein receive arterial tumor vessels from the dilated periportal arteries

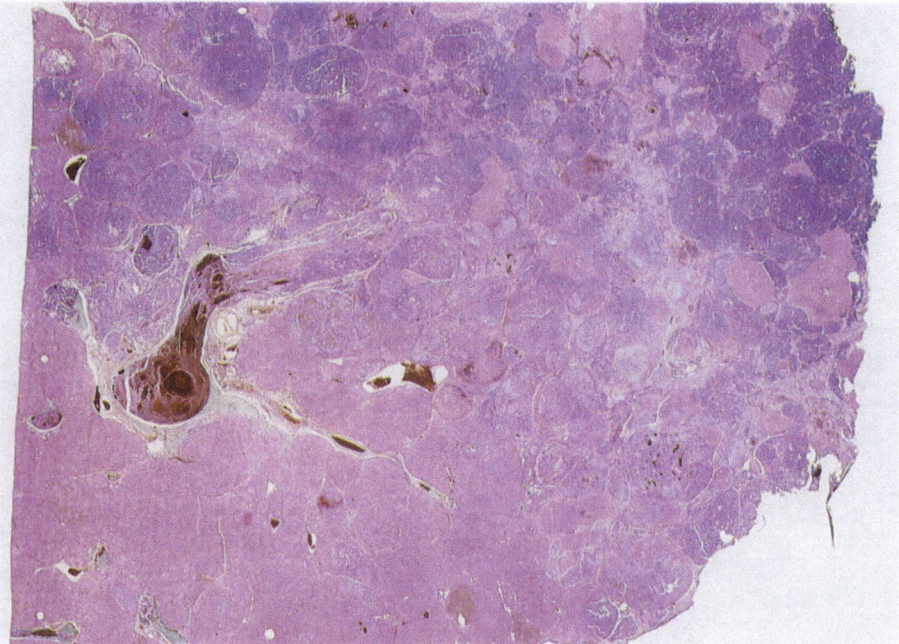

Fig. 1.8. Same case. Numerous tumor nodules are seen around the portal vein, which is filled with a massive tumor thrombus. HE, × 1

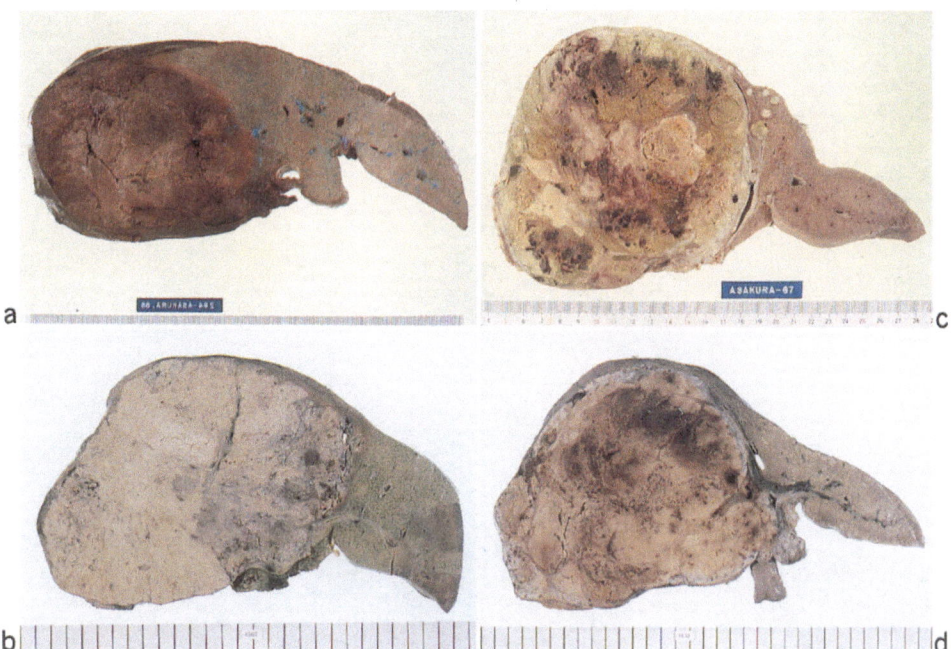

Fig. 1.9. Expansive HCC without associated cirrhosis. The tumors are sharply demarcated and the capsule is distinct (**a, b**) or thin (**c, d**)

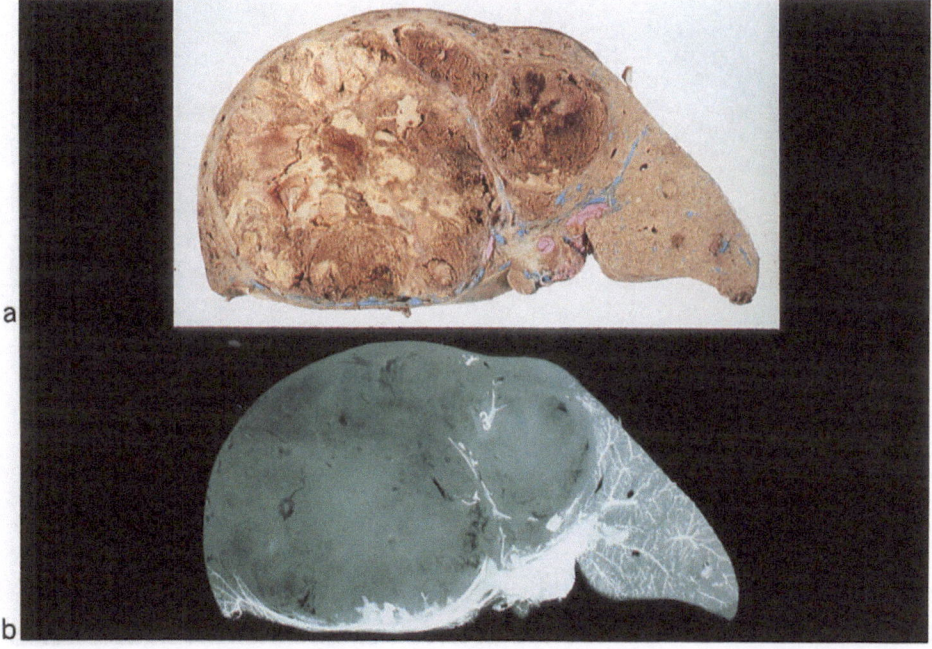

Fig. 1.10a, b. Expansive HCC without associated cirrhosis. The tumor is growing by merging with daughter nodules. Arteries and portal veins in the old capsules are seen as the blood vessels in the fibrous septa within the tumor (**a**). The tumor is hypovascular due to marked necrosis (**b**)

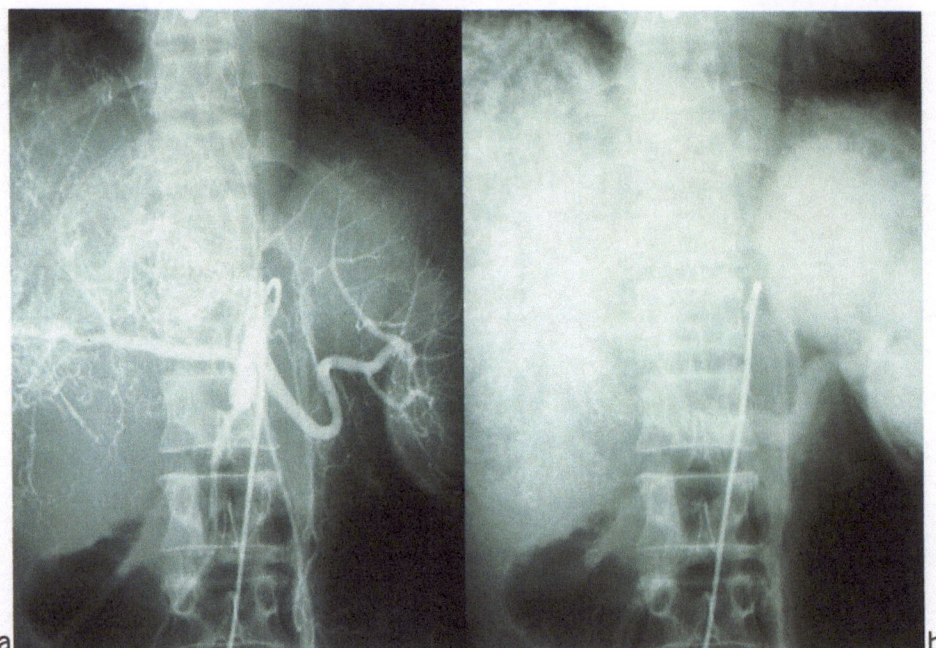

Fig. 1.11a, b. Celiac angiogram of expansive HCC. A hypervascular area in the right lobe in the arterial phase (**a**) corresponds to the marked tumor stain in the capillary phase (**b**)

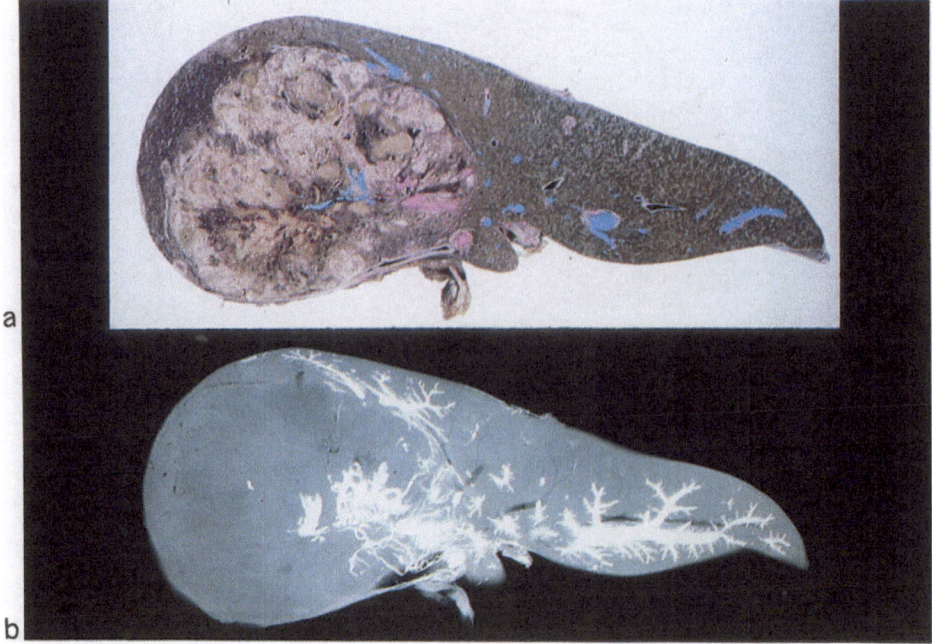

Fig. 1.12a, b. Postmortem angiogram of the same case. Portal veins (*blue*) are observed within the tumor and this finding suggests that the tumor grew by merging with neighboring tumor nodules (**a**). Most parts of the tumor are hypovascular due to necrosis (**b**)

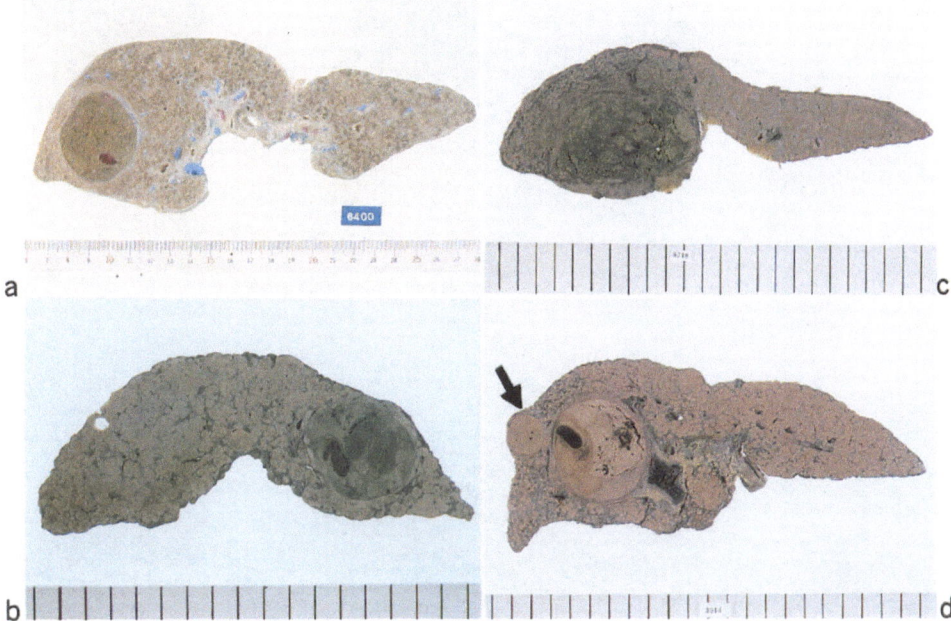

Fig. 1.13a–d. Expansive HCC, single nodular, with liver cirrhosis. The thin fibrous capsule is seen (encapsulated HCC). **d** A daughter nodule (*arrow*) is observed beside the encapsulated HCC

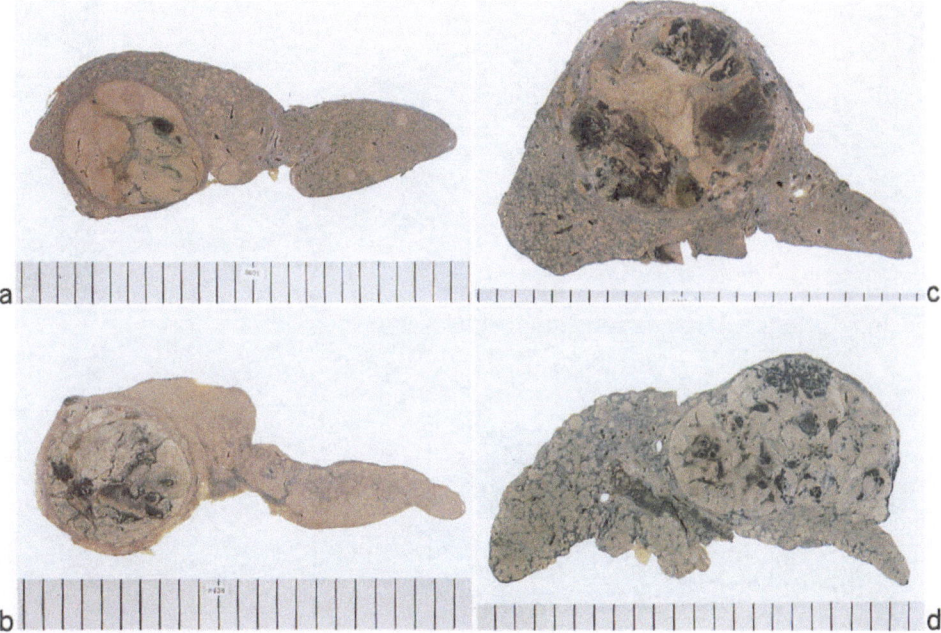

Fig. 1.14a–d. Expansive HCC, single nodular, with liver cirrhosis. A massive encapsulated HCC occupies the entire right or left hepatic lobe. Fibrous septa are seen in all tumors

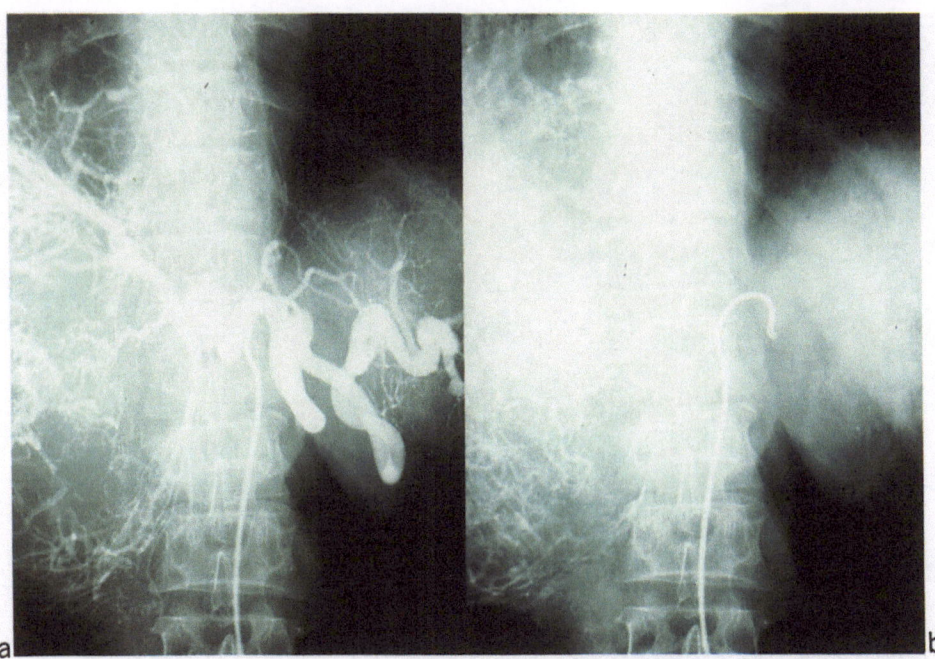

Fig. 1.15a, b. Celiac angiogram of massive, single nodular expansive HCC with liver cirrhosis. **a** Arterial phase: a large hypervascular area in the right hepatic lobe. **b** Capillary phase: the tumor stain corresponds to the hypervascular area in the arterial phase

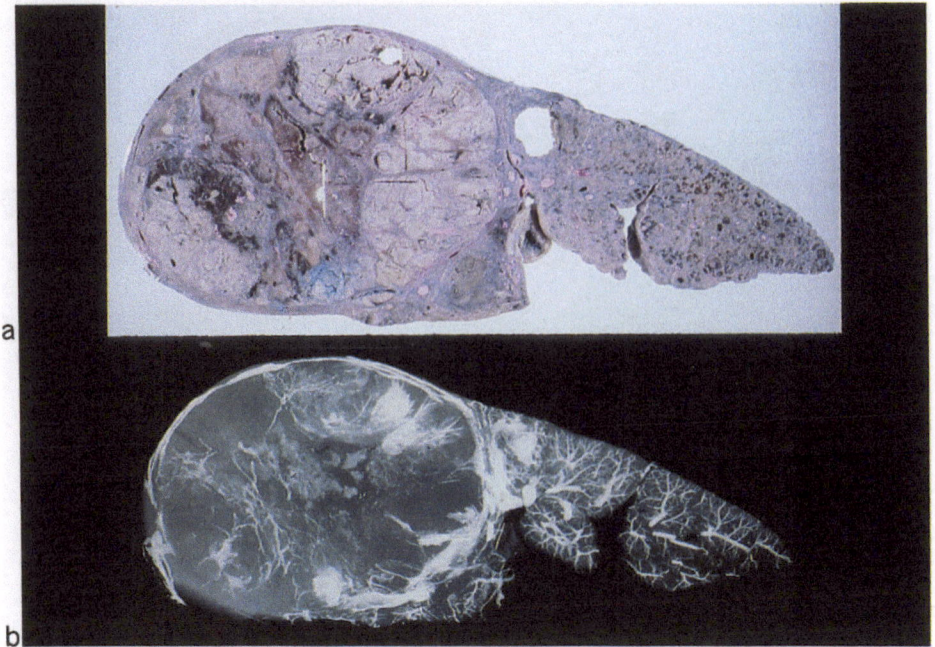

Fig. 1.16a, b. Same case. **a** Fibrous septa are observed in the tumor. **b** Soft X-ray finding: the vasculature of the tumor is different in each of the section divided by the fibrous septa

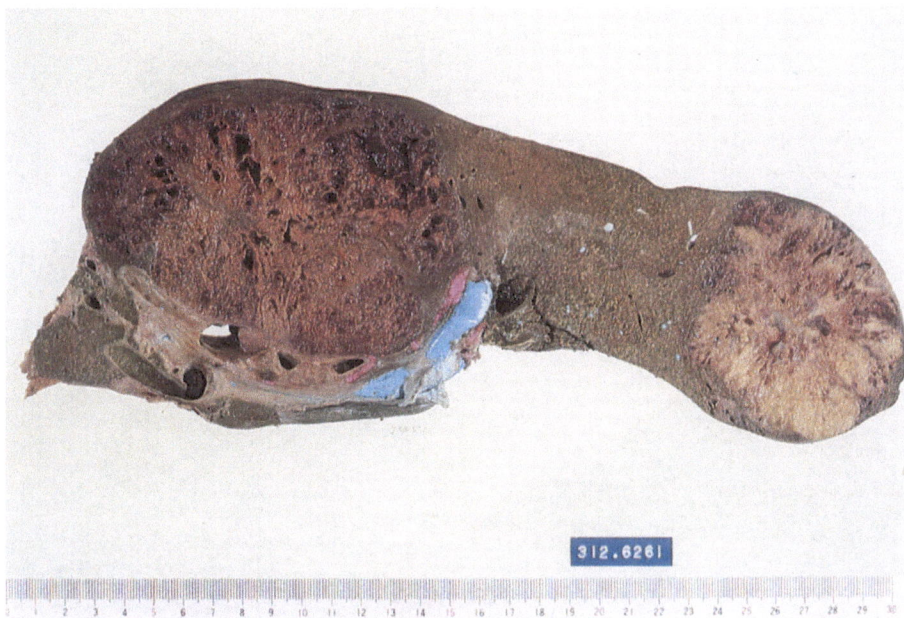

Fig. 1.17. Expansive HCC, multinodular, without liver cirrhosis. Highly necrotic tumors are located in the right and left hepatic lobes. No capsule is recognizable

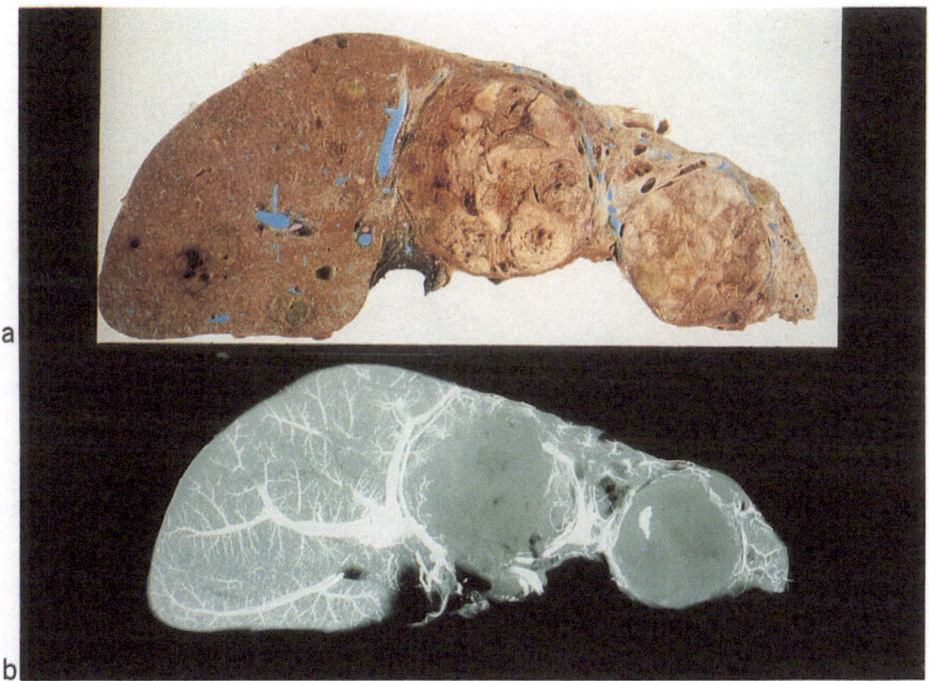

Fig. 1.18a, b. Expansive HCC, multinodular, without liver cirrhosis. **a** Two expansive tumors are located in the left lobe and intrahepatic metastases are seen in the right lobe. **b** Soft X-ray finding. Tumors are hypovascular

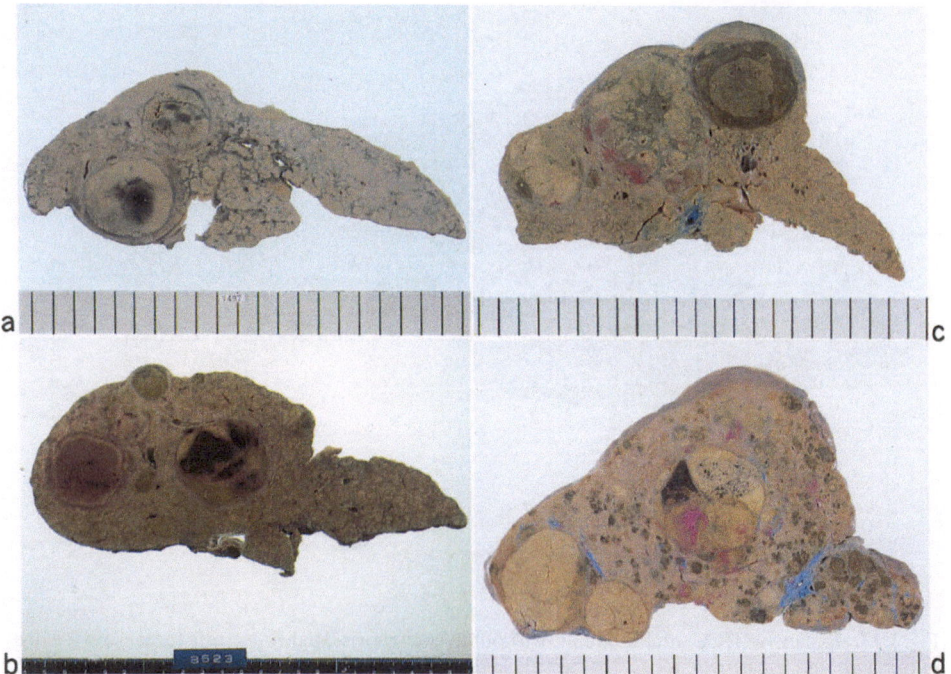

Fig. 1.19a–d. Expansive HCC, multinodular, with liver cirrhosis. Multiple well-demarcated tumors show various gross features

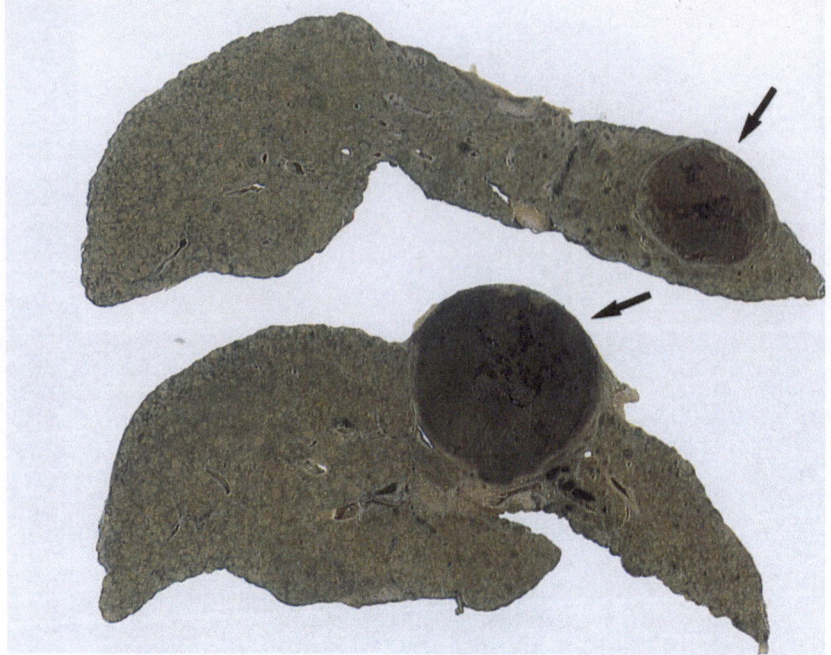

Fig. 1.20. Expansive type HCC, multinodular, with liver cirrhosis. Two encapsulated tumors are seen in different liver slices (*arrows*). Tumors are greenish in color due to marked bile production (so-called green hepatoma)

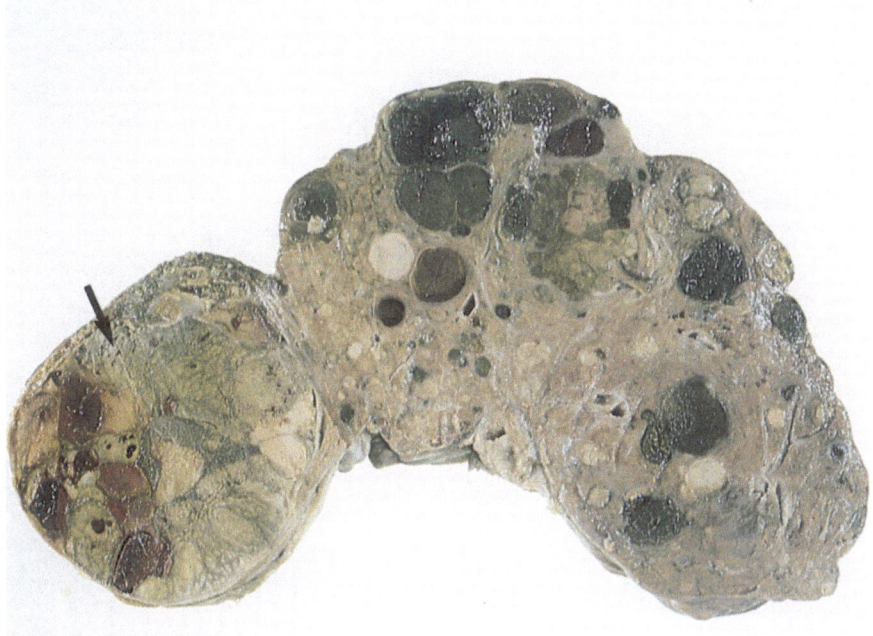

Fig. 1.21. Expansive HCC, multinodular, with liver cirrhosis. Possible primary tumor (*arrow*) in the right hepatic lobe and many intrahepatic metastases in the left lobe.

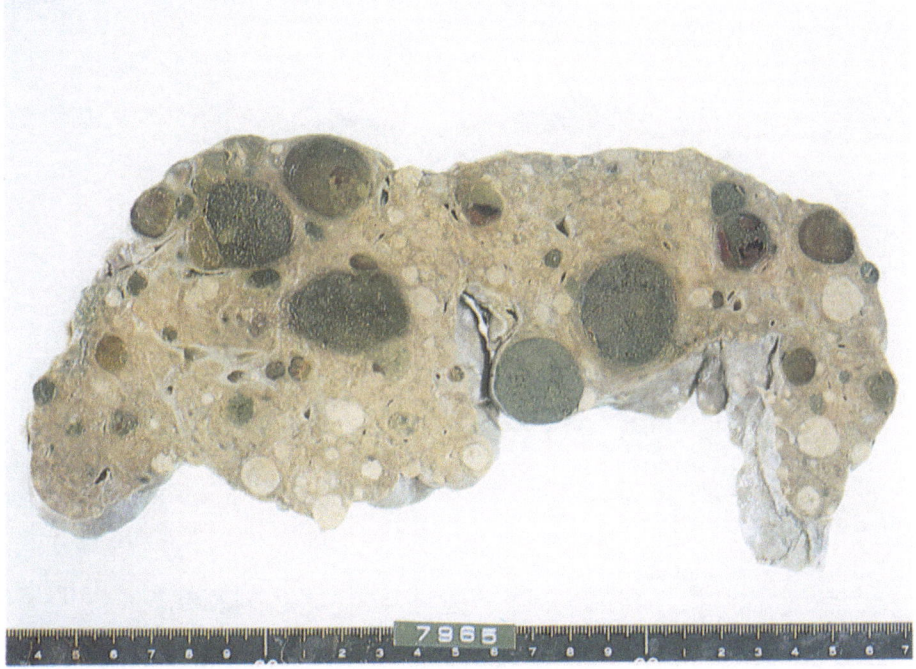

Fig. 1.22. Different slice in the same case. Numerous tumors of varying size are distributed throughout the liver

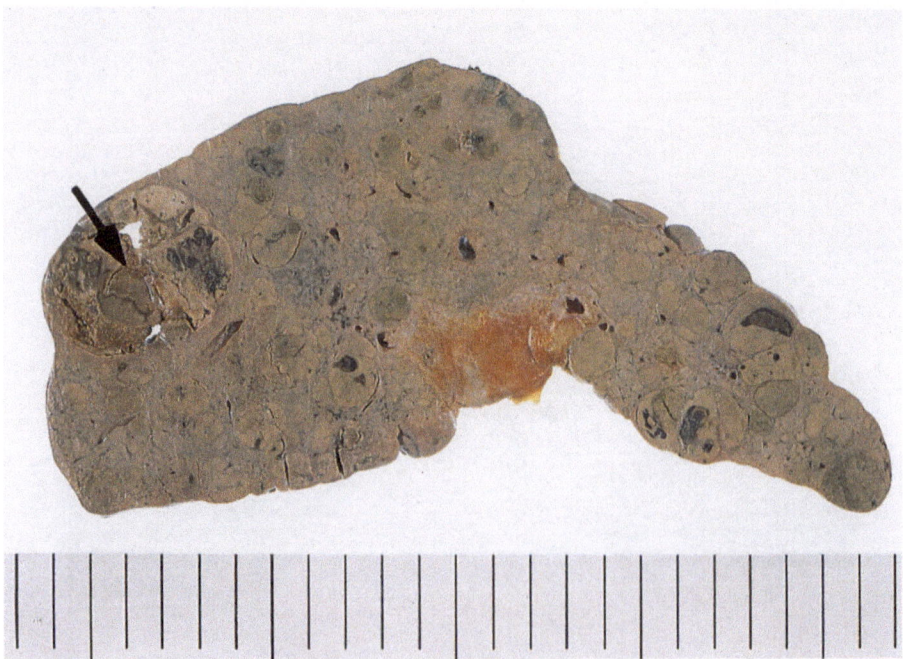

Fig. 1.23. Expansive HCC, multinodular, with liver cirrhosis. Primary focus (*arrow*) in the right hepatic lobe and numerous intrahepatic metastases

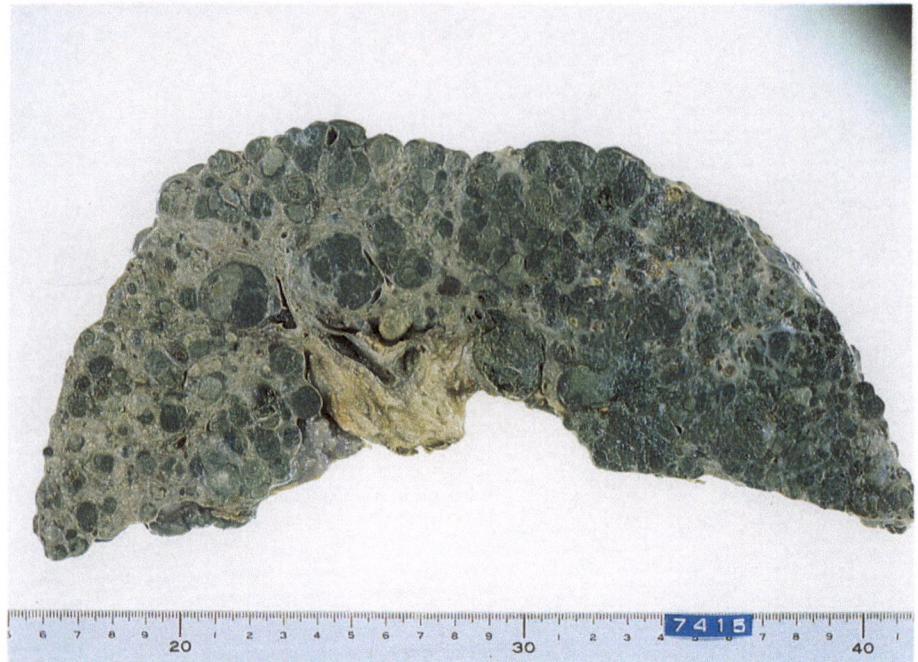

Fig. 1.24. Type of HCC intermediate between multinodular expansive type and diffuse type. There are a few tumors greater than 2 cm in diameter among numerous minute tumor nodules diffusely scattered throughout the liver

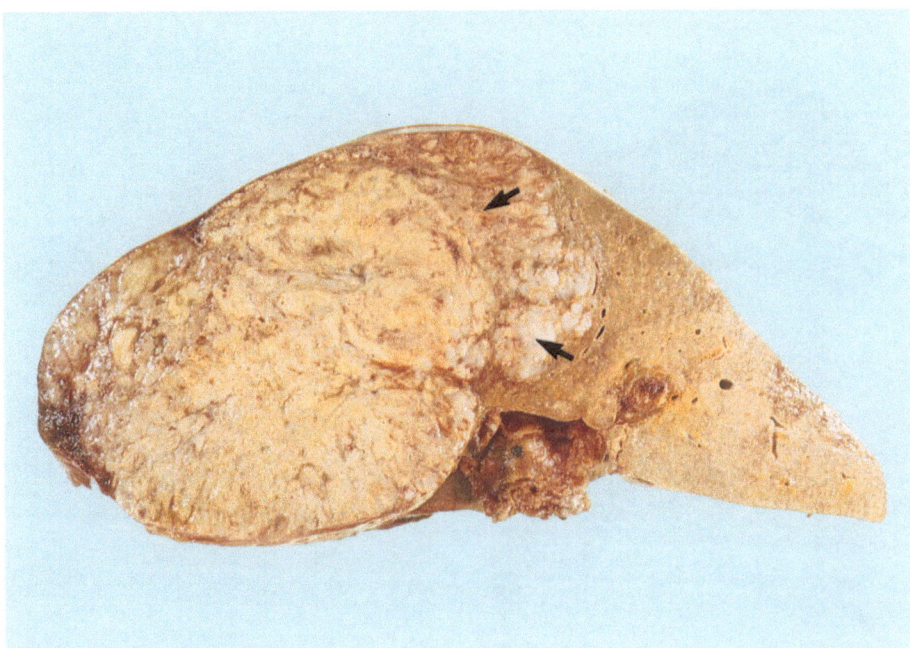

Fig. 1.25. Mixed expansive and infiltrative HCC, single nodular, massive, without liver cirrhosis. Infiltrative tumor growth (*arrows*) is seen beside the main tumor

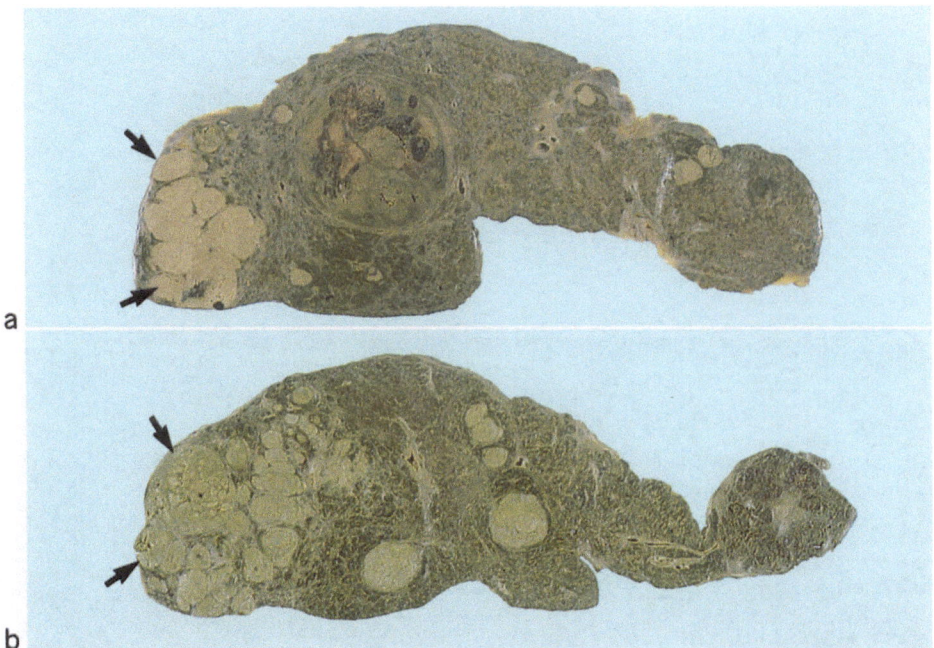

Fig. 1.26a, b. Mixed expansive and infiltrative HCC, single nodular, with liver cirrhosis. **a** Coexistence of well-encapsulated tumor and infiltrative tumor growth (*arrows*). **b** Marked tumor thrombi of the portal vein (*arrows*) with perivascular tumor infiltrates

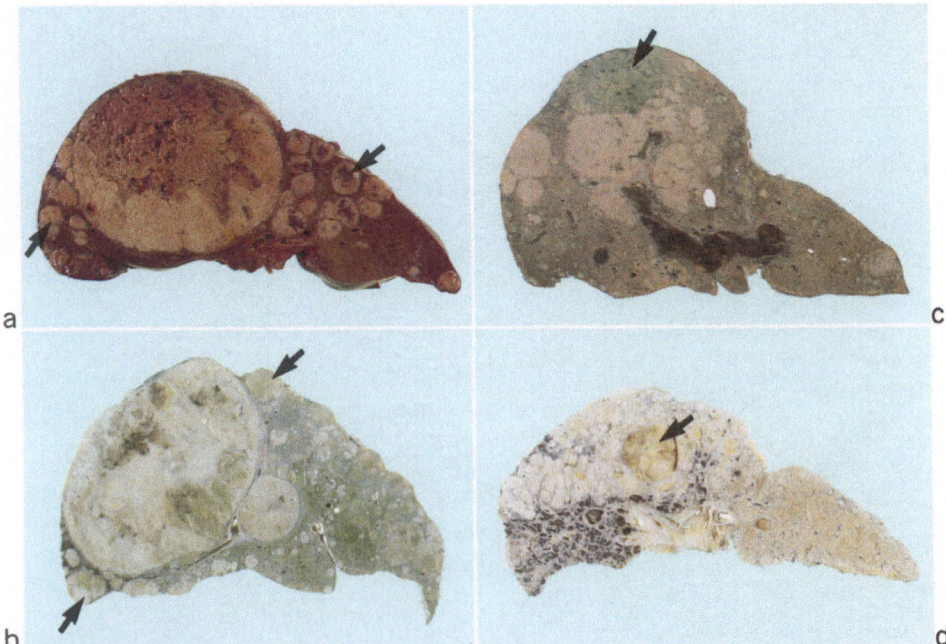

Fig. 1.27a–d. Mixed expansive and infiltrative HCC, single nodular, with liver cirrhosis. **a, b** Large expansive HCC in the right hepatic lobe with many intrahepatic metastases (*arrows*). **c, d** Encapsulated HCC (*arrows*) with infiltrative tumor spread

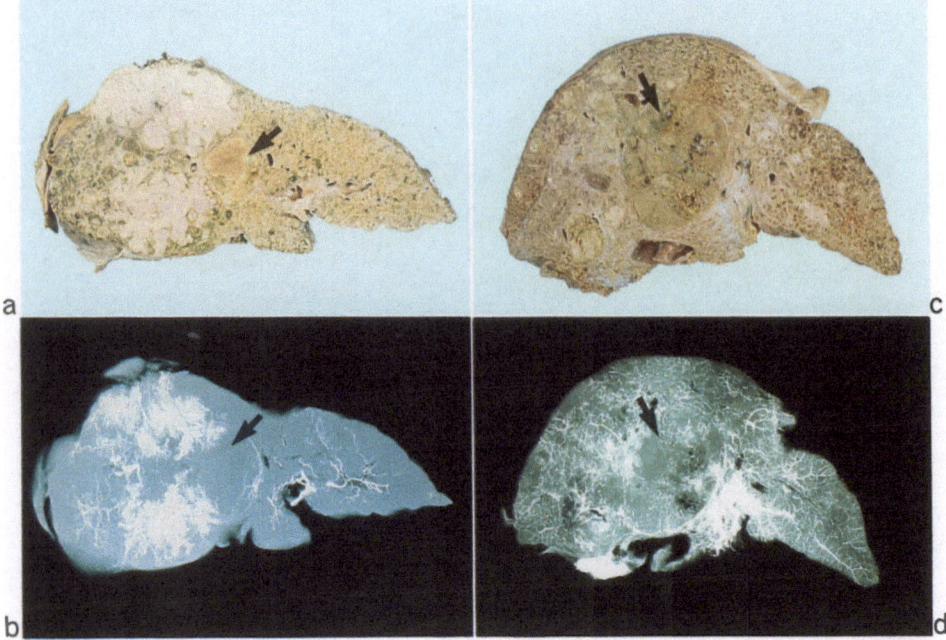

Fig. 1.28a–d. Mixed expansive and infiltrative HCC, single nodular, with liver cirrhosis. **a, c** Highly necrotic encapsulated tumors (*arrow*) with infiltrative tumor growth. **b, d** The encapsulated tumors are avascular or hypovascular (*arrow*), but the infiltrative tumors around the encapsulated ones are hypervascular

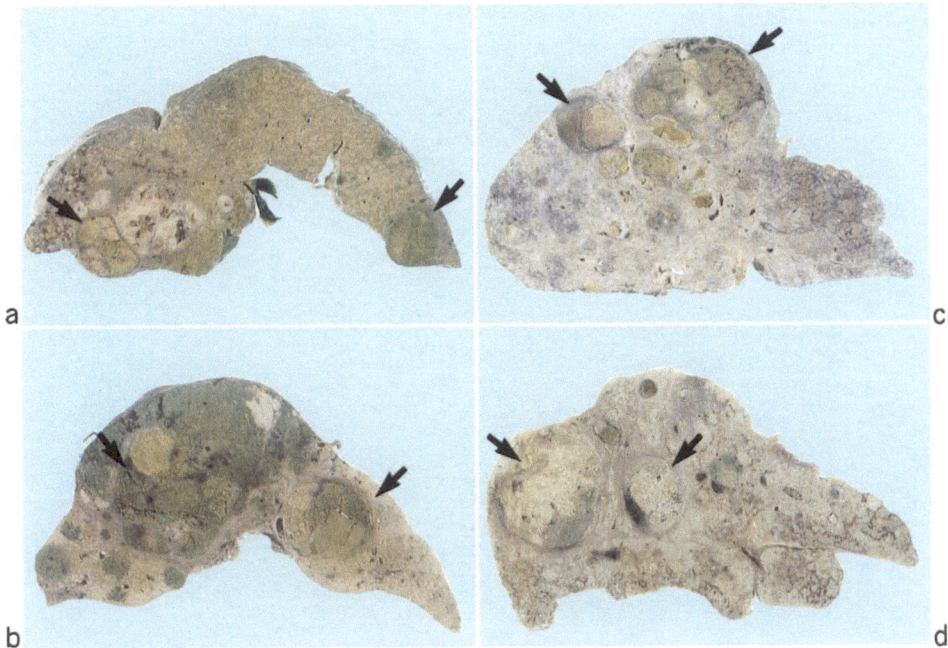

Fig. 1.29a–d. Mixed expansive and infiltrative HCC, multinodular, with liver cirrhosis. There are two encapsulated tumors (*arrows*) with infiltrative tumor growth

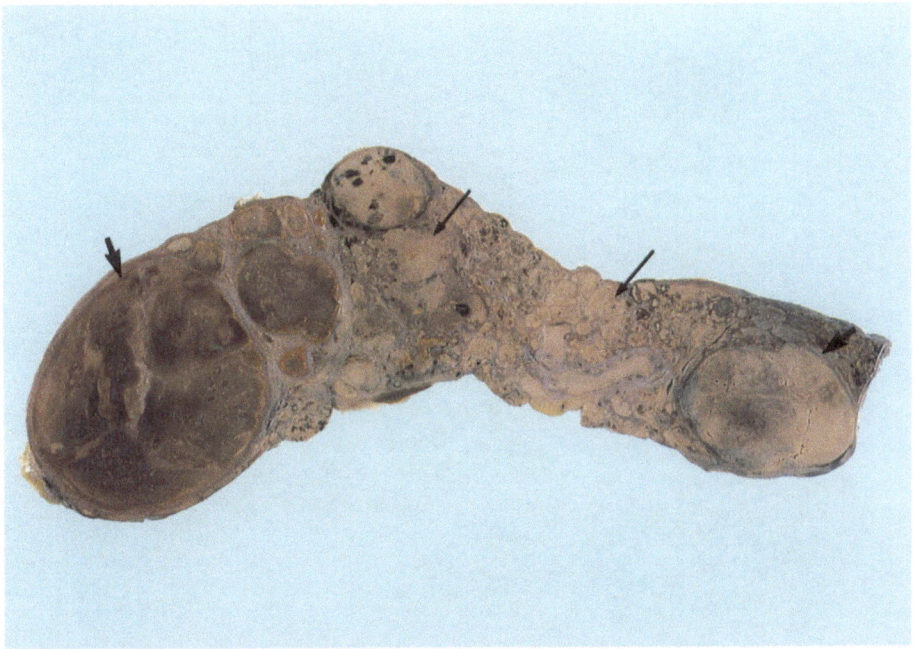

Fig. 1.30. Mixed expansive and infiltrative HCC, multinodular, with liver cirrhosis. Coexistence of well-encapsulated tumors (*thick arrow*) and infiltrative tumors (*thin arrows*)

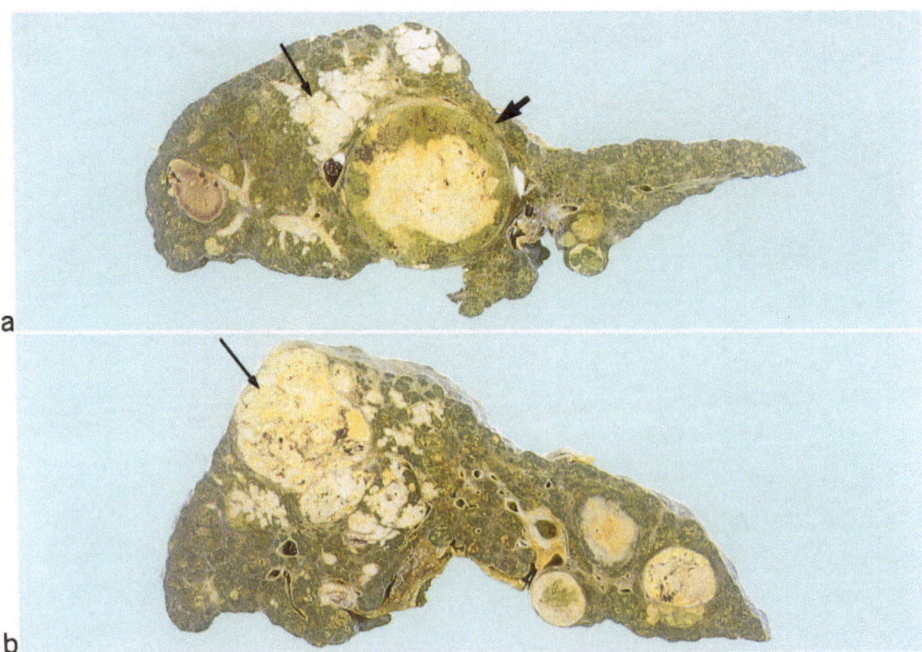

Fig. 1.31a, b. Mixed expansive and infiltrative HCC, multinodular, with liver cirrhosis. Highly necrotic encapsulated tumor (*thick arrow*) and infiltrative tumors (*thin arrow*)

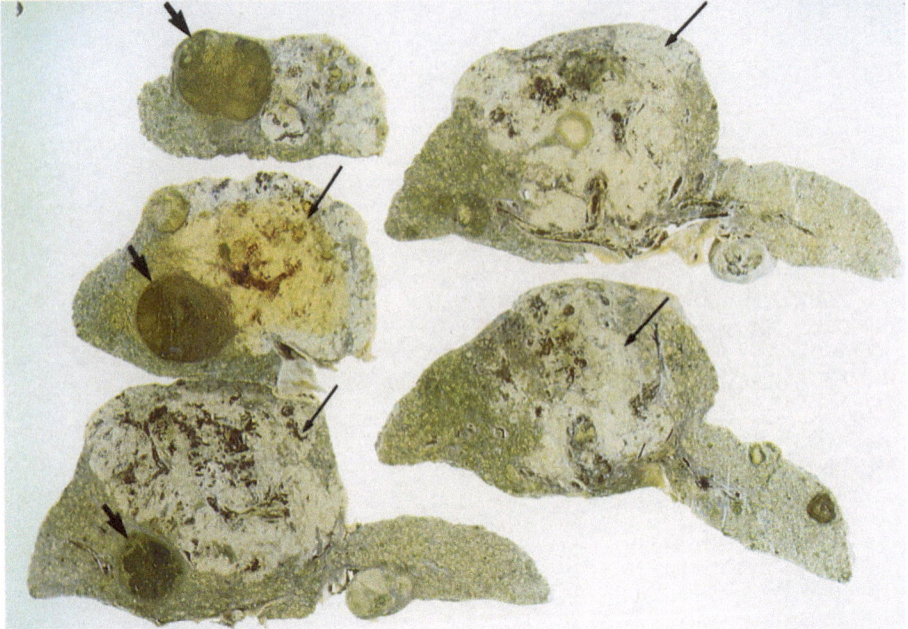

Fig. 1.32. Mixed infiltrative and expansive type HCC, multinodular, with liver cirrhosis. Well-encapsulated tumors (*thick arrows*) and infiltrative tumor spreads (*thin arrows*) are clearly visible in different liver slices

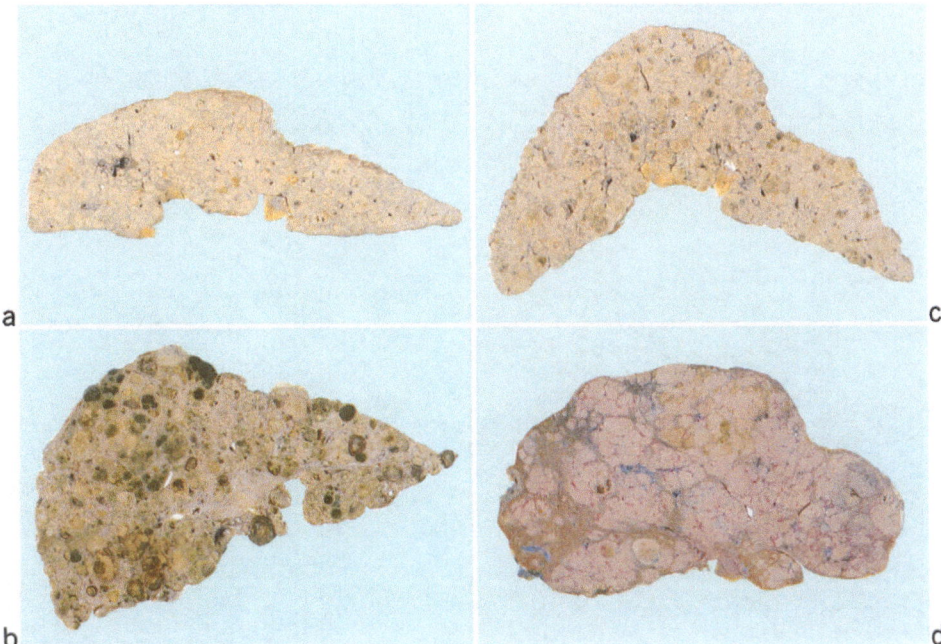

Fig. 1.33a–d. Diffuse HCC with liver cirrhosis. Numerous tumor nodules of similar size to cirrhotic nodules are scattered throughout the liver

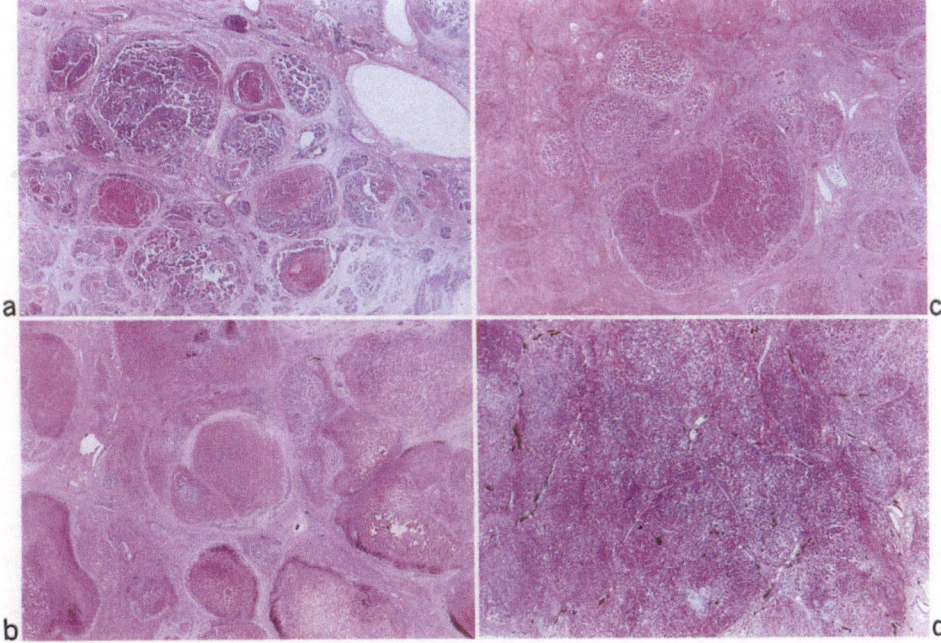

Fig. 1.34a–d. Same cases. **a–c** The tumors are proliferating as they replace the cirrhotic nodules. **d** Thin fibrous stroma is seen between tumor nodules. HE, × 20

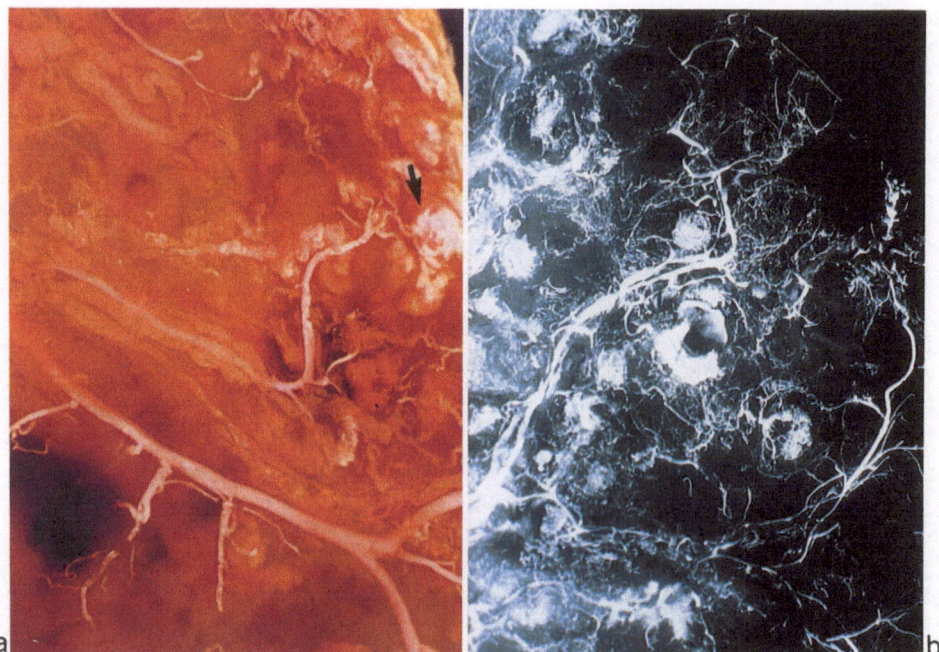

Fig.1.35a, b. Angioarchitecture of diffuse HCC. **a** Transparent preparation: an intrahepatic meta-static focus (*arrow*) receives the arterial tumor vessels. **b** Soft X-ray finding in the same case: the intrahepatic metastatic foci receive the arterial tumor vessels from the dilated periportal arteries

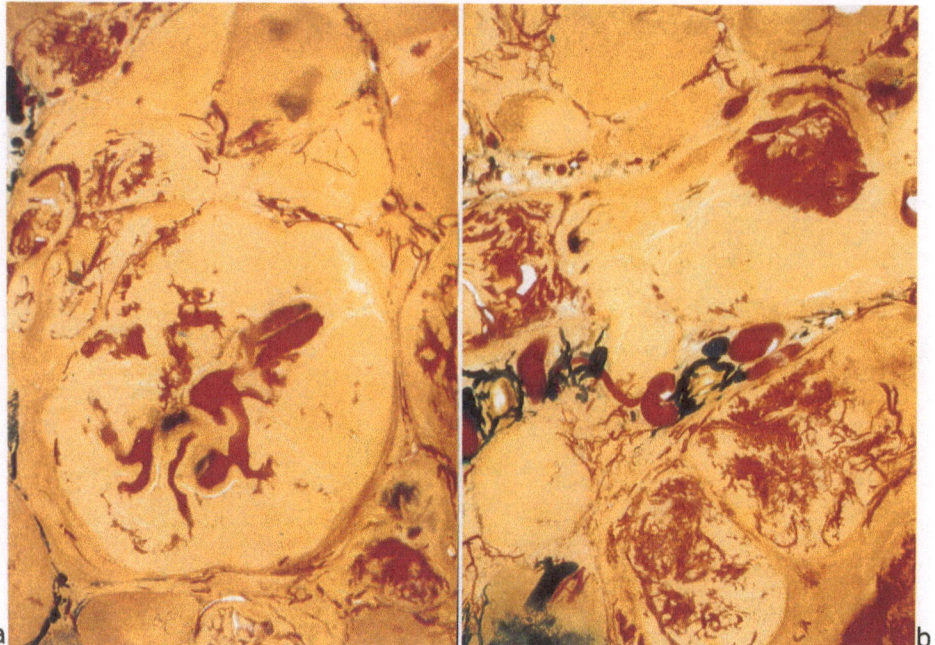

Fig. 1.36a, b. Transparent preparation of diffuse HCC. The vasculature of the tumor nodules consists solely of the arterial tumor vessels

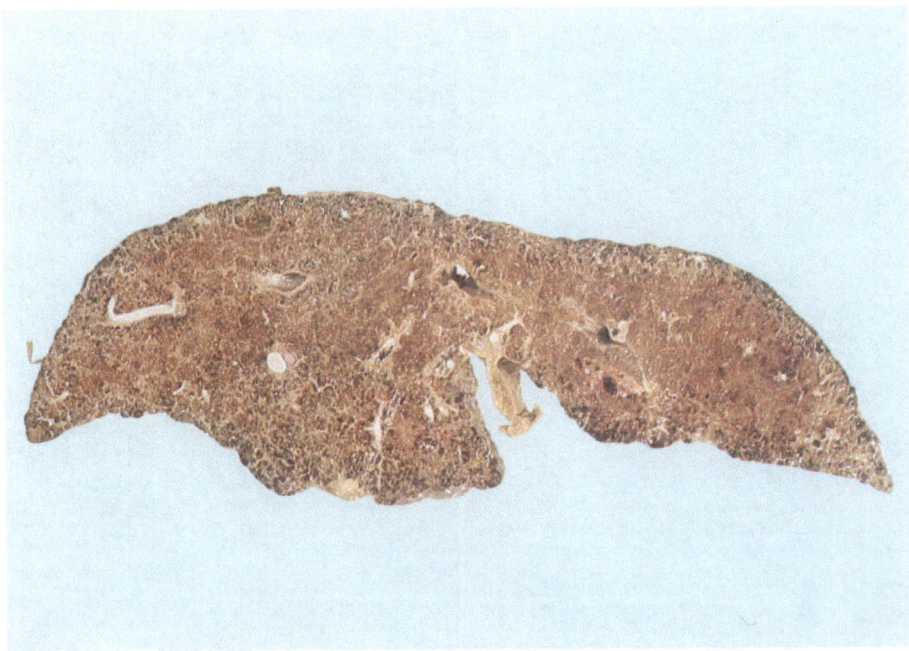

Fig. 1.37. Diffuse HCC. Grossly, the tumorous lesions are difficult to distinguish from the cirrhotic nodules

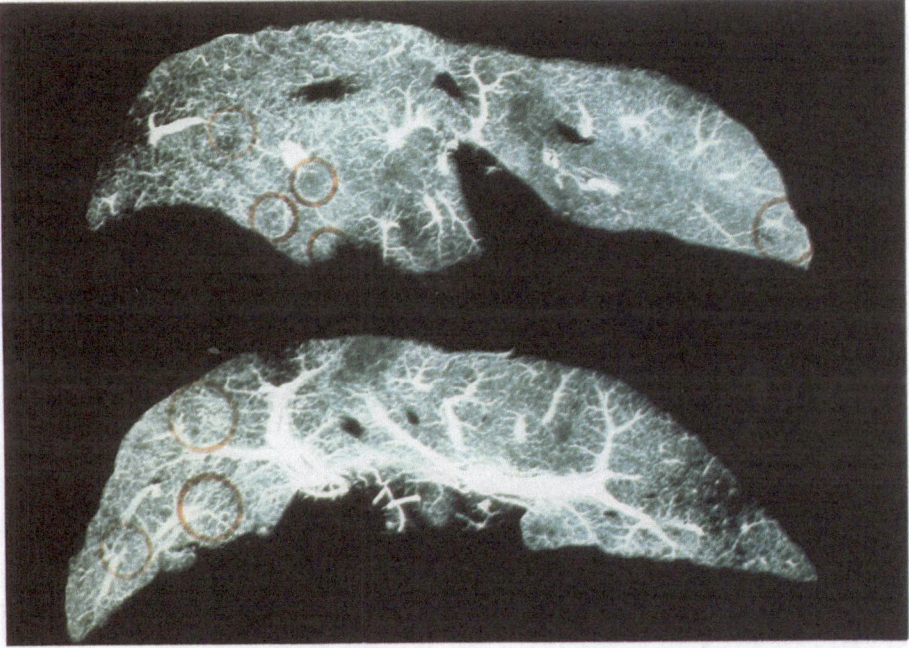

Fig. 1.38. Soft X-ray finding in the same case. The minute tumors (*encircled*) present vasculature different from that of the cirrhotic nodules. They are hypervascular or hypovascular

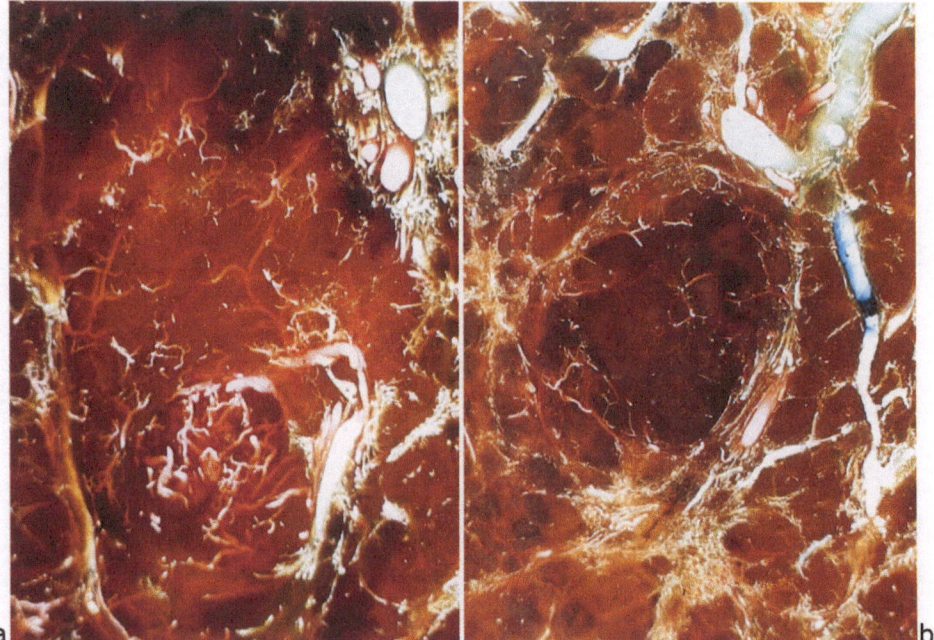

Fig. 1.39a, b. Transparent preparation of the same case. The arterial blood vessels are dominant, even in minute tumor nodules: *red*, artery; *blue*, portal vein

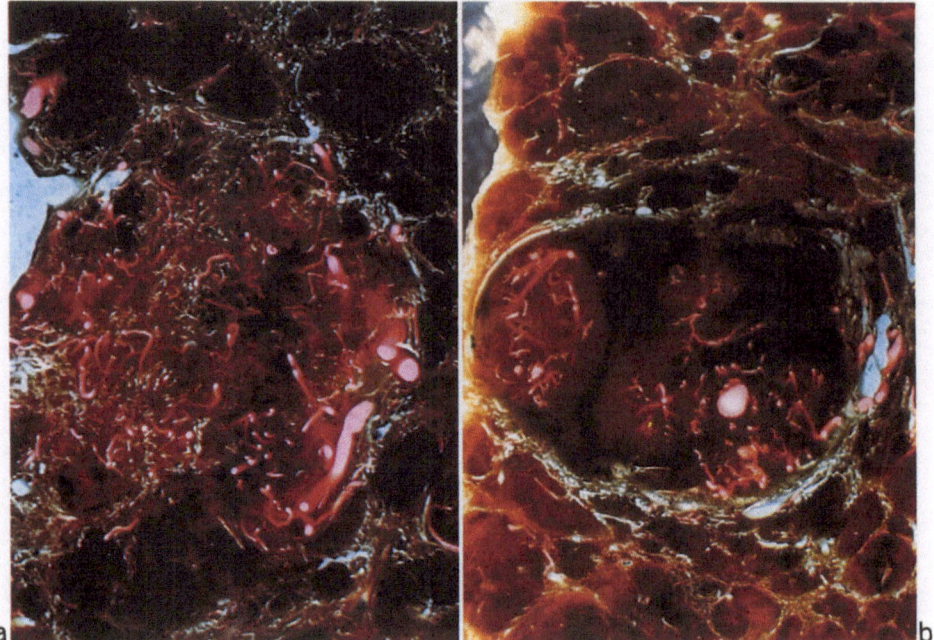

Fig. 1.40a, b. Transparent preparation of the same case. **a** A few portal vein branches remain in some nodules. **b** Compressed portal vein branches are seen only in the periphery of some tumor nodules

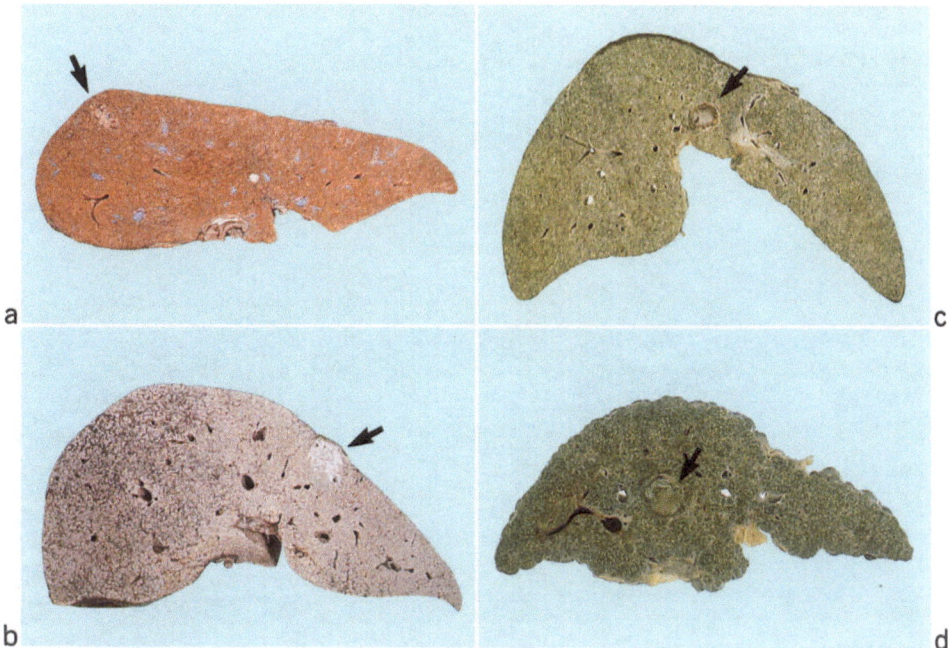

Fig. 1.41a–d. Small liver cancer (*arrows*). **a, b** Infiltrative type. **c, d** Encapsulated expansive tumor nodules. The tumors are less than 2 cm in diameter

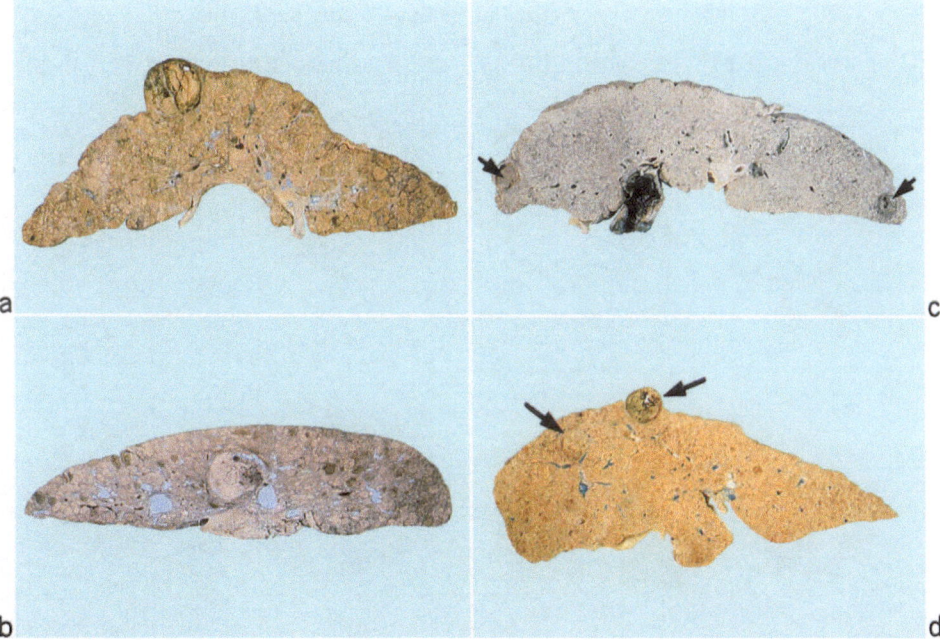

Fig. 1.42a–d. Small liver cancer. **a, b** Solitary tumor of expansive type. **c, d** Multiple tumors (*arrows*)

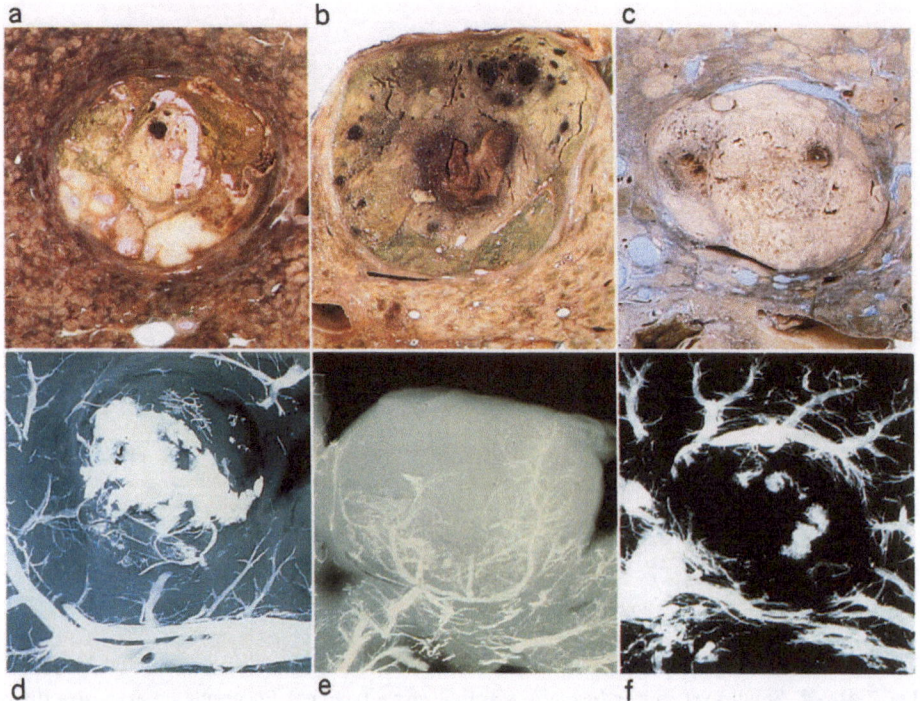

Fig. 1.43a–f. Gross features (**a–c**) and soft X-ray findings (**d–f**) in small liver cancer. The encapsulated tumor nodules have fibrous septa and each tumor shows different vasculature

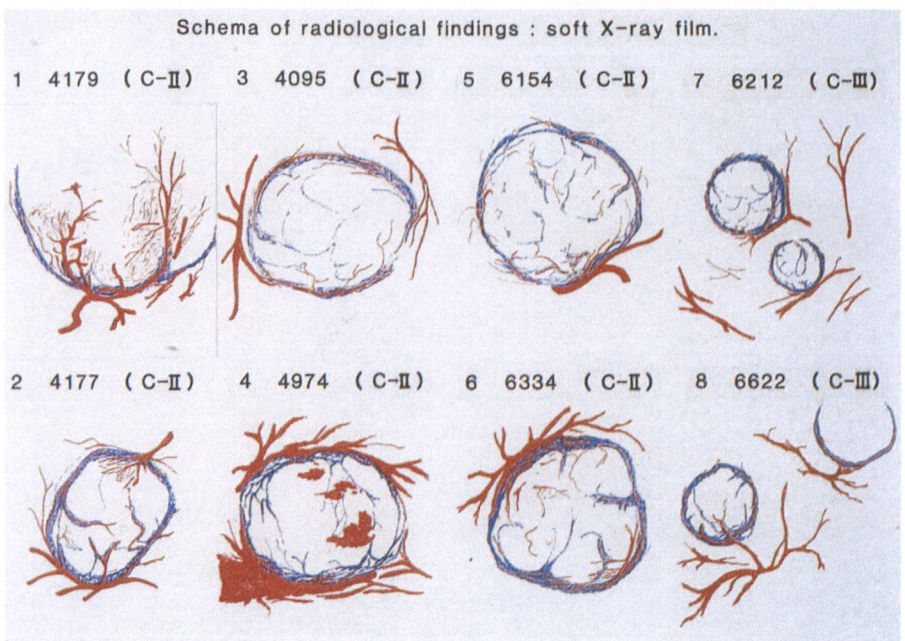

Fig. 1.44. Examples of angioarchitecture of small liver cancer

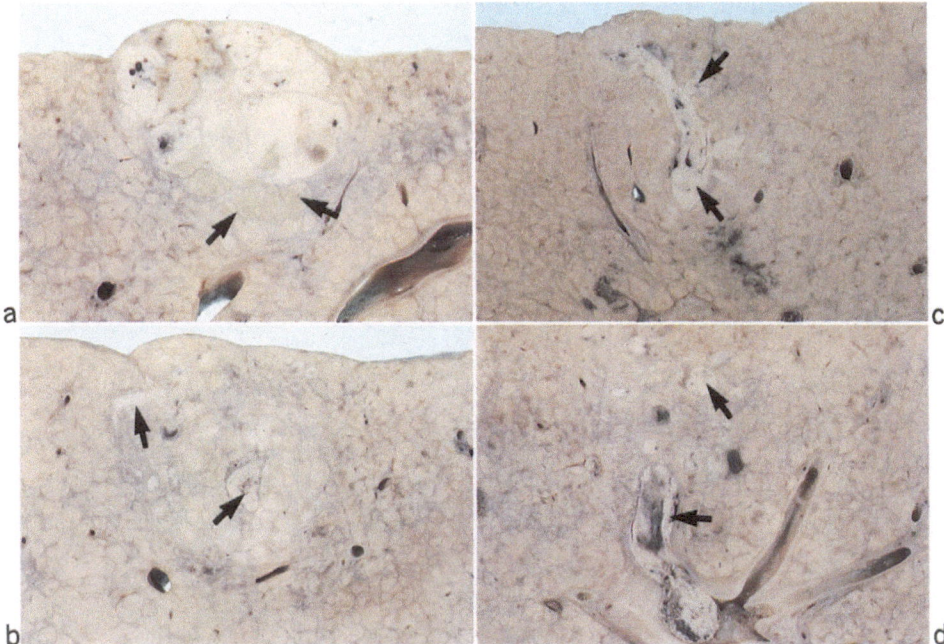

Fig. 1.45a–d. Infiltrative small liver cancer 1.5 cm in diameter. **a** The tumor is not encapsulated. **b–d** Tumor thrombi of the portal vein branches (*arrows*)

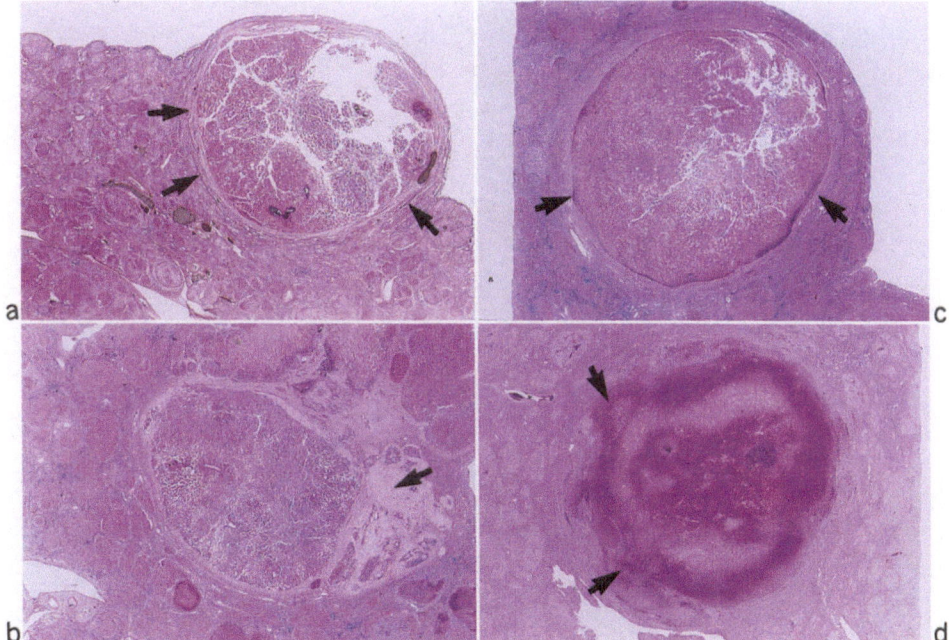

Fig. 1.46a–d. Small liver cancer. **a–c** The tumors are enclosed by fibrous capsule (*arrows*). **d** Small liver cancer of the expansive type with infiltrative growth in places (*arrows*). HE, × 1

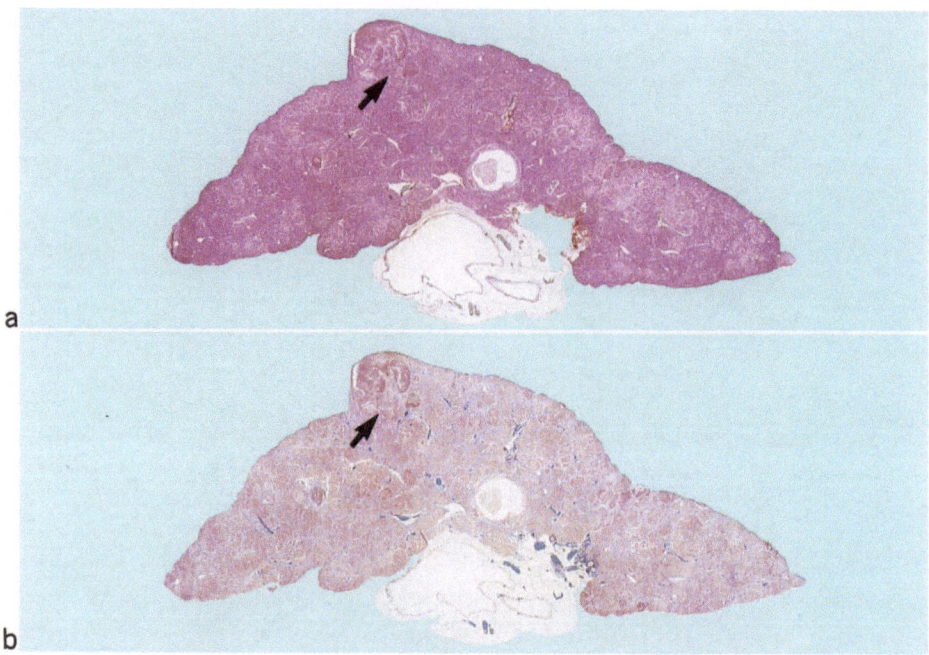

Fig. 1.47a, b. Expansive small liver cancer with liver cirrhosis. Solitary tumor nodule 2 cm in diameter (*arrow*) without capsule. **a** HE, **b** Azan-Mallory

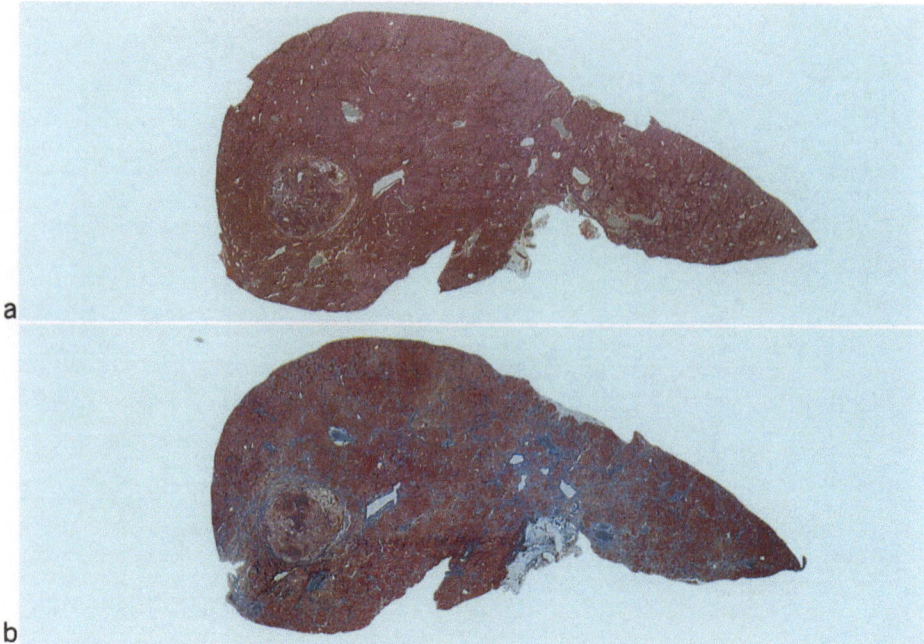

Fig. 1.48a, b. Expansive small liver cancer with liver cirrhosis. Solitary tumor nodule of 2 cm in diameter in the right hepatic lobe with fibrous capsule. **a** HE, **b** Azan-Mallory

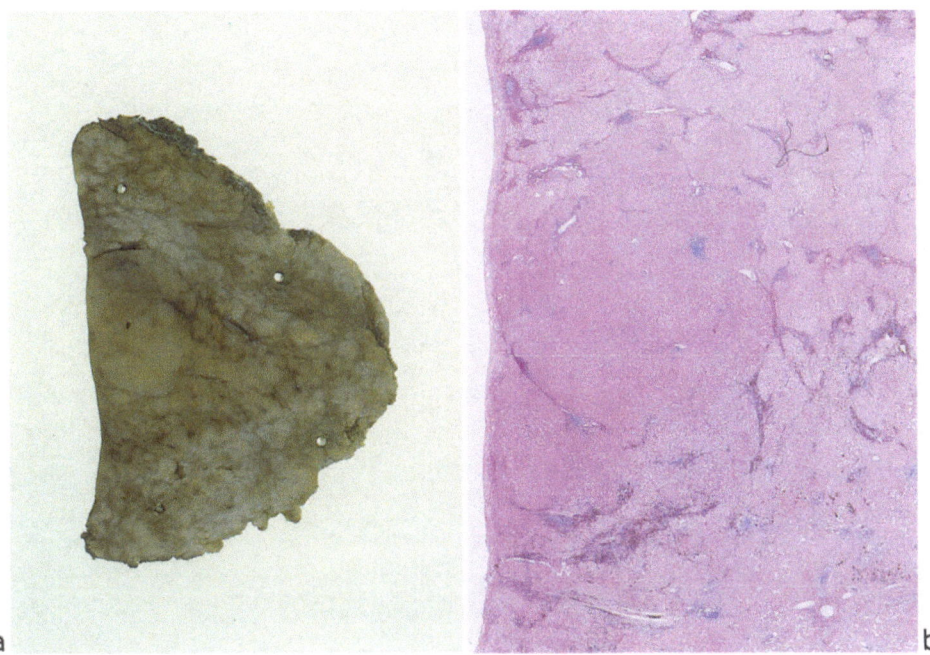

Fig. 1.49a, b. Infiltrative small liver cancer, resected case. **a** Ill-defined tumor of 1.8 cm maximum diameter. **b** The tumor-nontumor boundary is obscure. HE, × 1

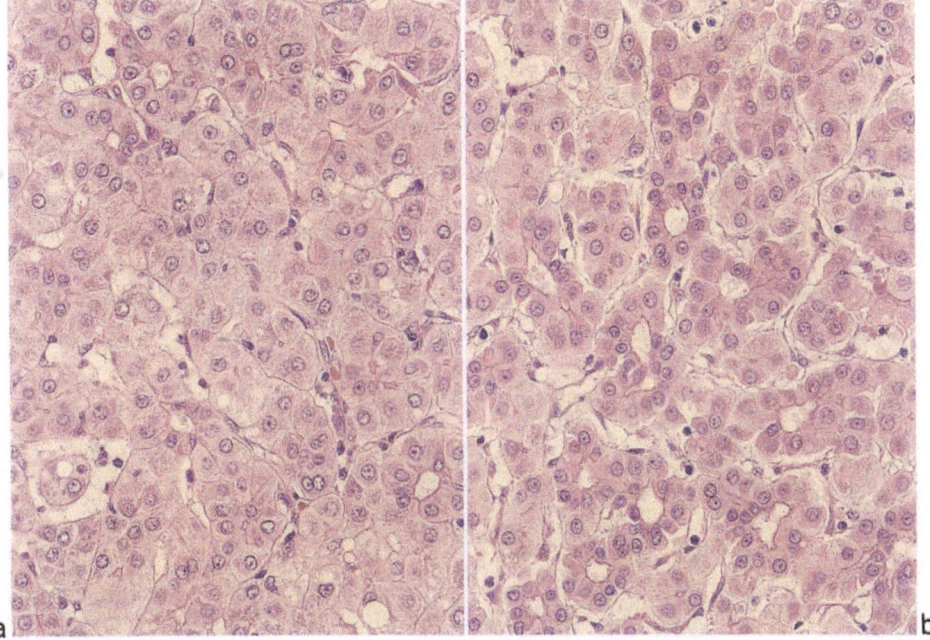

Fig. 1.50a, b. Histological features in the same case. **a** The tumor is highly differentiated, corresponding to Edmondson-Steiner grade I carcinoma. **b** Occasional glandular structure in the same tumor. HE, × 200

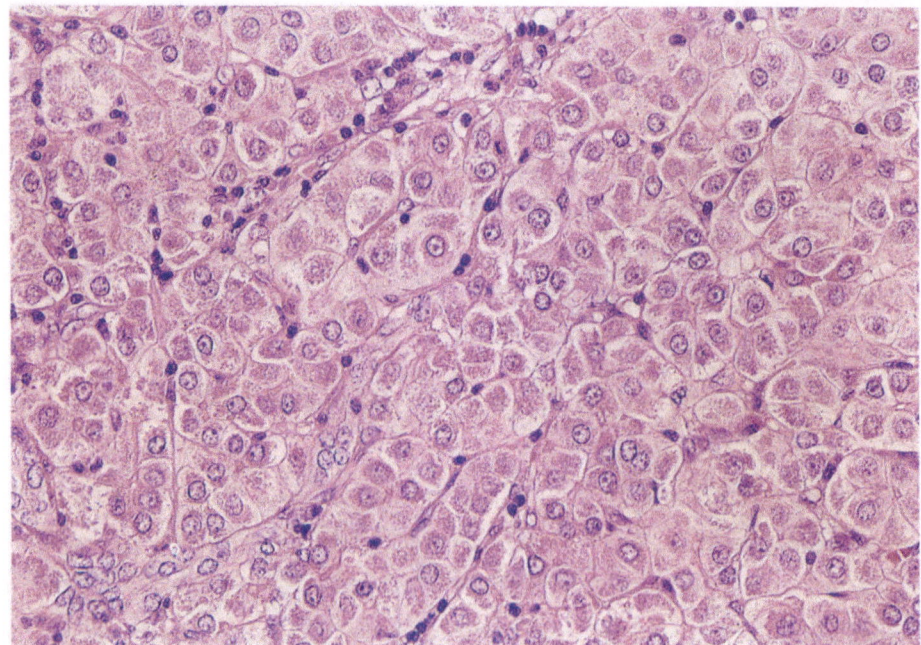

Fig. 1.51. Same case. Well-differentiated hepatocellular carcinoma proliferating in a solid fashion. HE, × 200

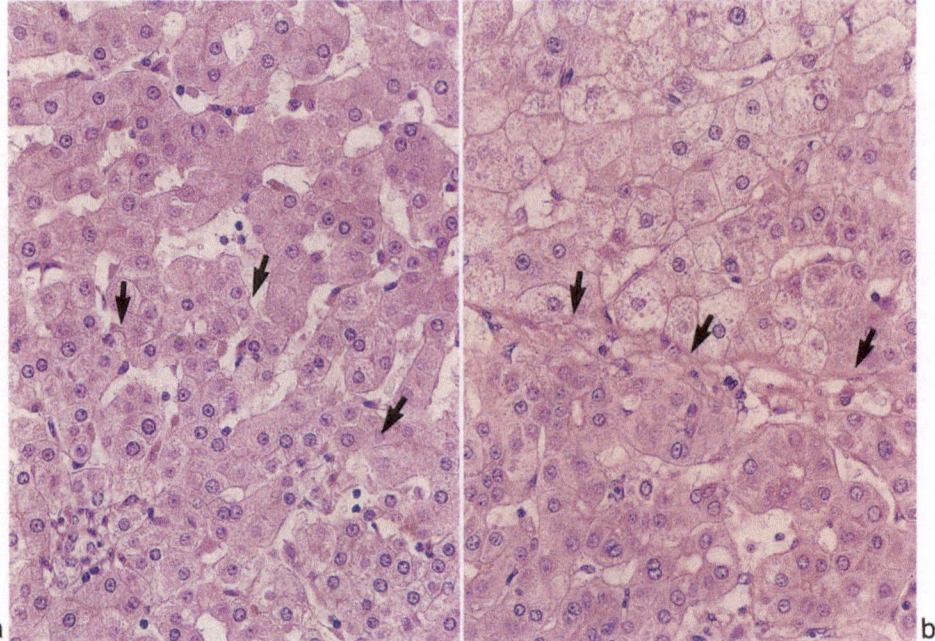

Fig. 1.52a, b. Same case. Highly differentiated tumor cells are proliferating as they replace the hepatocytes at the tumor-nontumor boundary (*arrows*). HE, × 200

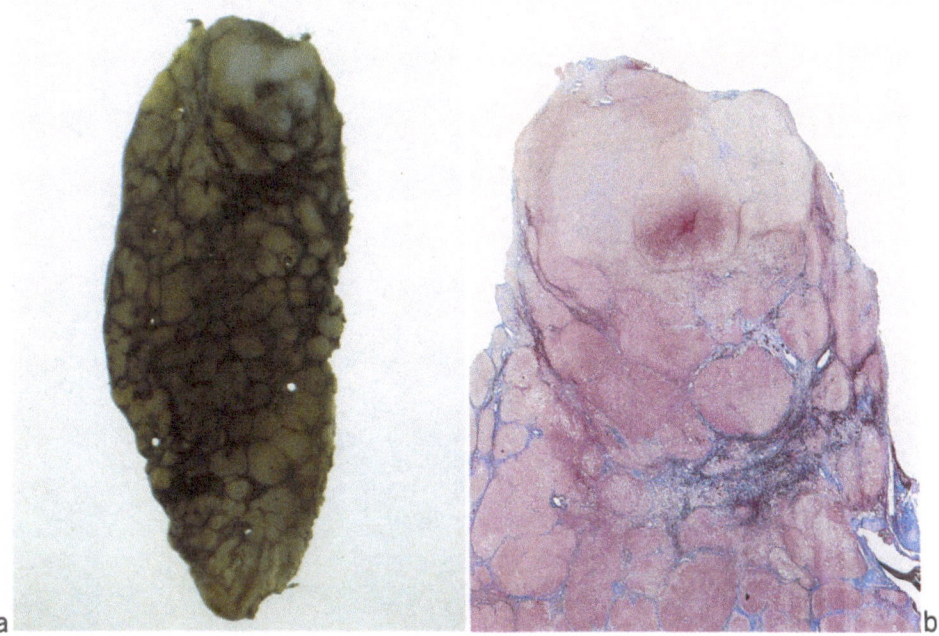

Fig. 1.53a, b. Resected infiltrative small liver cancer with various histologic patterns. **a** An ill-defined minute tumor 1.8 cm in diameter occurring in a cirrhotic liver. **b** The tumor is not encapsulated. HE, × 1

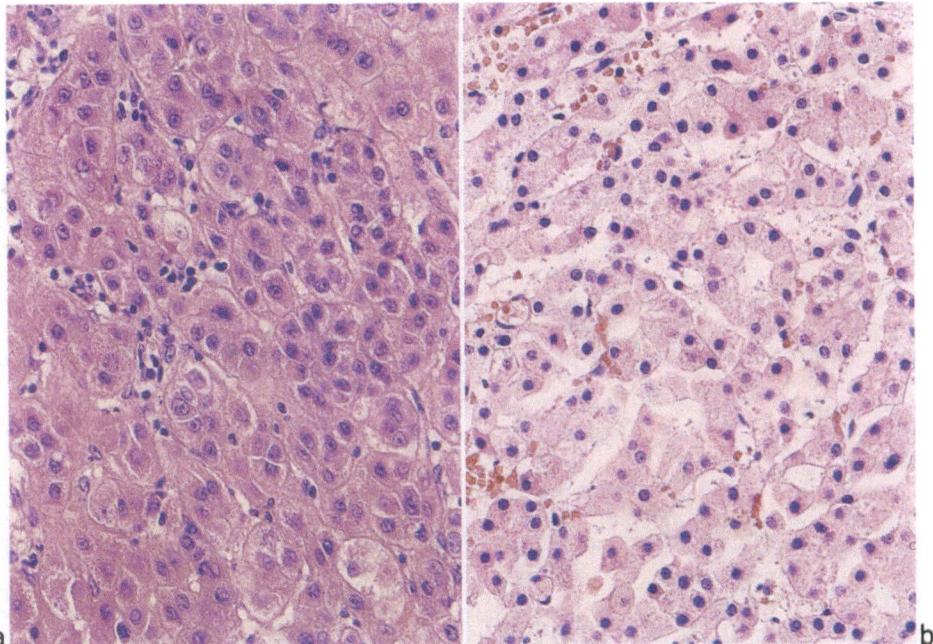

Fig. 1.54a, b. Same case. **a** Moderately differentiated hepatocellular carcinoma (Edmondson-Steiner grade II). **b** Highly differentiated carcinoma (grade I). HE, × 200

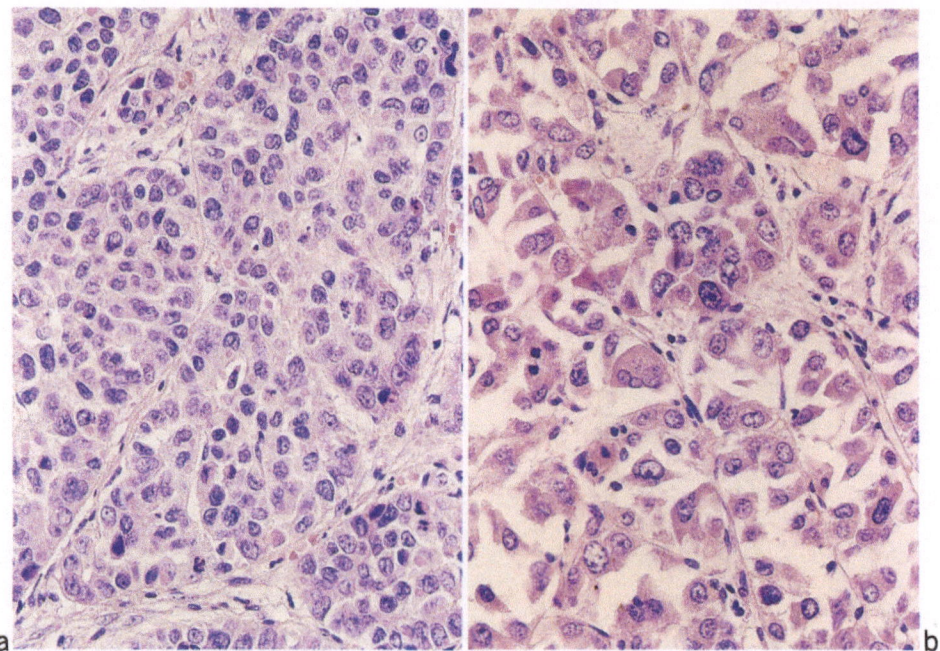

Fig. 1.55a, b. Same case. **a** Poorly differentiated carcinoma (grade IV). **b** Pleomorphic carcinoma (grade III). HE, × 200

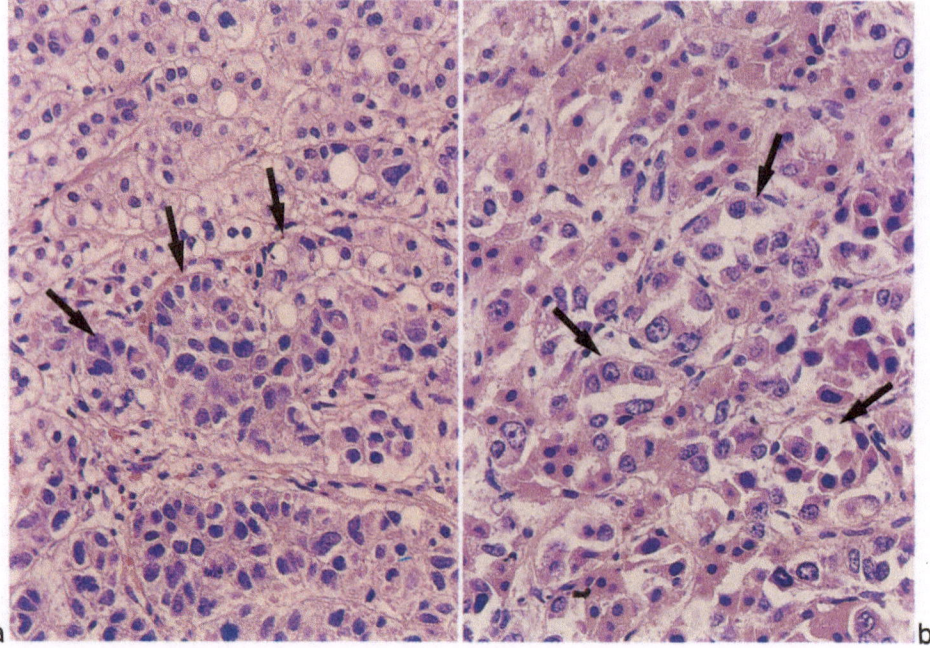

Fig. 1.56a, b. Same case. **a** Grade III carcinoma is replacing grade II carcinoma at the boundary (*arrows*). **b** Cancer cells of grade IV carcinoma are proliferating in the blood spaces of grade II carcinoma (*arrows*). HE, × 200

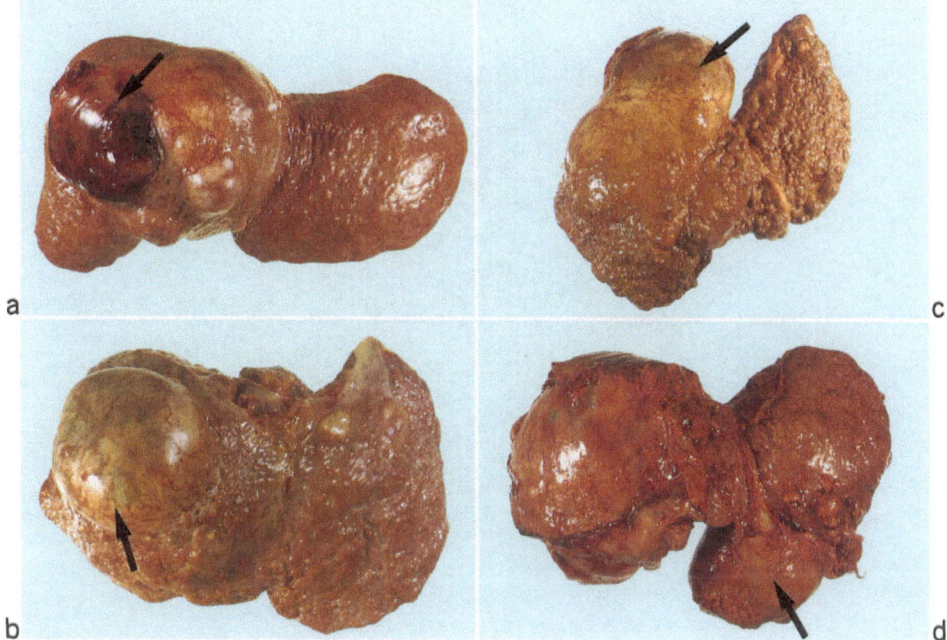

Fig. 1.57a–d. Pedunculated HCC type I. Spherical tumors (*arrows*) protrude from the liver capsule

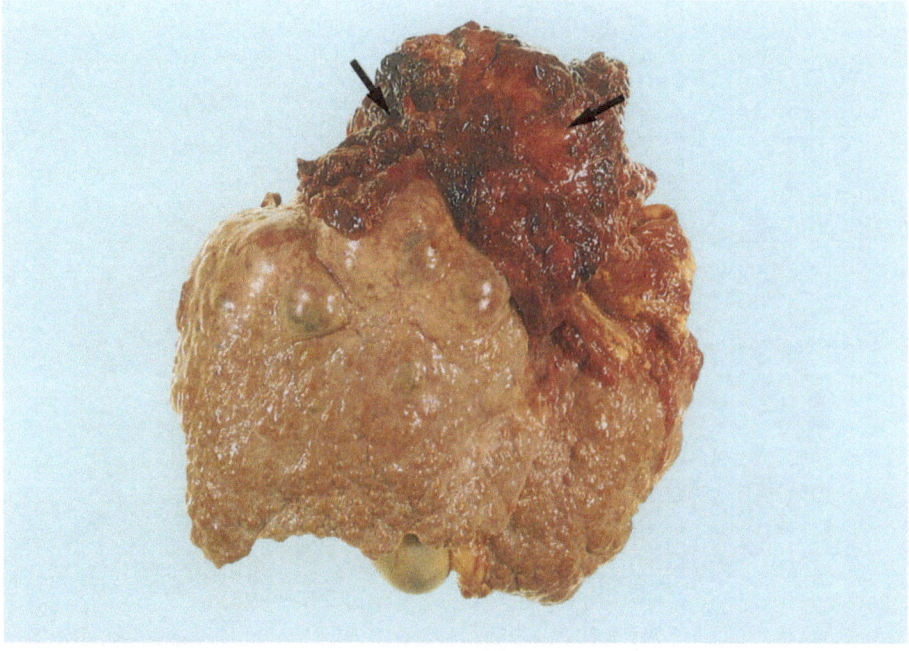

Fig. 1.58. Pedunculated HCC type I. Marked extrahepatic proliferation of the tumor (*arrows*)

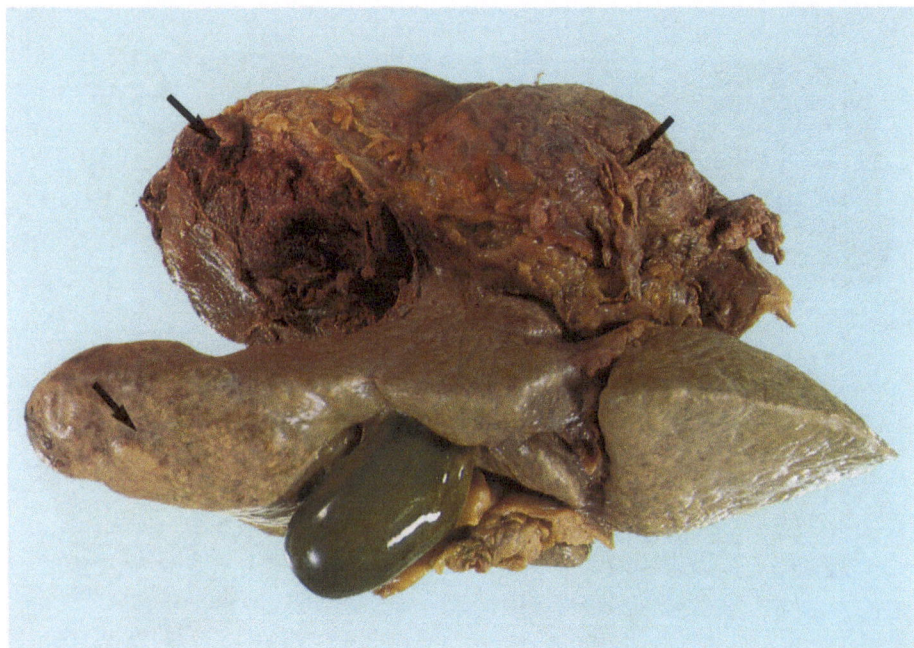

Fig. 1.59. Pedunculated HCC type I. Highly necrotic pedunculated tumor (*arrows*)

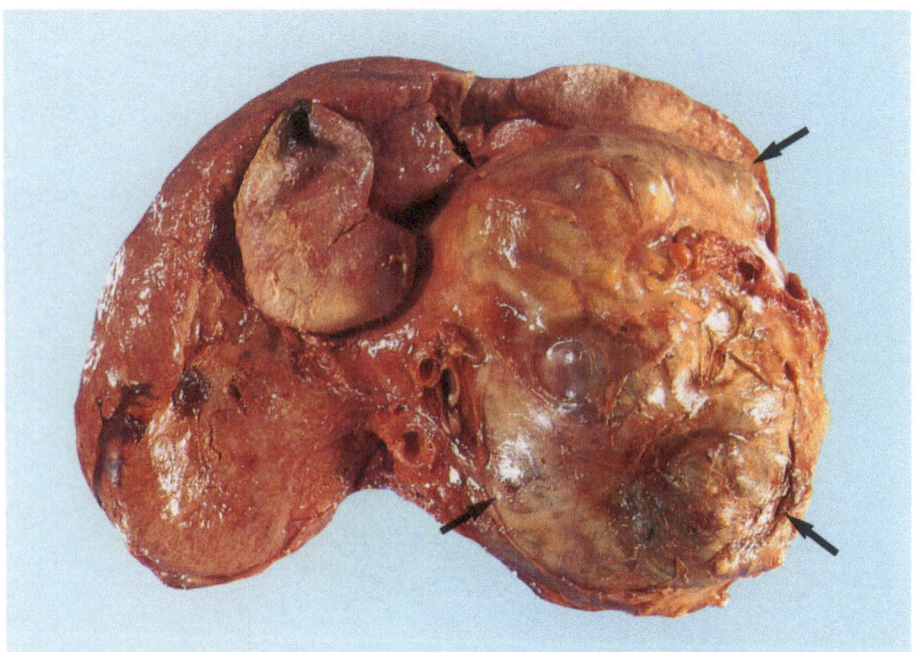

Fig. 1.60. Pedunculated HCC type II. Huge tumor with the possibility of origin in an accessory lobe (*arrows*)

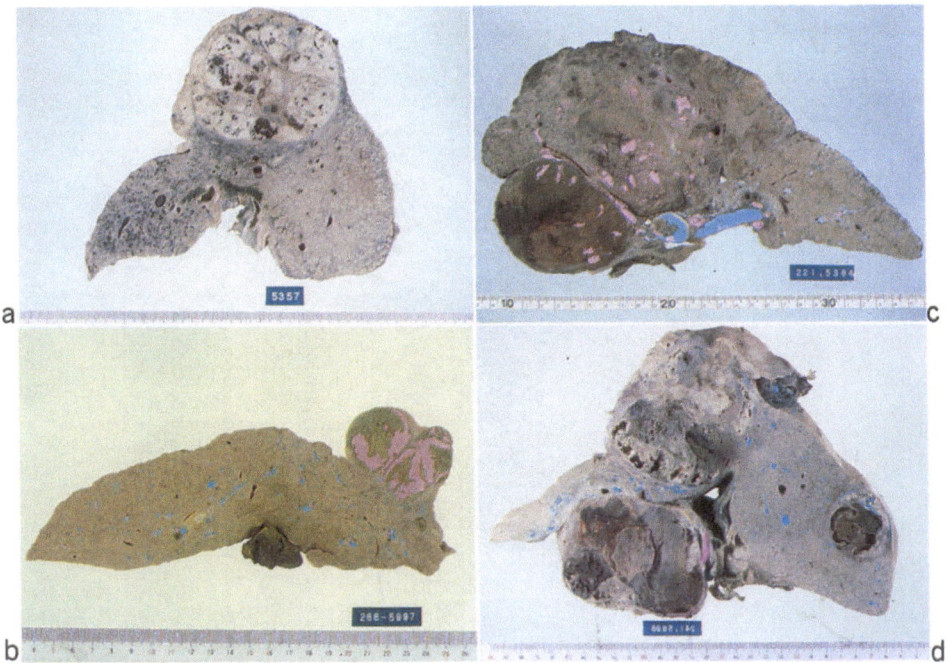

Fig. 1.61a–d. Pedunculated HCC type I. The tumors grow to form a large hemispheric protrusion from the surface of the liver

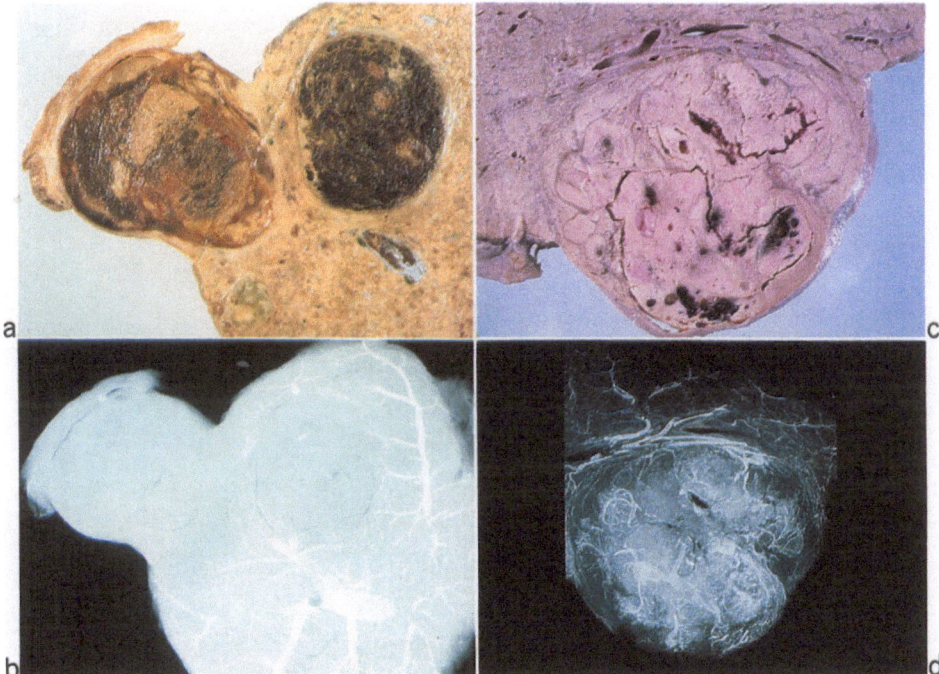

Fig. 1.62a–d. Pedunculated HCC type I. **a, b** Hypovascular pedunculated tumor. **c, d** Hypervascular pedunculated tumor (**b, d** soft X-ray)

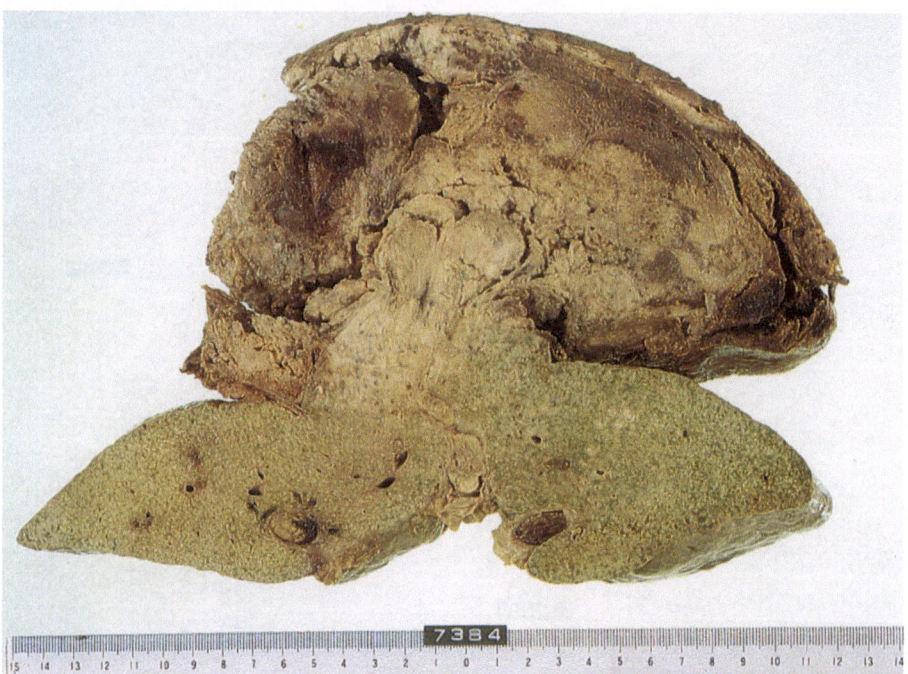

Fig. 1.63. Pedunculated HCC type I. The pedunculated tumor is highly necrotic

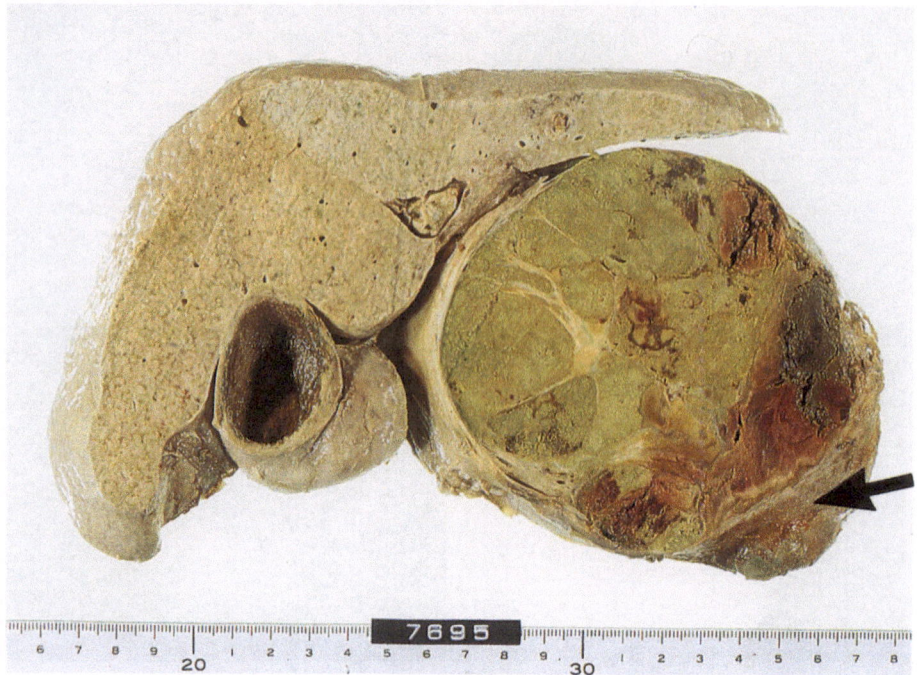

Fig. 1.64. Pedunculated HCC type II. High possibility of origin in an accessory lobe (*arrow*). Same case as Fig. 1.6

Chapter 2
Histological Features and Classification of Hepatocellular Carcinoma

Basically, the histological structure of HCC resembles that of the normal liver, in that the tumor parenchyma comprises a liver cell cord-like (trabecular) structure and the stroma consists of a sinusoid-like blood space lined by a single layer of endothelial cells.

Edmondson and Steiner [9] divided HCC into grades I–IV according to the degree of differentiation of the tumor, using Broders' classification [59] as a basis, and their classification has been widely employed in Japan since the study of the relationship between AFP and histological differentiation of HCC began in the early 1970s. The WHO classification [60] was proposed in 1978 and has since obtained worldwide currency. We have employed a slightly modified version of the WHO classification.

Edmondson-Steiner Classification of HCC

Grade I carcinoma. This type of HCC is the most differentiated and consists of tumor cells arranged in a thin trabecular pattern (Fig. 2.1). Grade I carcinoma is not seen as the sole type in any specimen of this carcinoma but only occurs locally predominantly in grade II.

Grade II carcinoma. Although the tumor cells show a marked resemblance to normal hepatic cells, the nuclei are larger and more hyperchromatic than usual. The cytoplasm, however, is abundant and acidophilic. The acinar structure is frequently associated with the trabecular pattern (Fig. 2.2).

Grade III carcinoma. The nuclei are usually larger and more hyperchromatic than in grade II. The nuclei occupy a relatively greater proportion of the cell. Bile and acinar formation are noted less frequently. Tumor giant cells are most numerous in this type (Fig. 2.3).

Grade IV carcinoma. This type of HCC is the most poorly differentiated. The nuclei are intensely hyperchromatic and occupy a great part of the cell. The cytoplasm varies in amount; it is often scanty and contains fewer granules. The growth in the liver is more medullary and the trabeculae are difficult to find; many of the cell masses seems to lie loosely and without cohesion. Bile is extremely rare in this type (Figs. 2.4, 17, 18).

Present Authors' Classification of HCC

Trabecular (sinusoidal) type
Tumor cells grow in cords of variable thickness separated by prominent sinusoids lined by flat endothelial cells. The endothelial cells, although commonly inconspicuous, may sharply define the trabeculae. Fibrous connective tissue is absent between tumor cords and cells but a few collagen fibers may sometimes be detected in the sinusoidal walls (figs. 2.5–8). When, as in some cases, there is wide and irregular dilatation of the sinusoids, tumor cells may be grouped around the vascular spaces in rosette arrangements, which at first glance resemble glands.

Pseudoglandular (acinar) type
A variety of gland-like structures may be seen (Figs. 2.9–12). Canaliculi, with or without bile, are often recognizable and may be dilated into gland-like spaces. Larger cystic spaces, lined by a layer of cells, are apparently formed by central degeneration and breakdown in otherwise solid trabeculae. The contents of the gland-like spaces may be fat-filled macrophages, fibrinous exudates, cellular debris, or homogeneous colloid-like material, in which case there may be some resemblance to thyroid follicles. The contents may be PAS-positive but should not be mistaken for mucus. The basic trabecular pattern with intervening sinusoids often remains detectable.

Compact (solid) type
The pattern is basically trabecular but the tumor cells apparently grow in solid masses and the sinusoids are rendered inconspicuous by compression (Figs. 2.13, 14).

Scirrhous (sclerosing) type
Areas with abundant fibrous stroma separating cords of tumor cells are most often seen following radiation, chemotherapy, or transhepatic arterial embolization therapy (Figs. 2.15, 16) [61]. HCC of such appearance should be distinguished from cholangiocarcinoma and metastatic tumors (Fig. 2.16).

Free-cell type
This type corresponds to Edmondson-Steiner grade IV carcinoma. Tumor cells lack a mutual contact (Figs. 2.17, 18).

Sarcomatous type
The existence of a sarcomatous appearance has been reported sporadically [62–68]. In many such cases, it is difficult to decide whether the sarcomatous appearance is caused by sarcomatous change of part of the HCC or by the coexistence of HCC and sarcoma. We found 14 cases (3.9%) of sarcomatous appearance among 355 consecutive autopsy cases of HCC (Figs. 2.19–23). Clinically, HCCs with sarcomatous appearance are characterized by undetectable or low serum levels of AFP and a high incidence of extrahepatic metastasis. Histologically, the tumor is comprised mainly of spindle-shaped cells and partly of multinucleated bizarre giant cells, and a transitional form between a trabecular arrangement and a sarcomatous appearance is observed in some cases. Immunohistochemically, sarcomatous tumor cells

are frequently found to be positive for keratin, albumin, AFP, and/or fibrinogen. These results strongly suggest that the sarcomatous appearance represents sarcomatous change of HCC rather than coexistence of HCC and sarcoma. Regarding the development of the sarcomatous change, it may be inferred that morphological alteration is induced by various factors, including chemotherapy.

Cytological and Other Variants of HCC

The following cytological and other variants of HCC (Figs. 2.24–36) have also been recorded: pleomorphic HCC, clear cell HCC, tumor cells with little cytoplasm, spindle-shaped tumor cells, bile production, glycogen, fat, cytoplasmic inclusions, such as reticular hyalin (Mallory body) and globular hyalin, sarcoid-like reaction, and extramedullary hematopoiesis.

Giant cell HCC
Multinucleated or single-nucleus giant cells are frequently observed in HCC (Figs. 2.24–26). Although the basic trabecular structure is retained in most HCC of the giant-cell type, pleomorphic giant cells have poor mutual contact. Giant cell HCC is considered relatively less differentiated and is grade III carcinoma in the Edmondson-Steiner classification.

Clear cell HCC
Occasionally, HCC consisting exclusively of clear cells is encountered (Figs. 2.27, 28). Buchanan and Huvos [69] described that clear cells constituted 30%–100% of tumor cells in 13 of 150 cases of HCC. Wu et al. [70] reported favorable prognosis in HCC of the clear cell type. The clear cytoplasm contains abundant glycogen. Sasaki et al. [71] described two cases of clear cell carcinoma of the liver associated with hypoglycemia and hypercholesterolemia and postulated a diverted glucose metabolism of the tumor tissue in the direction of lipogenesis and/or glycogenesis. Clear cell HCC with associated hypoglycemia was also described by Ross and Kurian [72] and McFadzean and Yeung [73].

Cytoplasmic hyaline inclusions
It is common to find that HCC cells contain various intracytoplasmic hyalins (Fig. 2.31). These can be divided into four types: PAS-positive or -negative globular hyalin. PAS-negative reticular hyalin, and ground-glass hyalin

The *reticular hyalins* and most *PAS-negative globular hyalins* are histochemically and ultrastructurally indistinguishable from Mallory's alcoholic hyalins [74]. It is well known that Mallory bodies are seen in the liver in various diseases, including HCC [75-83], and Mallory bodies in HCC have been widely studied [81, 86–89]. We found reticular hyalin and PAS-negative globular hyalin in 15.7% and 9.5% of 146 consecutive autopsy cases of HCC, respectively, and they coexisted in four cases. Ultrastructurally, reticular hyalin and PAS-negative globular hyalin are seen as fibrillar deposits with no limiting membrane and are indistinguishable from classic Mallory bodies. Light-microscopic differentiation between reticular hyalin and PAS-negative globular hyalin depends on whether the margin of fibrillar deposits is regular or irregular at the ultrastructural level.

Diastase-resistant *PAS-positive inclusions* are occasionally observed in HCC [84, 85]. They were seen in 6 (4.1%) of 146 consecutive autopsy cases of HCC in our series. They are brightly stained with eosin and are round to oval in shape. They are 3–30 μm in diameter and are usually seen in groups. All such inclusions in our series were negative for alpha-1-antitrypsin.

Stromeyer et al. [90] first described the *ground-glass inclusions*, which were seen as non-membrane-bound fibrillar materials and reacted with antifibrinogen. We found similar inclusions in 3 (2.0%) of 146 consecutive autopsy cases of HCC and all of them reacted with antifibrinogen. In all three cases, the endoplasmic reticulum exhibited varying degrees of dilatation and contained fine fibrillar material, and extremely dilated endoplasmic reticula were seen as the inclusions. We believe that ground-glass inclusions are the result of the accumulation of secreted protein, mainly fibrinogen, in endoplasmic reticulum showing cystic dilatation due to the disturbance of secretory function of HCC cells.

Sarcoid-like reaction
The sarcoid-like reaction within malignant tumors or in the regional lymph nodes that drain an area involved with malignant tumors has long been recognized [91]. However, it is believed to be rare in HCC [92, 93]. We have encountered only two cases of HCC with granulomatous reaction in cancerous tissue among the 439 consecutive autopsy cases in our series (Figs. 2.33–36). Granulomas are characterized by epithelioid cells, Langhans-type giant cells, and varying numbers of lymphocytes, of which most are seen within the tumor but a few in tumor thrombi of the portal veins. In these cases, there was no evidence of tuberculosis or systemic sarcoidosis. Regarding the pathogenesis of the sarcoid-like reaction in HCC, there are two proposals: (1) a tissue response mechanism against a malignant tumor, including an immunological mechanism, and (2) nonspecific, fortuitous phenomena [92]. We consider a nonspecific reaction to metabolic or disintegration products of HCC to be the most likely answer.

Extramedullary hematopoiesis
It is not unusual to find extramedullary hematopoiesis in HCC tissue, because the liver is one of the hematopoietic organs. We found foci of extramedullary hematopoiesis in cancerous tissue in 4 (3.4%) of 116 consecutive autopsy cases of HCC, and the hematopoietic cells were mostly nucleated red blood cells.

Calcification of HCC
Calcification is rarely found in necrotized areas of HCC. We found varying degrees of calcification in the necrotized area of 2 of the 329 cases.

Histology of Small Liver Cancer

It has been noted that resected and autopsy cases of minute liver cancer are more differentiated than advanced cases, and HCC often contains tumor cells of two or more different histological types. It is rather rare to encounter tumors which are histologically uniform, as shown in Figs. 1.54–56.

We found an inverse correlation between the presence of extremely well-differentiated HCC, corresponding to Edmondson-Steiner's grade I carcinoma, and overall tumor size, as shown in Table 2.1. Furthermore, the proportion of the HCC composed of extremely well-differentiated tumor cells appeared to diminish as the diameter of the tumor increased.

Of four tumors less than 1 cm in diameter, three consisted solely of extremely well-differentiated HCC cells, as shown in Figs. 1.50–52. By contrast, moderately to poorly differentiated elements of the HCC tended to increase concomitantly with tumor size. These findings were not significantly correlated to the association of liver cirrhosis. Together with the observation that poorly differentiated elements of the HCC appeared to be replacing the well-differentiated elements of the same tumor, as shown in Fig. 1.56, these findings suggest that many cases of HCC may begin as small, extremely well-differentiated lesions which develop less differentiated elements at a later stage. Indeed, the development of such poorly differentiated areas may be at least partially responsible for the enlargement of some tumors.

Following recent progress in diagnostic imaging techniques, including ultrasonography, increasing numbers of minute liver tumors have been detected and surgically resected. Minute liver tumors resected because of suspected HCC include borderline lesions such as adenomatous regenerative nodules, which may be difficult to distinguish from HCC. In fact, it is frequently difficult to distinguish extremely well-differentiated HCC from the adenomatous regenerative foci which may be seen in the cirrhotic liver. Thus, it is presumed that some cases of HCC develop from borderline lesions such as adenomatous regenerative nodules.

The demonstration of more than one histological grade even in very small solitary HCC may also be relevant to the issue of the unicentric or multicentric origin of HCC. The fact that two or more HCC nodules of different histological types can occur separately within a single liver has been used to support the possibility of a multicentric origin of HCC.

Table 2.1. Resected HCC cases with different histological grading in a single tumor nodule (smaller than 5 cm in diameter)

Case	Age (years)	Sex	LC	Size of tumor (cm)	Histological grading[a]			
1	58	M	−	0.7 × 0.6	I			
2	65	M	+	0.7 × 0.7	I			
3	51	M	+	0.8 × 0.7	I			
4	54	M	+	0.8 × 0.8	I	II		
5	62	M	+	1.2 × 1.2	I	II		
6	47	M	+	1.4 × 1.4	I	II		
7	75	M	+	1.5 × 1.5	I	II		
8	65	F	+	1.6 × 1.4	I	II	III	IV
9	62	M	+	1.9 × 1.8	I	II	III	
10	49	M	−	2.0 × 2.0	I	II		
11	57	F	+	2.4 × 2.2		II	III	
12	54	M	+	2.5 × 2.2	I	II	III	
13	51	M	+	2.5 × 2.2		II	III	
14	61	M	+	2.5 × 2.5	I	II		
15	69	M	−	3.2 × 3.2		II	III	
16	58	M	−	3.5 × 2.0		II	III	
17	56	M	−	3.5 × 3.0		II	III	
18	50	M	+	3.5 × 3.0		II	III	
19	52	M	+	4.0 × 4.0		II	III	
20	46	M	+	4.0 × 4.0		II	III	
21	46	M	+	5.0 × 3.0		II	III	
22	52	M	+	5.0 × 4.0		II	III	
23	56	M	+	5.0 × 4.0		II	III	

LC Liver cirrhosis
[a] Edmondson-Steiner's classification

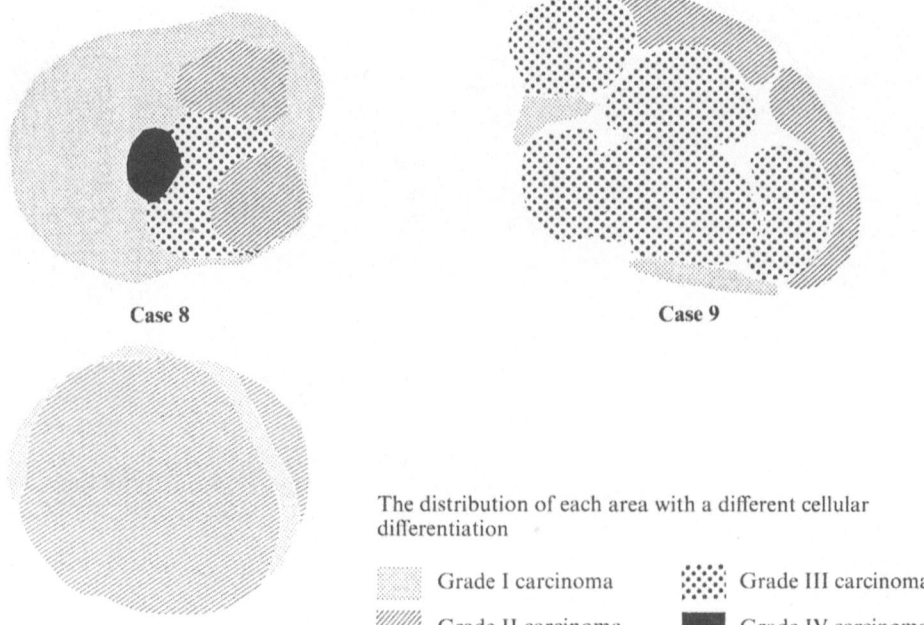

Case 8

Case 9

Case 14

The distribution of each area with a different cellular differentiation

▨ Grade I carcinoma   ⣿ Grade III carcinoma

▨ Grade II carcinoma   ■ Grade IV carcinoma

The relationship between the histological grade of HCC and tumor size

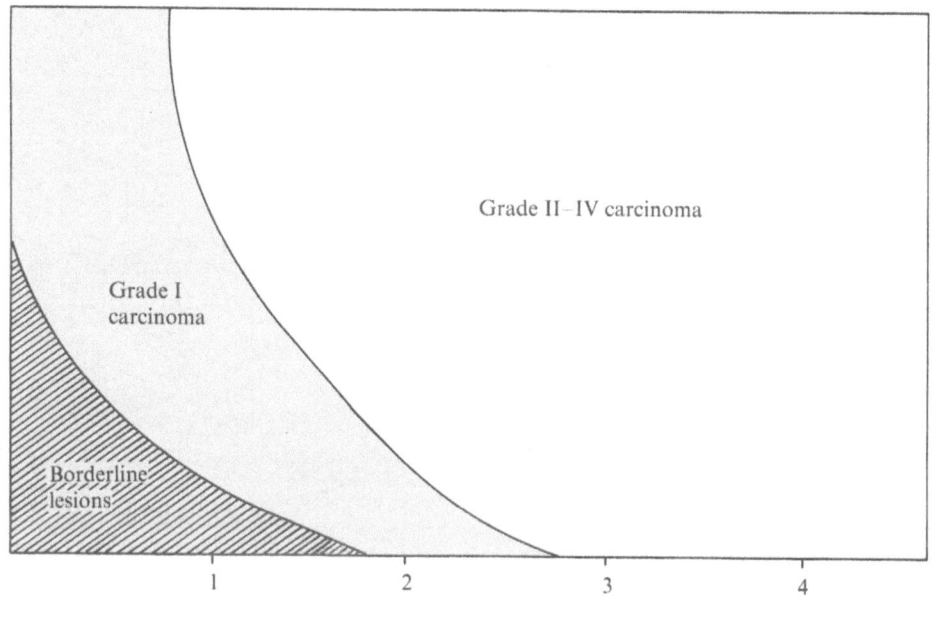

Diameter of tumor (cm)

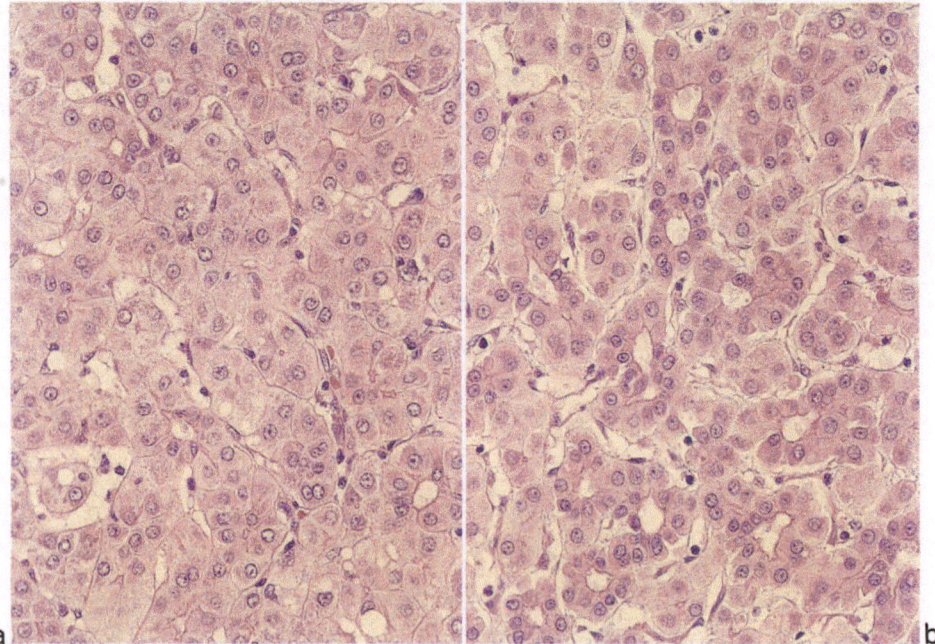

Fig. 2.1a, b. Well-differentiated HCC. **a** Highly differentiated tumor with a thin trabecular pattern. **b** Well-differentiated tumor. The cells show more atypism than those in **a**. HE, × 200

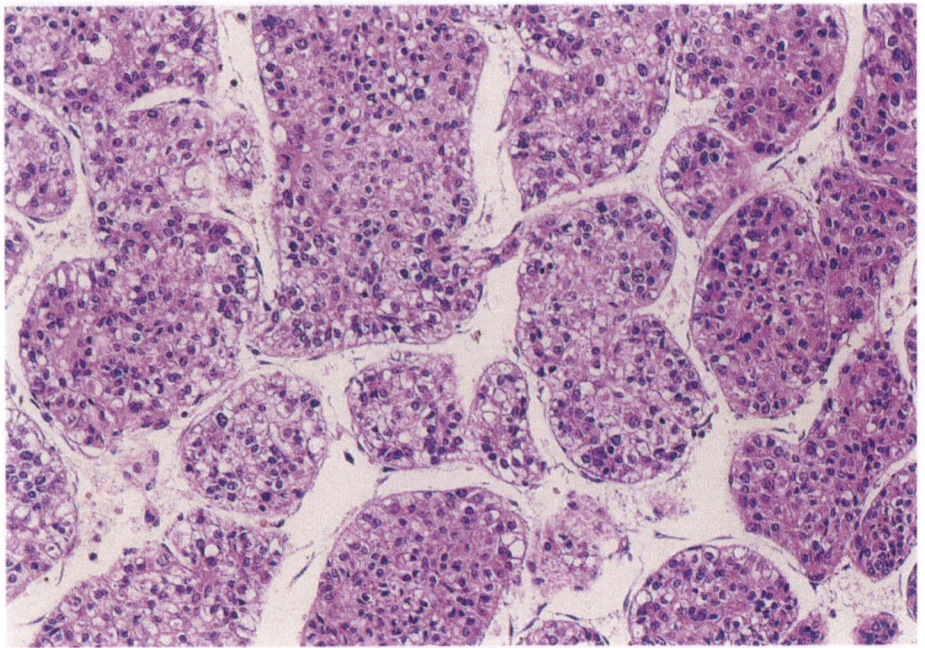

Fig. 2.2. Poorly differentiated tumor (grade IV carcinoma, *arrows*) replacing moderately differentiated tumor. HE, × 200

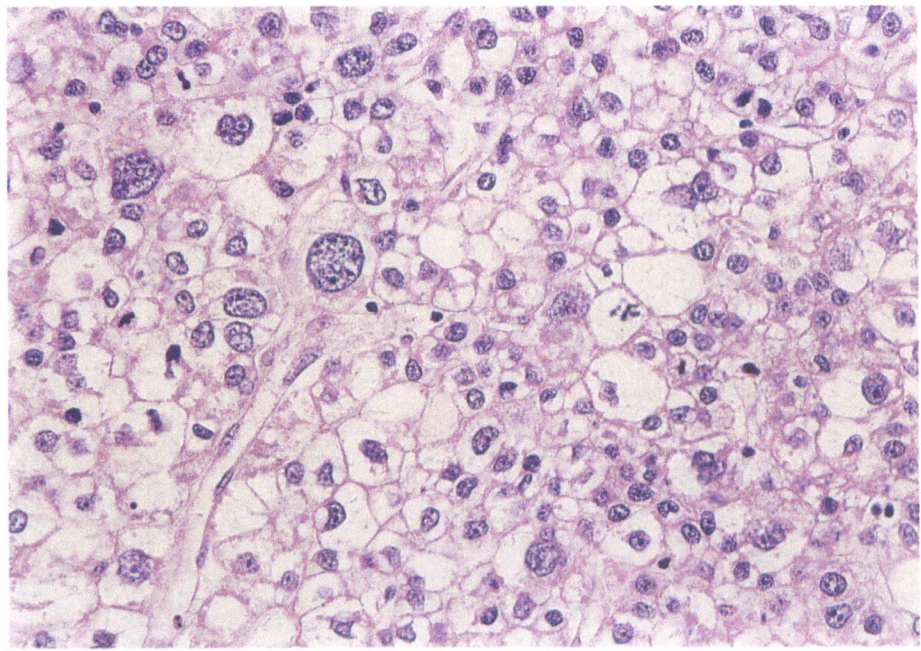

Fig. 2.3. Pleomorphic HCC (grade III carcinoma). Tumor shows marked pleomorphism and a solid growth pattern. HE, × 200

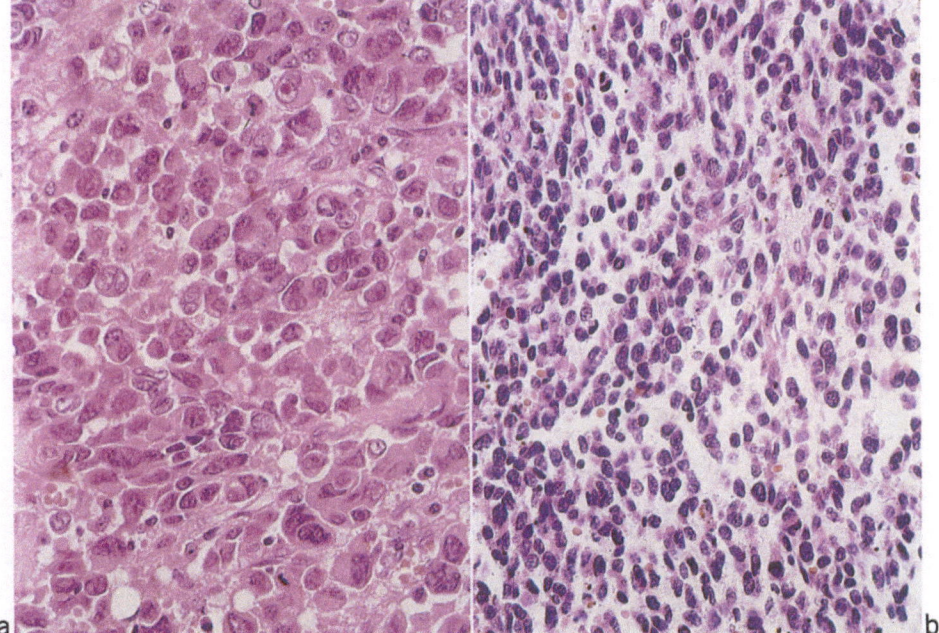

Fig. 2.4a, b. Poorly differentiated HCC (grade IV carcinoma). Tumor is hypercellular without showing any arrangement. Tumor cells lack a mutual contact (free-cell type). HE, × 200

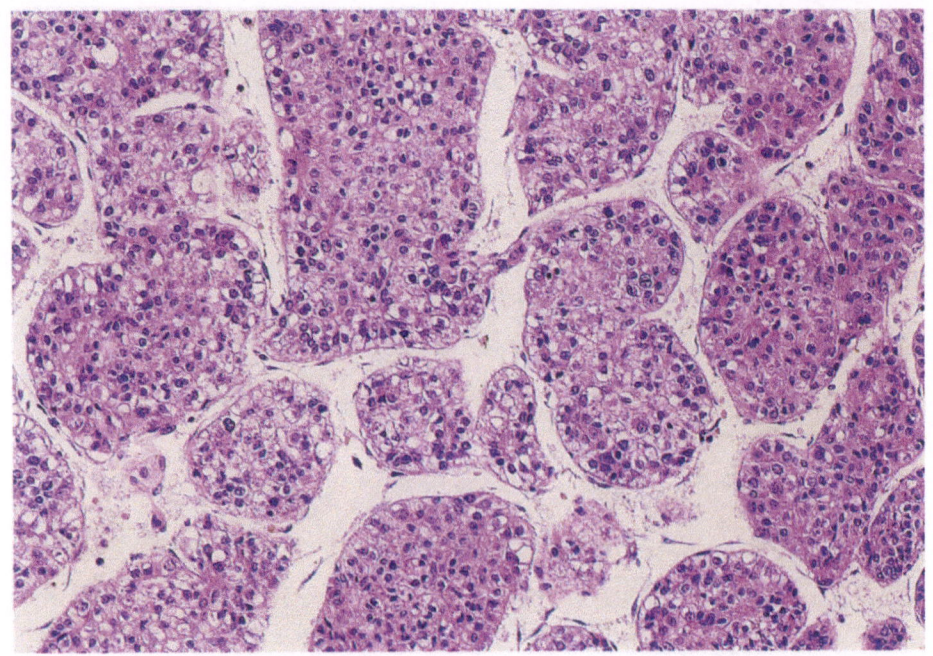

Fig. 2.5. Moderately differentiated HCC showing a typical trabecular pattern. HE, × 100

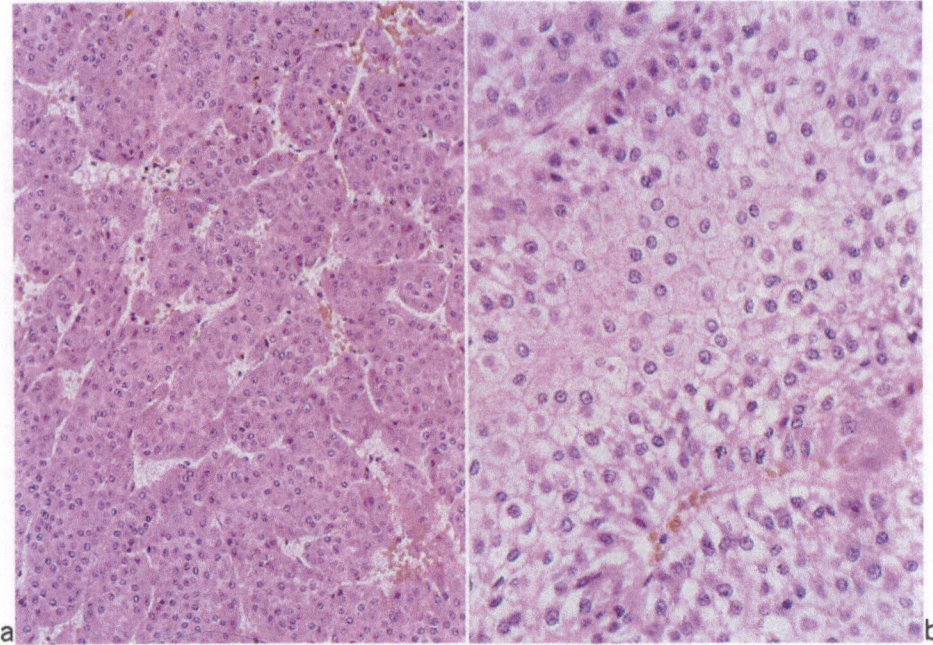

Fig. 2.6a, b. Moderately differentiated HCC. **a** Typical trabecular pattern. **b** Tumor cells with a thick trabecular pattern showing a paving-stone arrangement. HE, × 100

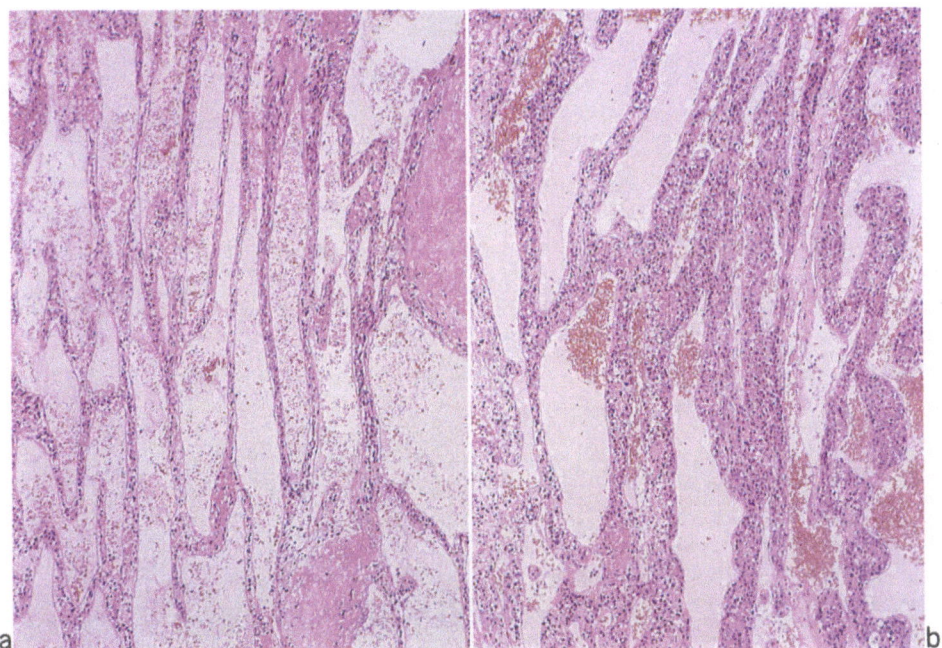

Fig. 2.7a, b. Histological features of tumor thrombus of the portal vein. Thin long trabeculae in direction of bloodstream are characteristic (finger-like colum pattern). HE, × 50

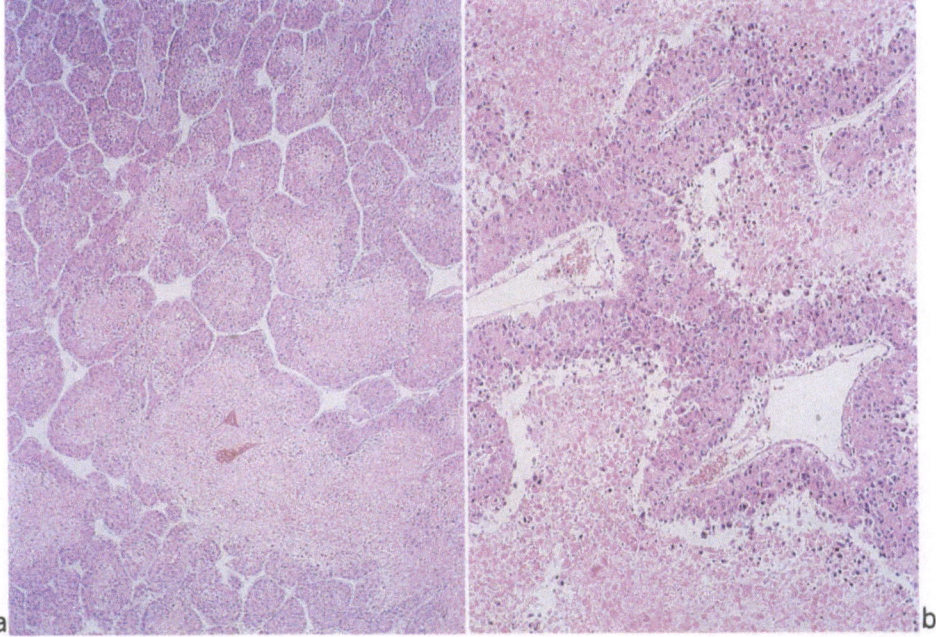

Fig. 2.8a, b. Tumor thrombus of the portal vein showing marked necrosis in the center of the trabeculae. HE; **a** × 50, **b** × 100

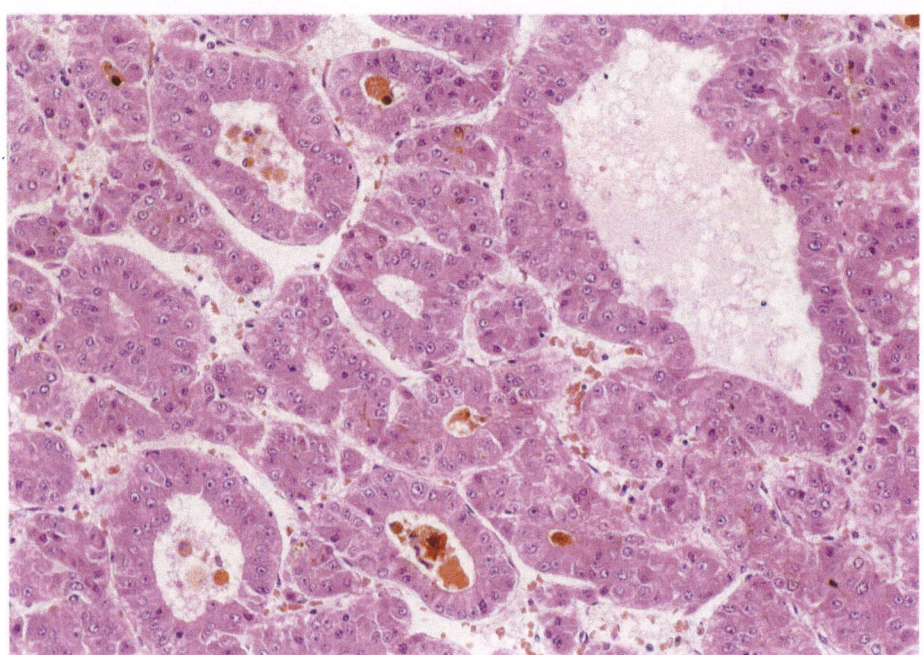

Fig. 2.9. Pseudoglandular HCC with bile production. HE, × 100

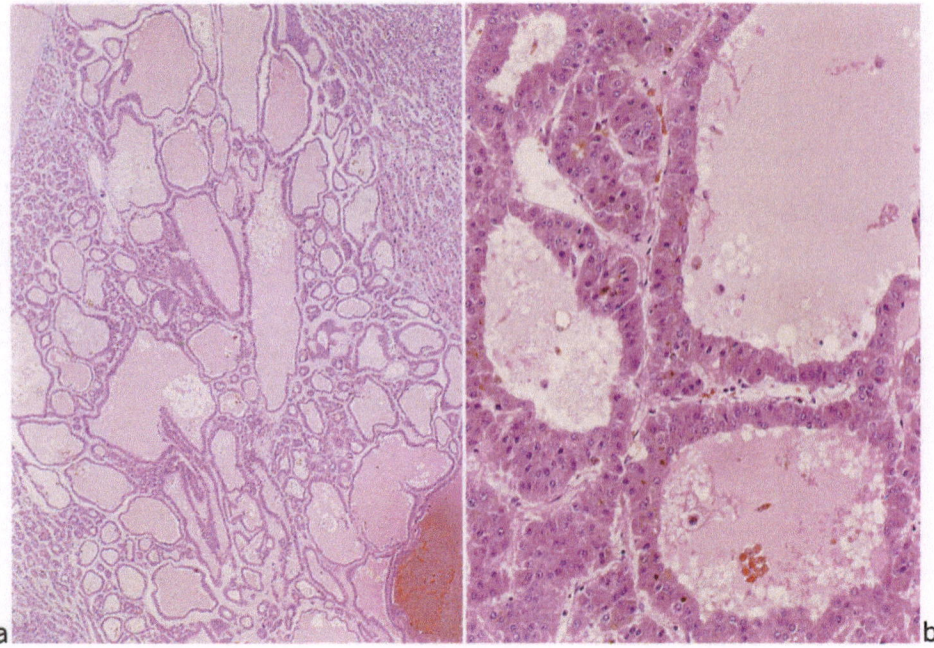

Fig. 2.10a, b. Pseudoglandular HCC showing thyroid-gland-like appearance. HE; **a** × 20, **b** × 50

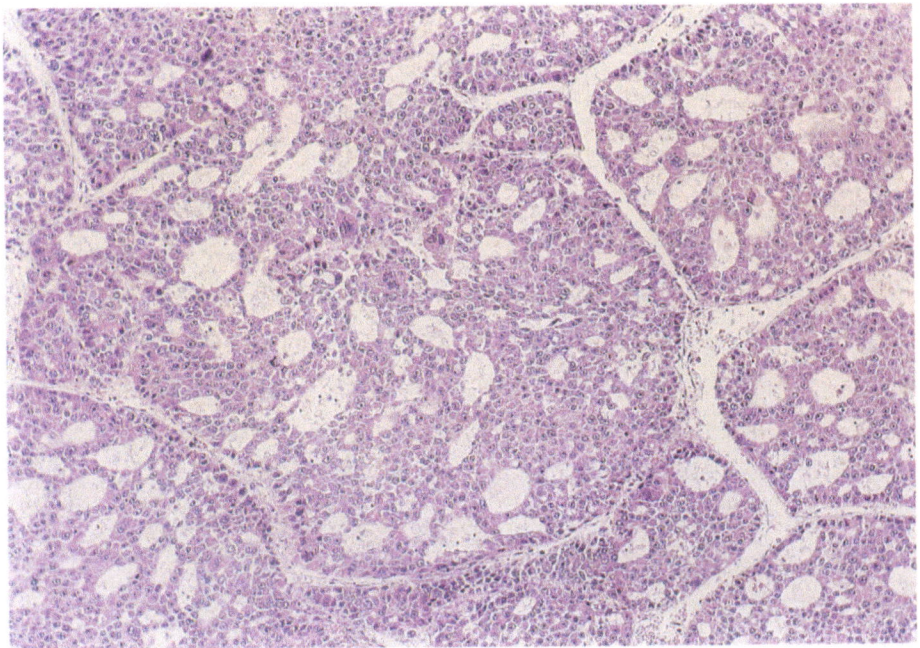

Fig. 2.11. Pseudoglandular HCC showing adenoid cystic pattern. HE, × 50

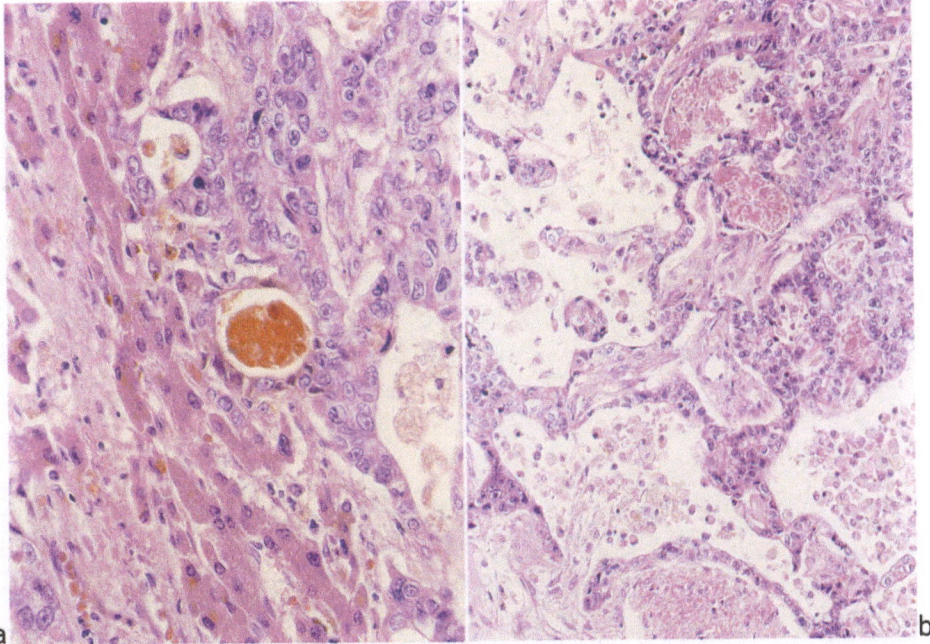

Fig. 2.12. a Tumor-nontumor boundary of pseudoglandular HCC. **b** Tumor thrombus of the portal vein in the same case. The pseudoglands are markedly dilated and show a papillary pattern in part. HE; **a** × 100, **b** × 50

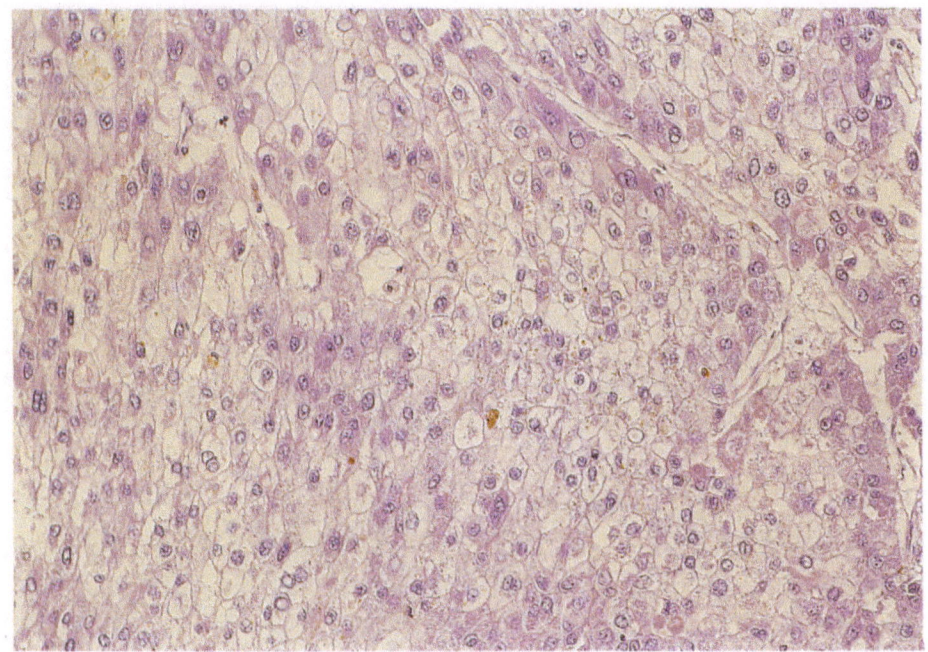

Fig. 2.13. HCC with a compact growth pattern. HE, × 100

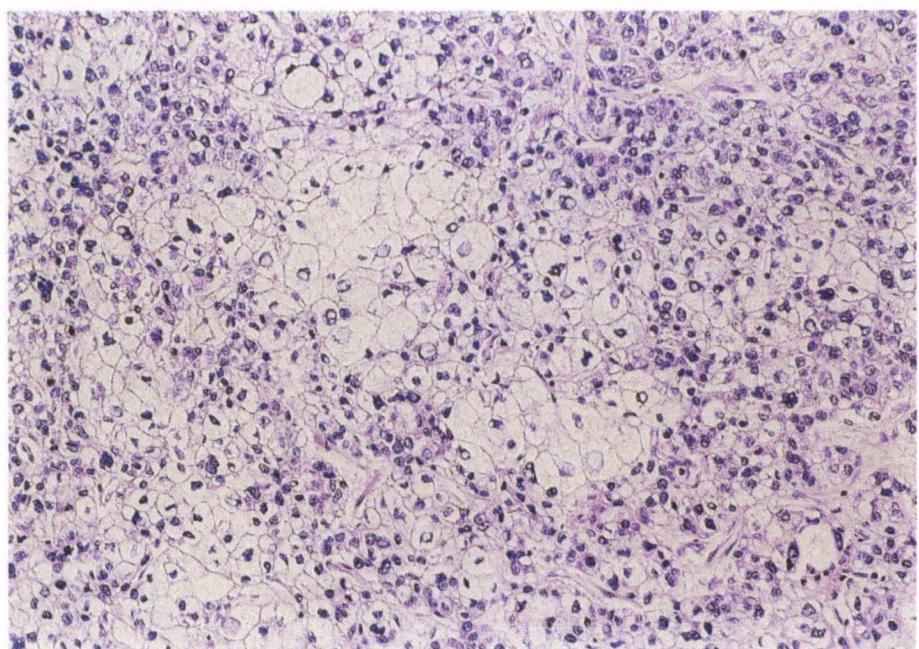

Fig. 2.14. Clear cell HCC with a compact growth pattern. HE, × 100

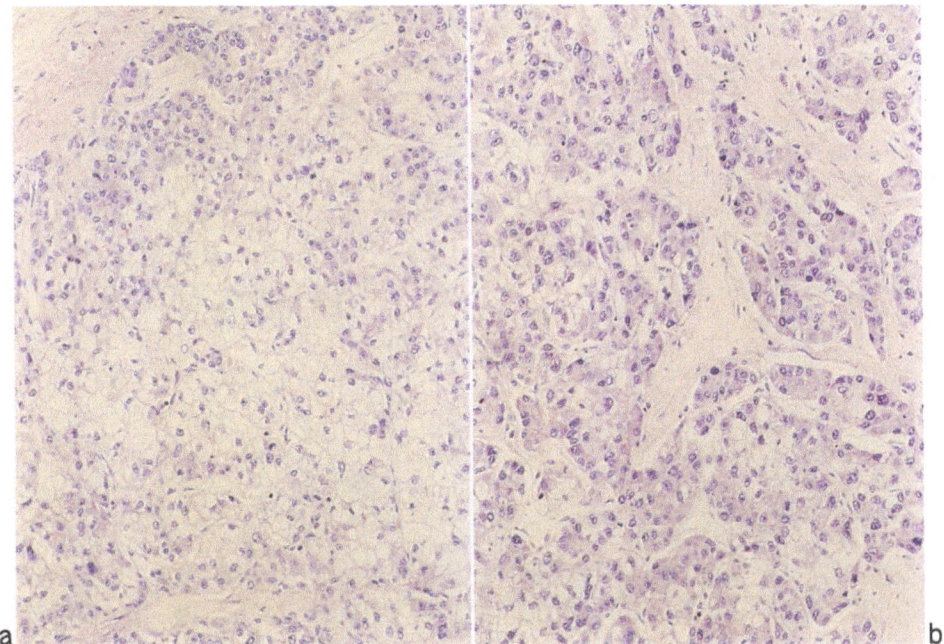

Fig. 2.15. **a** Clear cell HCC showing a compact growth pattern. **b** Scirrhous HCC. HE, × 50

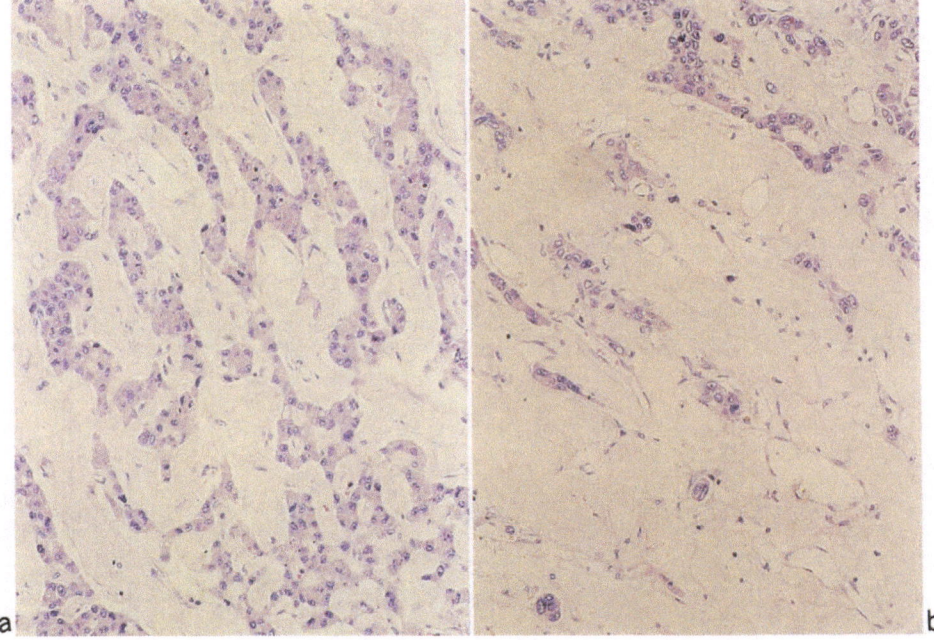

Fig. 2.16a, b. Scirrhous HCC. Hyalinized fibrous stroma is dominant. Blood spaces remain as capillary vessels in the stroma. HE, × 50

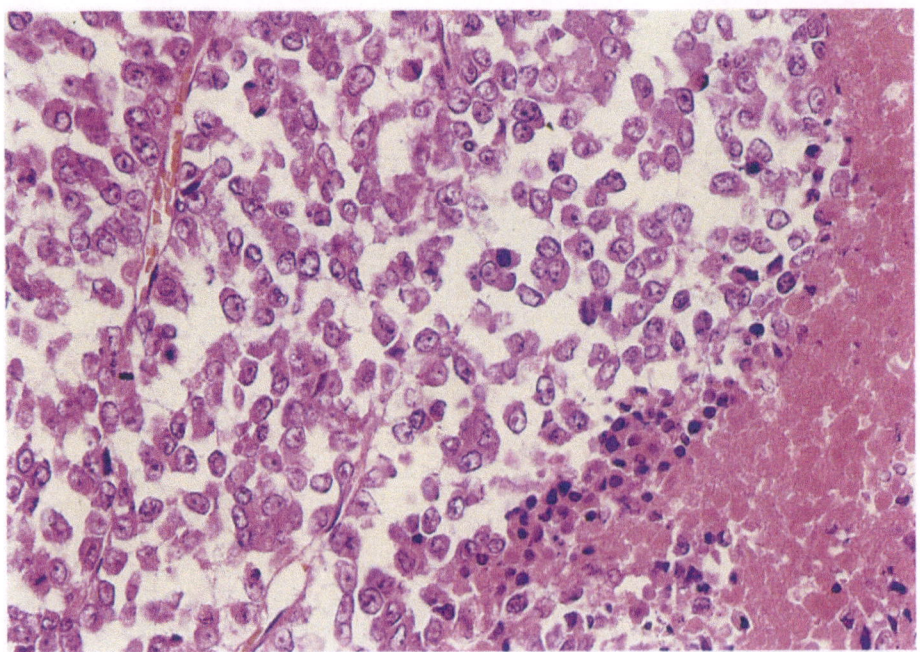

Fig. 2.17. Poorly differentiated free-cell HCC. Tumor cells lack a mutual adherence. HE, × 200

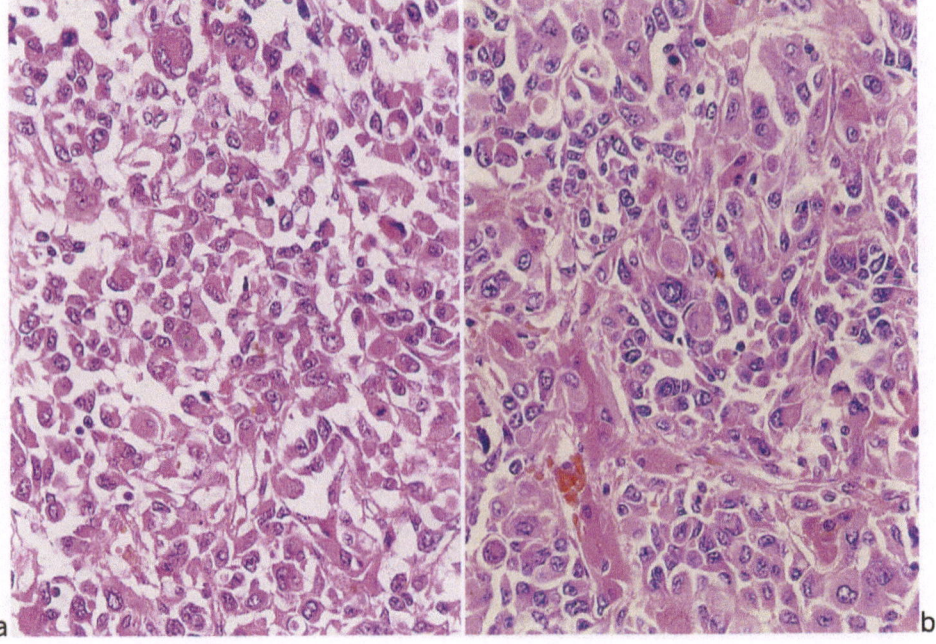

Fig. 2.18a, b. Poorly differentiated HCC showing pleomorphism. **a** Tumor cells show marked pleomorphism including multinucleated giant cells, and lack a mutual adherence. **b** Tumor cells of free-cell type proliferate in the sinusoids of the noncancerous area. HE, × 100

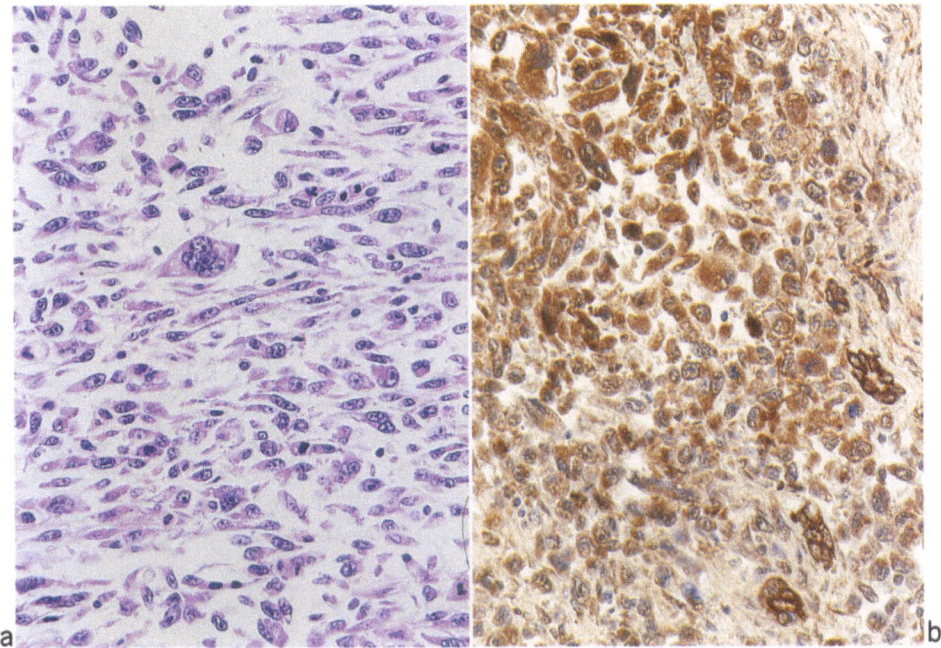

Fig. 2.19a, b. HCC of sarcomatous appearance. **a** The tumor cells are spindle-shaped with occasional multinucleated giant cells. **b** The sarcomatous tumor cells are positive to keratin. **a** HE, **b** Avidin-Biotin peroxidase method; × 100

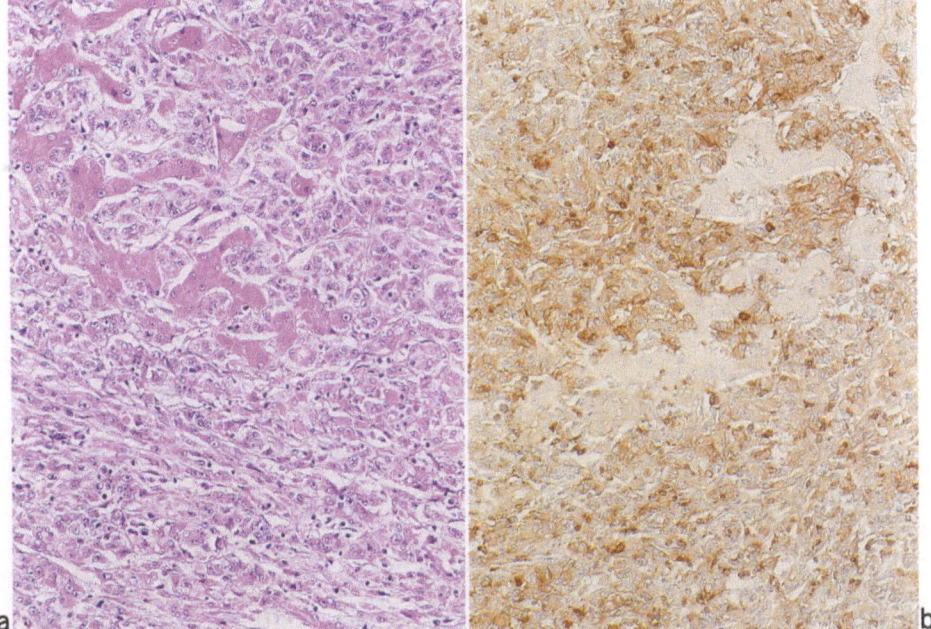

Fig. 2.20a, b. HCC of sarcomatous appearance. **a** Pleomorphic tumor cells grow in the sinusoids and liver cell cords are highly atrophic. **b** Tumor cells in the sinusoids are positive to vimentin, but hepatocytes are negative. **a** HE, **b** Avidin-Biotin peroxidase method; × 50

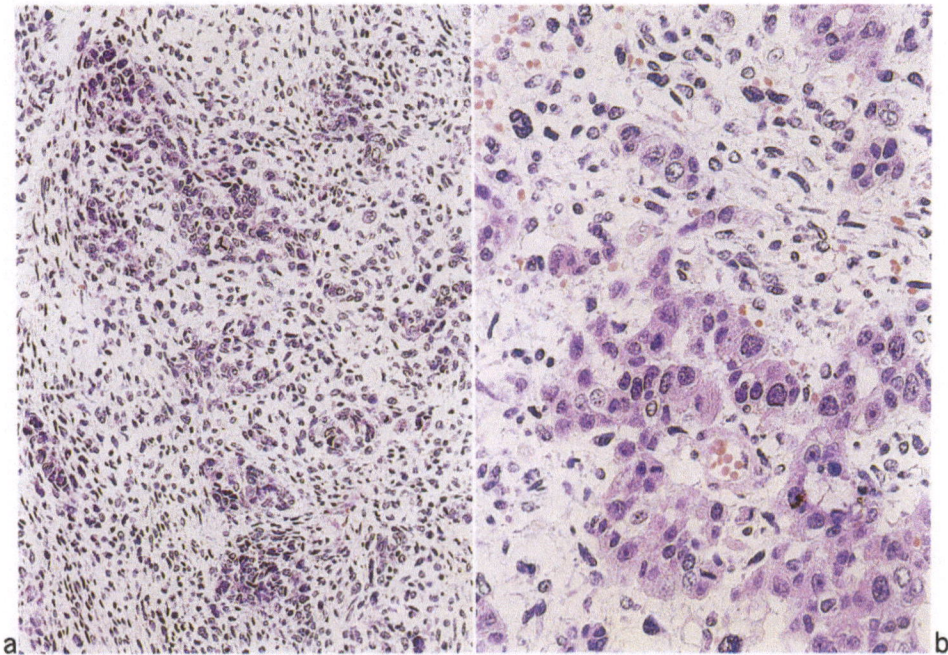

Fig. 2.21a, b. HCC with sarcomatous change. Vague trabecular pattern remains in sarcomatous area. HE; **a** × 100, **b** × 200

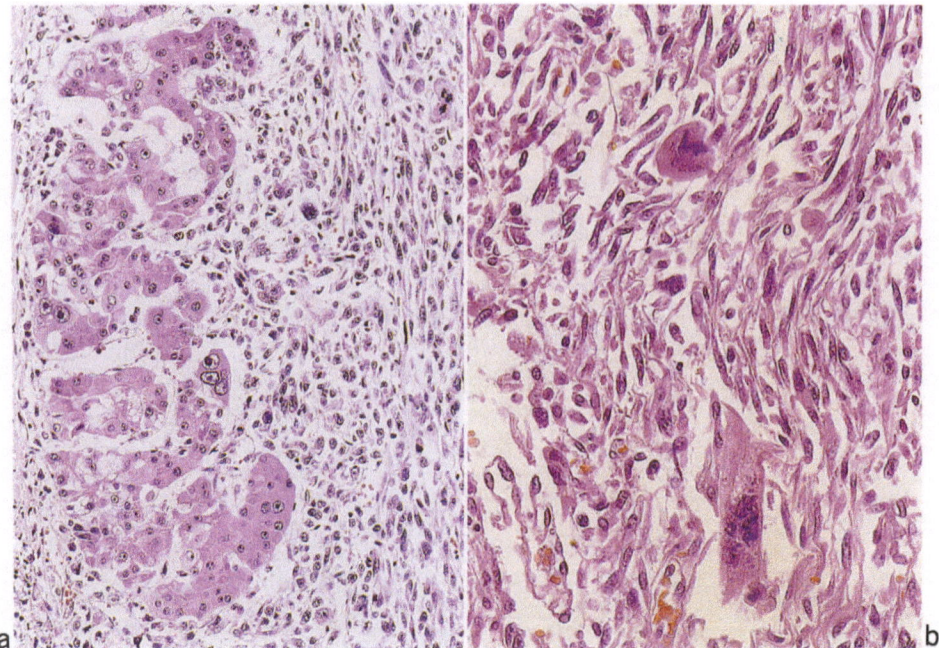

Fig. 2.22a, b. HCC with sarcomatous change. **a** Remnants of trabecular structure in sarcomatous area. **b** Sarcomatous HCC consists of spindle-shaped tumor cells with occasional bizarre multinuleated giant cells. HE; **a** × 100, **b** × 200

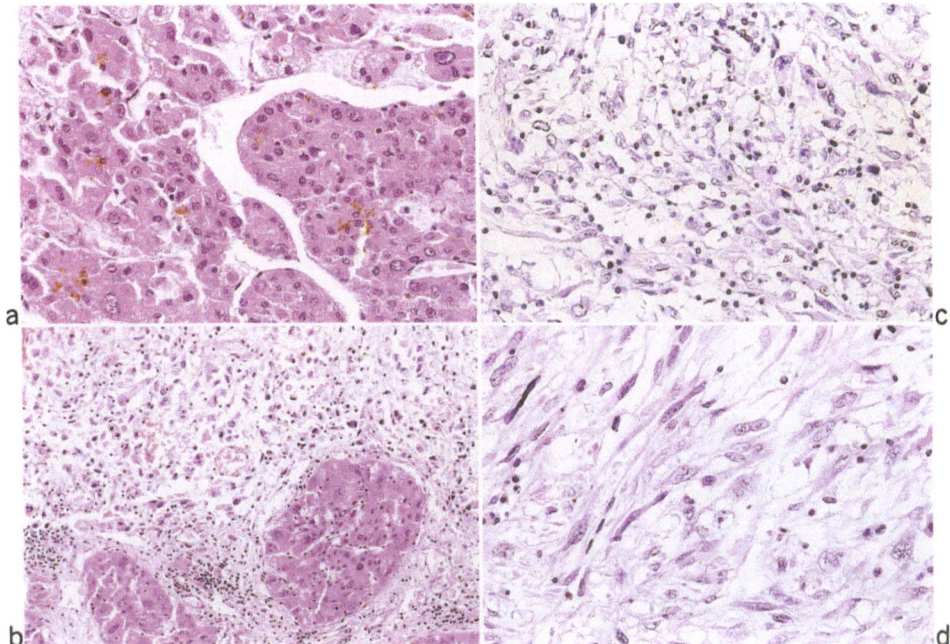

Fig. 2.23a–d. Sarcomatous change in pedunculated HCC **a, b** Remnants of trabeculae. **c, d** Sarcomatous change. HE; **a** × 100, **b, c** × 50, **d** × 100

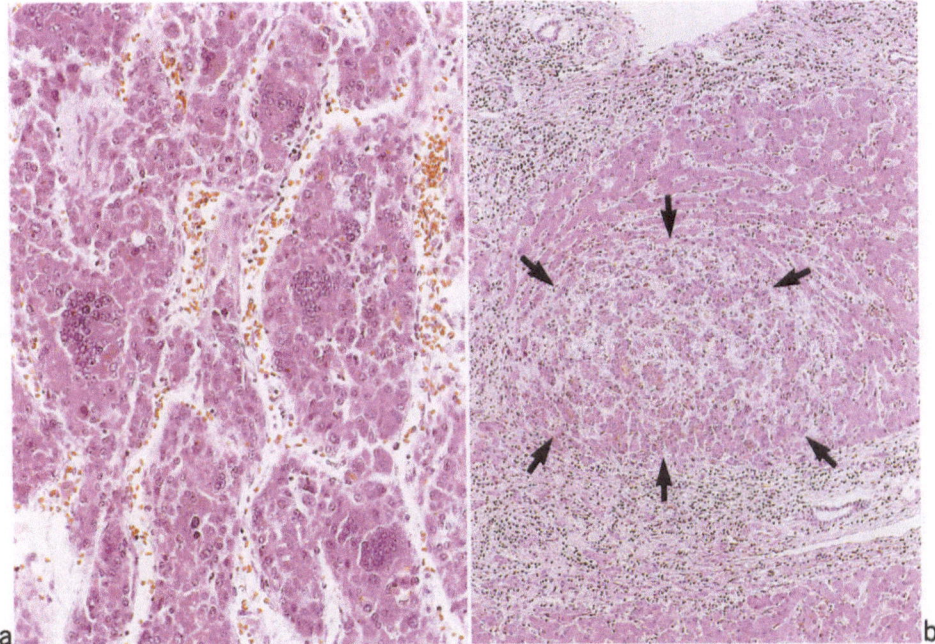

Fig. 2.24. a Giant cell HCC with a trabecular pattern (grade III carcinoma). **b** A minute metastatic focus (*arrows*) in the cirrhotic pseudolobule. HE; **a** × 100, **b** × 50

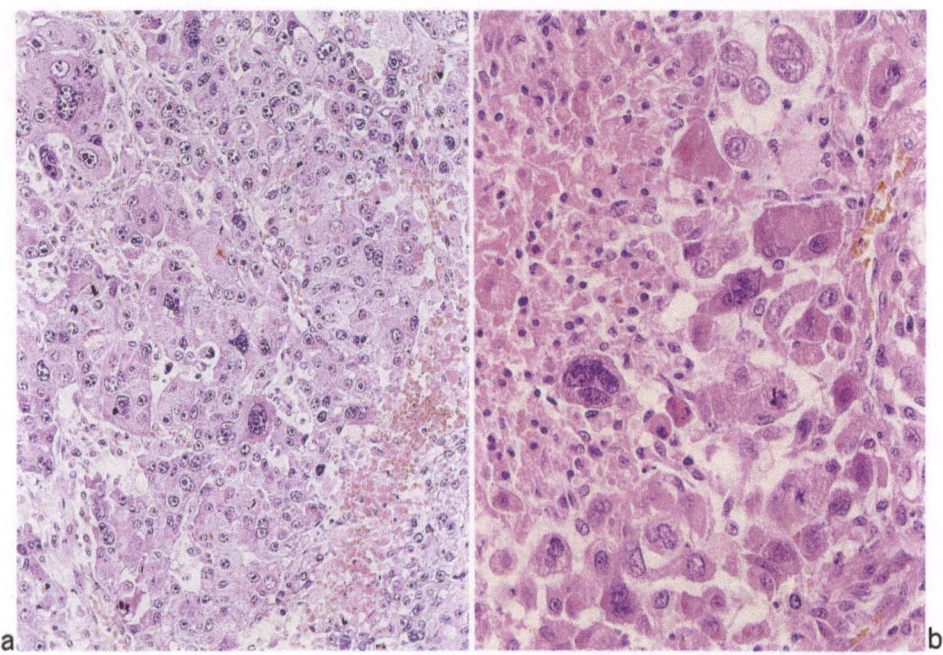

Fig. 2.25a, b. Giant cell HCC (grade III carcinoma). **a** Vague trabecular pattern. **b** Necrosis. HE; **a** × 100, **b** × 200

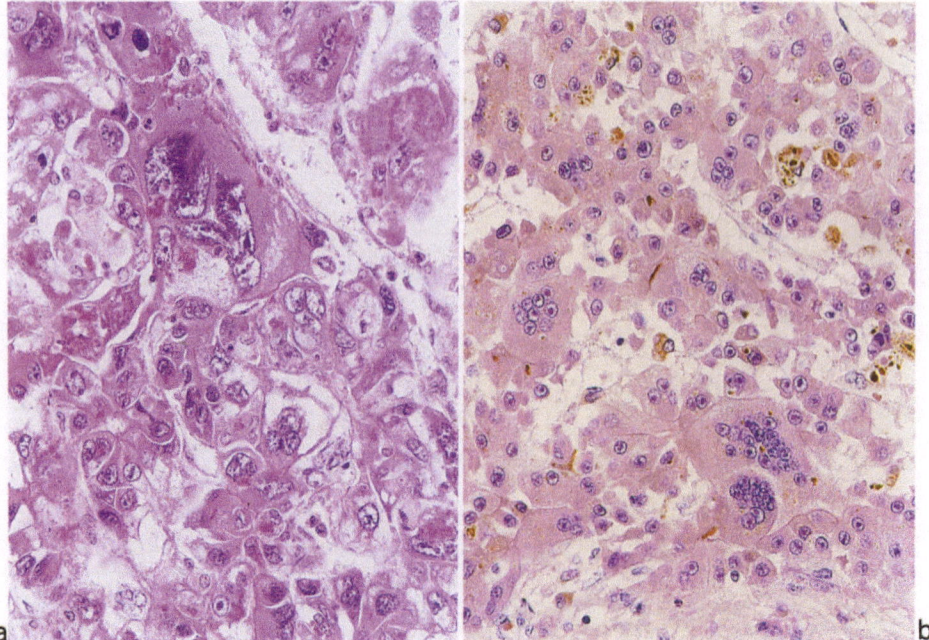

Fig. 2.26a, b. Giant cell HCC. **a** Bizarre multinucleated giant cells are prominent. **b** The nuclei of the giant cells are uniform in size. HE; **a** × 200, **b** × 100

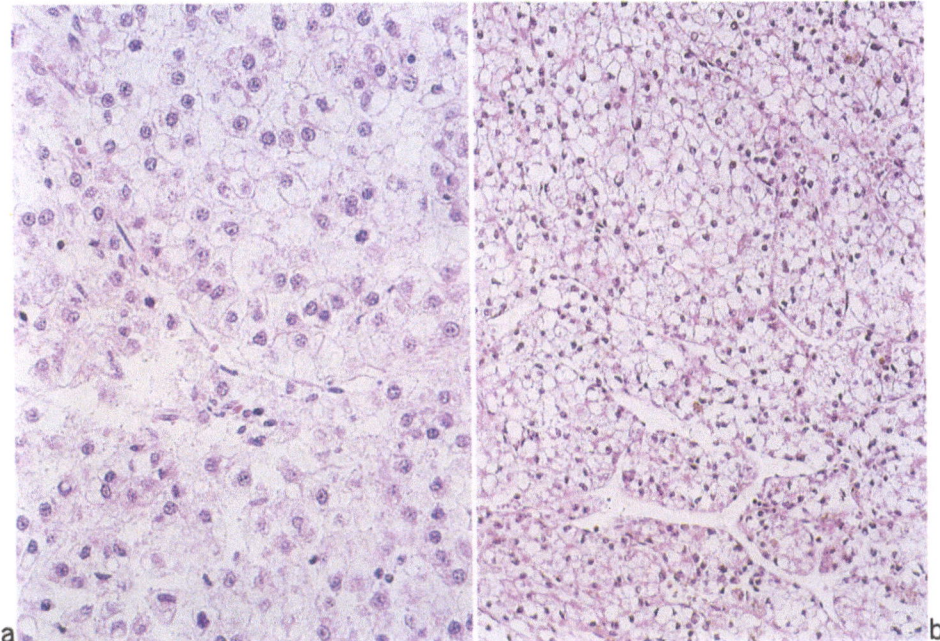

Fig. 2.27a, b. Clear cell HCC. HCC cells having clear cytoplasm show a trabecular arrangement. HE; **a** × 200, **b** × 100

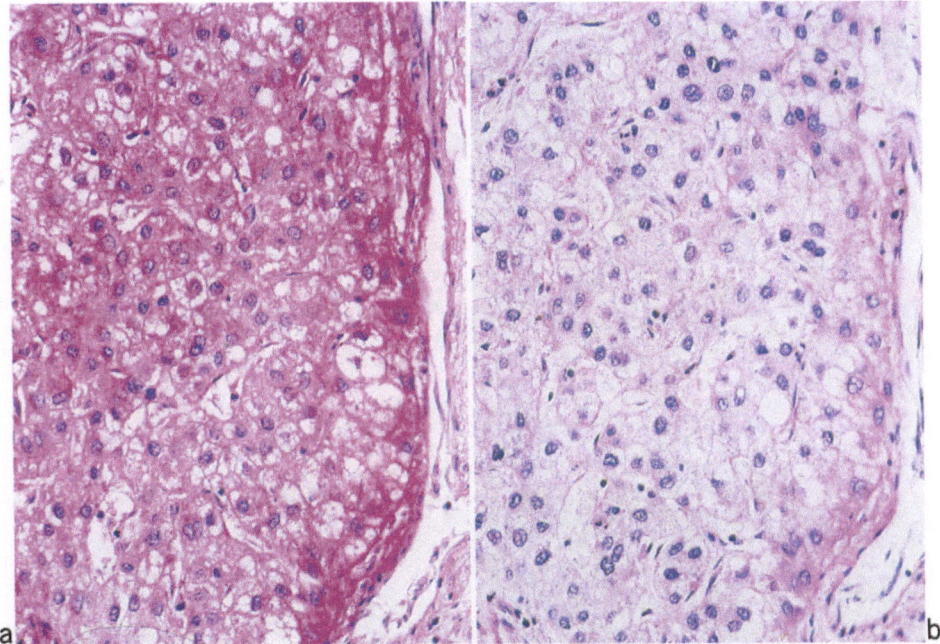

Fig. 2.28a, b. Clear cell HCC. **a** The tumor cells are strongly positive to PAS stain. **b** The PAS-positive reaction is digested by diastase. **a** PAS, **b** PAS with diastase digestion; × 200

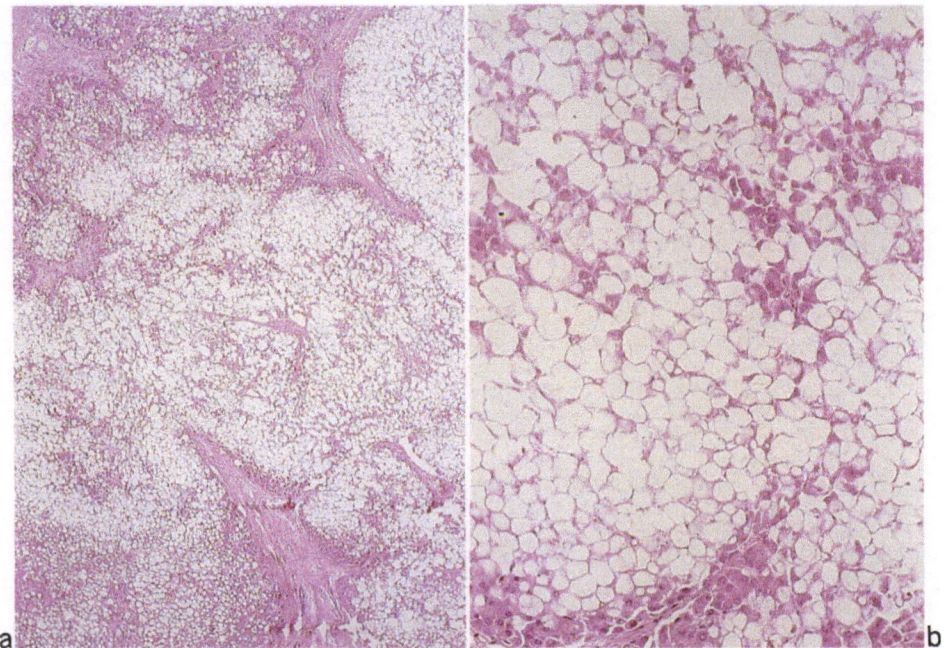

Fig. 2.29a, b. HCC with prominent fatty degeneration. HE; **a** × 50, **b** × 100

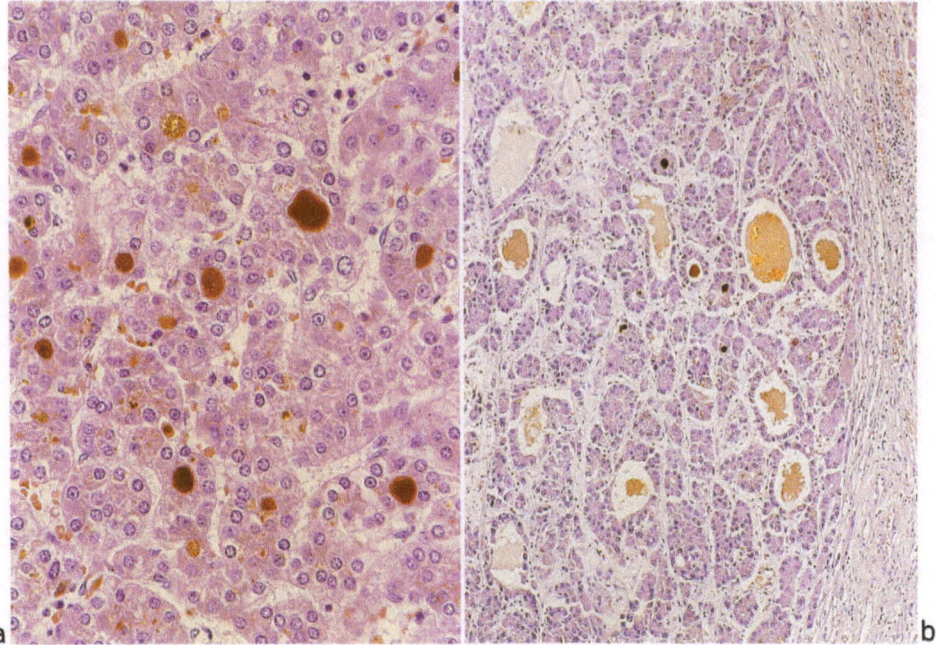

Fig. 2.30a, b. HCC with prominent bile production. HE; **a** × 100, **b** × 50

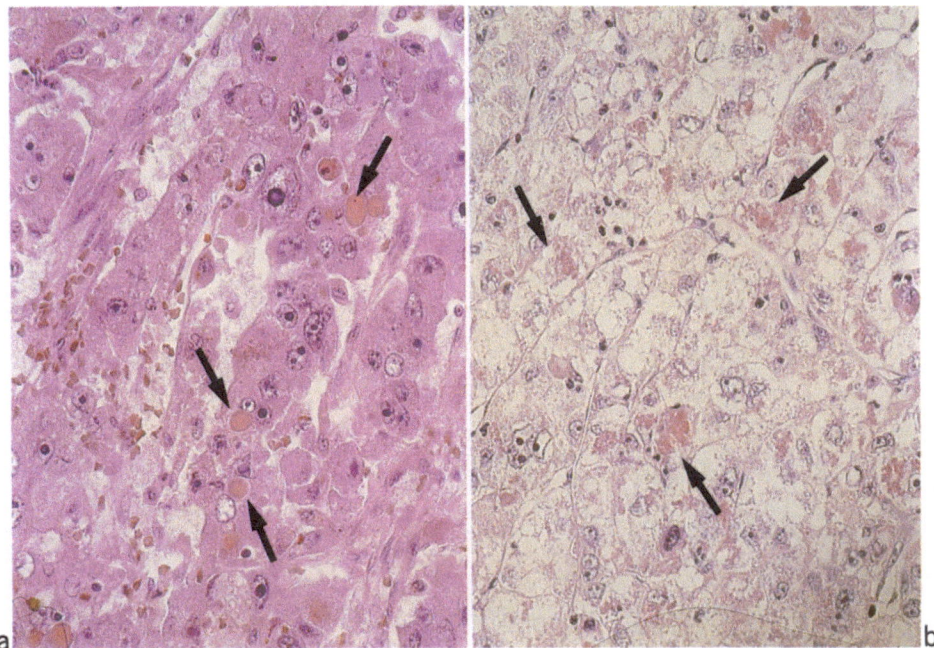

Fig. 2.31a, b. Intracytoplasmic hyalins in HCC. **a** Globular hyalin (*arrows*). **b** Mallory's hyalin (*arrows*). HE, × 200

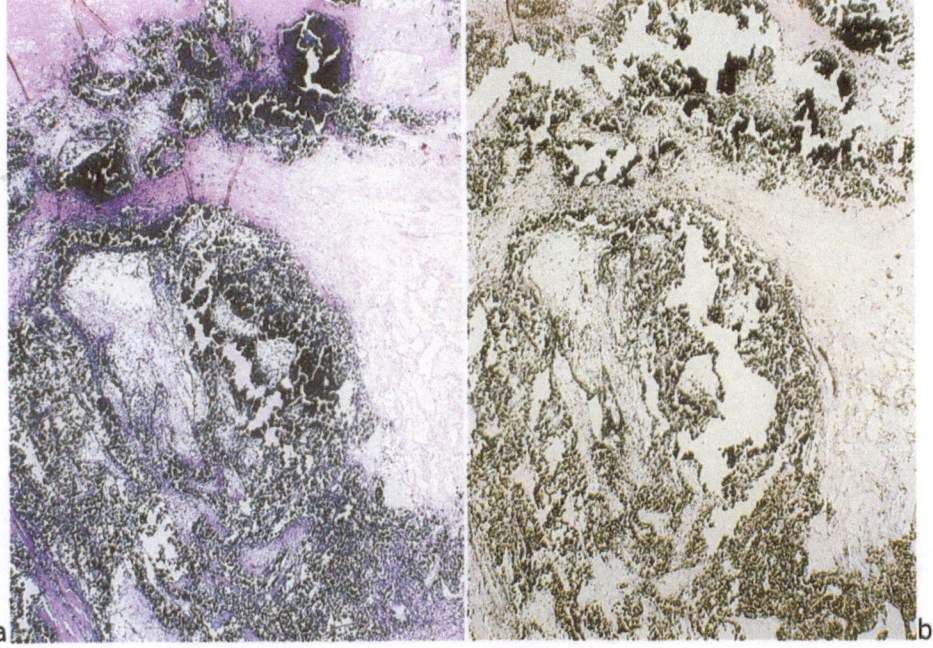

Fig. 2.32a, b. Calcification in necrotized HCC. **a** HE, **b** Kossa's stain; × 50

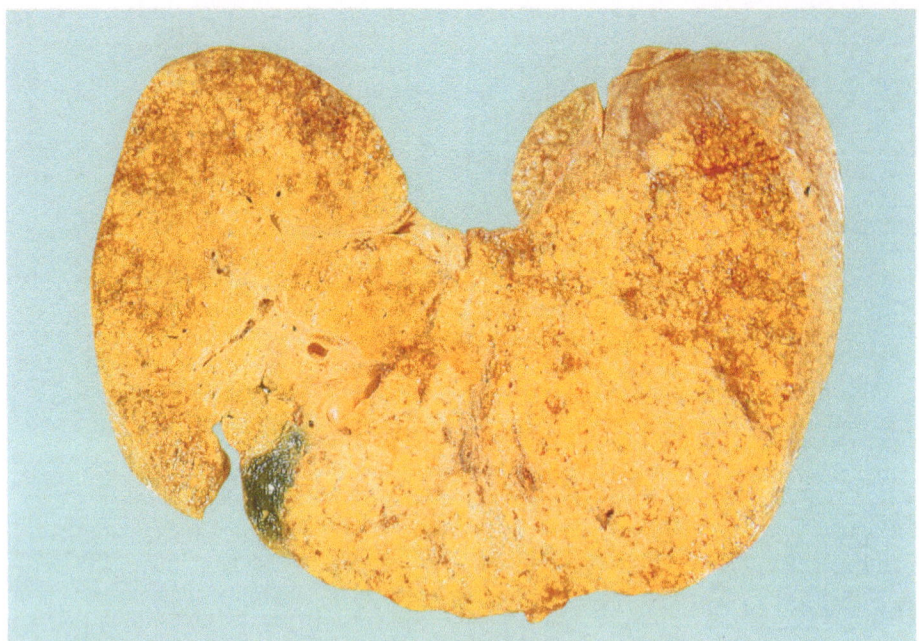

Fig. 2.33. HCC of diffuse type with sarcoid-like reaction

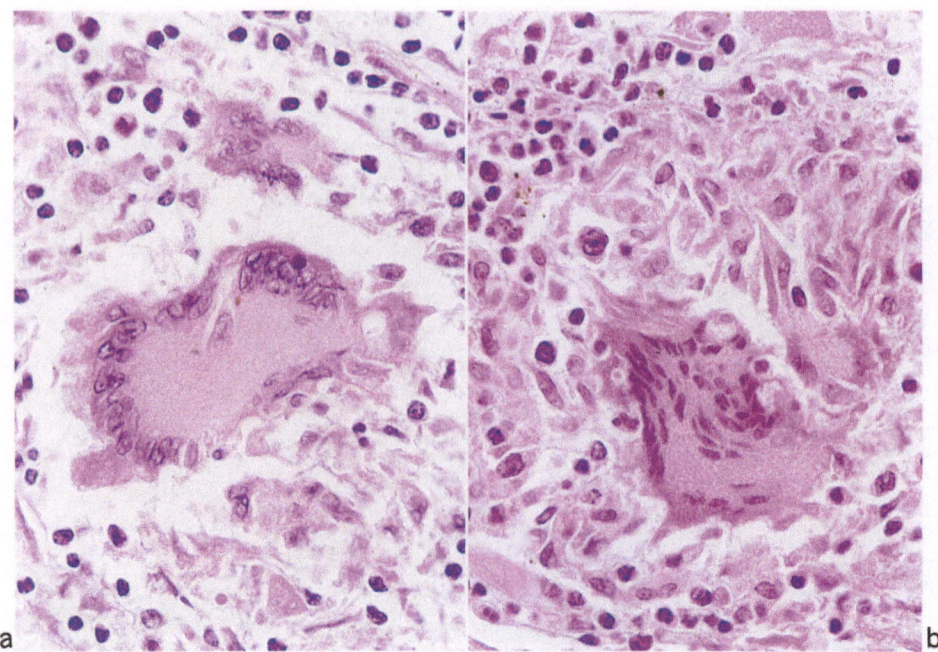

Fig. 2.34a, b. Same case. Langhans-type giant cells seen in granulomas within tumor. HE, × 200

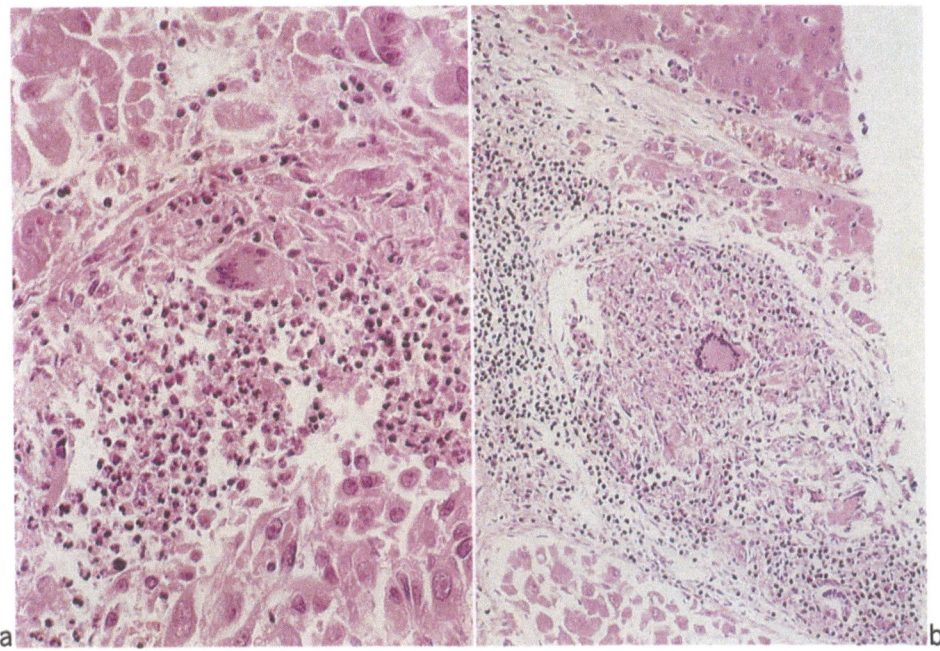

Fig. 2.35a, b. Same case. **a** Granulomatous reaction with Langhans-type giant cell in cancerous tissue. **b** Sarcoid-like granuloma seen in tumor thrombus of the portal vein. HE; **a** × 100, **b** × 50

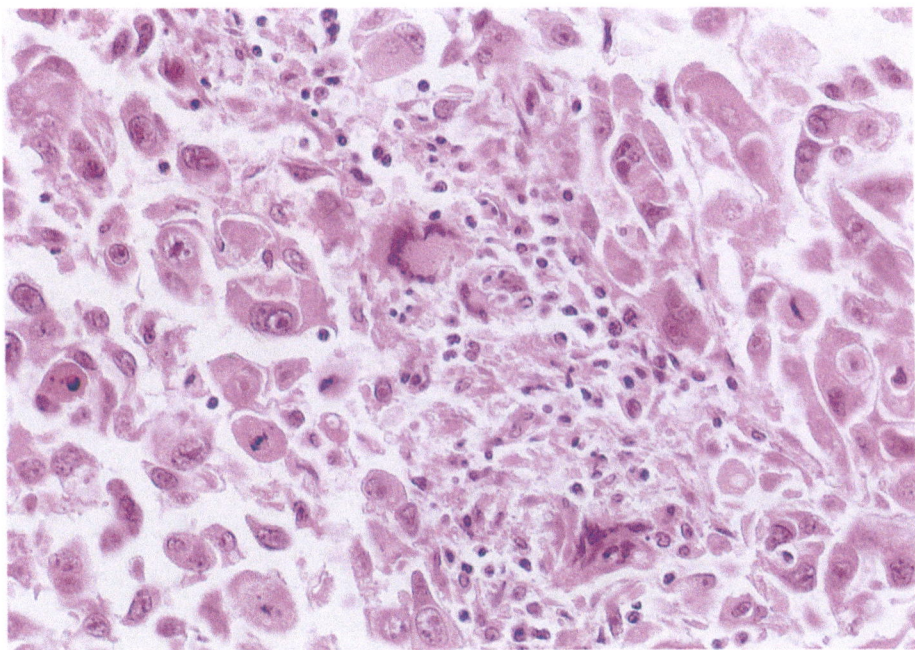

Fig. 2.36. Sarcoid-like granuloma within HCC of pleomorphic type. Langhans-type giant cell is characteristic. HE, × 200

Chapter 3
Ultrastructure of Hepatocellular Carcinoma

The ultrastructural features of HCC vary according to the degree of differentiation [94, 95]. When HCC is less differentiated, the nuclei increase in size and nuclear irregularity becomes more evident. Ultrastructurally, moderately or well-differentiated HCC can be distinguished from the poorly differentiated type by differences in the development of cellular organelles, the number of bile canaliculi, and the cellular attachment. In moderately to well-differentiated HCC, mitochondria and rough endoplasmic reticulum (rER) are well developed; the well-developed rER is believed to be evidence of the production of secretory proteins such as albumin. The Golgi apparatus and peroxisomes are evident, but remarkably decrease in number. In accordance with these findings, the smooth endoplasmic reticulum (sER) is also poorly developed. The formation of bile canaliculi and bile production are of value in the diagnosis of moderately to well-differentiated HCC, but it is occasionally difficult to diagnose poorly differentiated HCC ultrastructurally because of the sparse formation of bile canaliculi.

Trabecular HCC

In a normal liver, the cells occur in one-cell-thick plates, which are arranged in a radiating fashion from the central vein to Glisson's capsule, while two- to three-cell-thick plates are seen in a cirrhotic liver. In trabecular HCC, a structure reminiscent of normal liver cell cords is seen, but the plates vary irregularly in thickness, forming thin to thick trabeculae (Figs. 3.1–12).

The relationship between the blood space and the trabecular tumor nest is similar to that between the sinusoid and liver cell cords in a normal liver. Isomura and Nakashima [95], however, distinguished the blood space from the normal sinusoid by the sparsity of pores in the endothelial cells, the presence of intercellular junctions between the endothelial cells, and the existence of a basement membrane-like substance, in the subendothelial space of the blood space, which is seen as an either continuous or discontinuous membrane of up to several layers in thickness. The appearance of the basement membrane-like substance in HCC corresponds to capillarization of sinusoids in chronic hepatic lesions or liver cirrhosis [96]. Microvilli formation on the free surface in the subendothelial space becomes prominent when the HCC is well differentiated. The microvilli are, however, partly dependent on the amount of collagen in the subendothelial space. The number of microvilli is reduced in the collagen-rich space, which indicates that the exchange of material in the blood space in HCC may depend not only on the degree of differentiation of the tumor, but also on the amount of collagen in the blood space.

Pseudoglandular HCC

In pseudoglandular HCC (Figs. 3.13–16), the tumor forms a tubular structure to varying degrees. The tubules with microvilli on the free surface of the lumen are similar to normal bile canaliculi or bile canaliculi between tumor cells. In addition, the tubules occasionally contain an electron-dense substance, presumably bile, in the lumen. Thus, some of the tubules can be considered dilated bile canaliculi. The degree of development of microvilli varies, possibly according to the differentiation of the tumor. The microvilli vary in size, but we were unable to find any blebs, as seen in obstructive jaundice. The microfilaments are well developed in some tubules, but are sparse in others. In the lumen of the latter, myelin figures are evident, suggesting that such figures are formed by degeneration of the tumor cells.

Compact HCC

In compact HCC, the nucleus/cytoplasm ratio is high, the development of organelles is poor, cellular attachment is poor, and bile canaliculi are sparse. All these electron-microscopic findings suggest that tumors of the compact type are poorly differentiated. In general, compact HCC lacks the histological characteristics of HCC. The structure of the blood space between tumor cells, however, is similar to that seen in trabecular HCC. Therefore, the presence of a blood space-like structure may play an important role in electron-microscopic diagnosis.

Clear Cell HCC

Although Anthony [97] and Cameron [98] classified clear cell HCC as a specific type, it is not uncommon to encounter HCC consisting of clear cells in varying degrees. Ultrastructurally, HCC cells of the clear cell type contain abundant glycogen granules in their cytoplasm, or fat droplets in some cases (Figs. 3.17, 18).

Mallory Bodies in HCC Cells

Ultrastructurally, Yokoo et al. [99] classified alcoholic hyalins into three distinct morphological forms: *type I*, bundles of filaments in parallel arrays; *type II*, clusters of randomly oriented fibrils; *type III*, granular or amorphous substance containing only scattered remains of fibrils.

In HCC, globular hyalins are observed as either type I or type II inclusions (Fig. 3.19), and reticular hyalins are seen as type III inclusions accompanying type I inclusions in their periphery (Fig. 3.20). Tomimatsu [87] suggested that peroxisomes might be related to the formation of type I and type II inclusions, according to the evidence that they surrounded type I or type II inclusions in some cases (Fig. 3.19).

Ground-Glass Inclusions in HCC Cells

Stromeyer et al. [90] first reported ground-glass inclusions in HCC cells and described them as non-membrane-bound fibrillar material that reacted with antifibrinogen. We have found similar inclusions, but they were seen as membrane-bound fine fibrillar material. We consider that antifibrinogen-positive ground-glass inclusions are the result of the accumulation of fibrinogen in endoplasmic reticulum showing cystic dilatation.

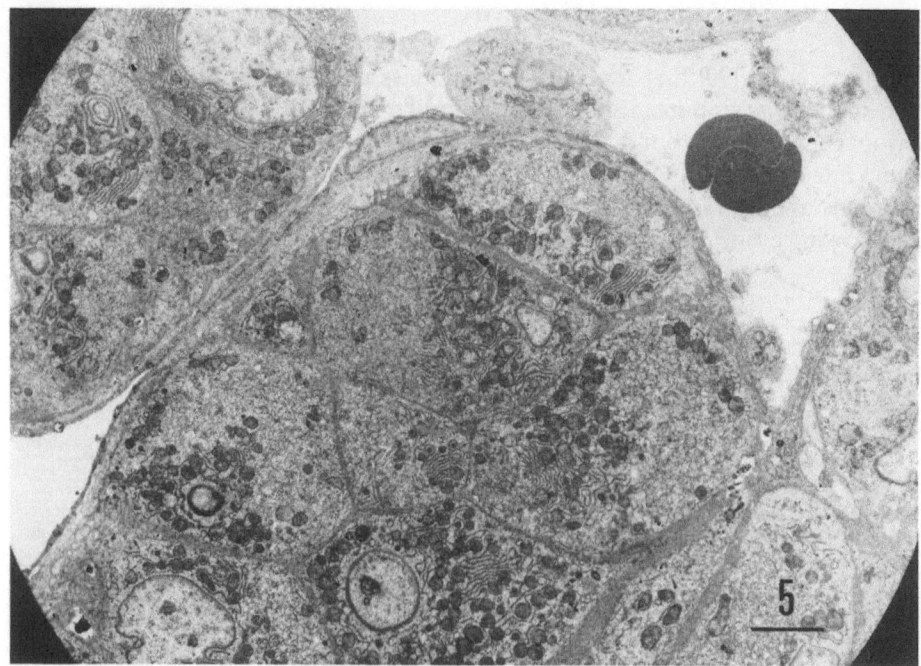

Fig. 3.1. Trabecular HCC, well-differentiated. The tumor cells are surrounded by a single layer of endothelial cells

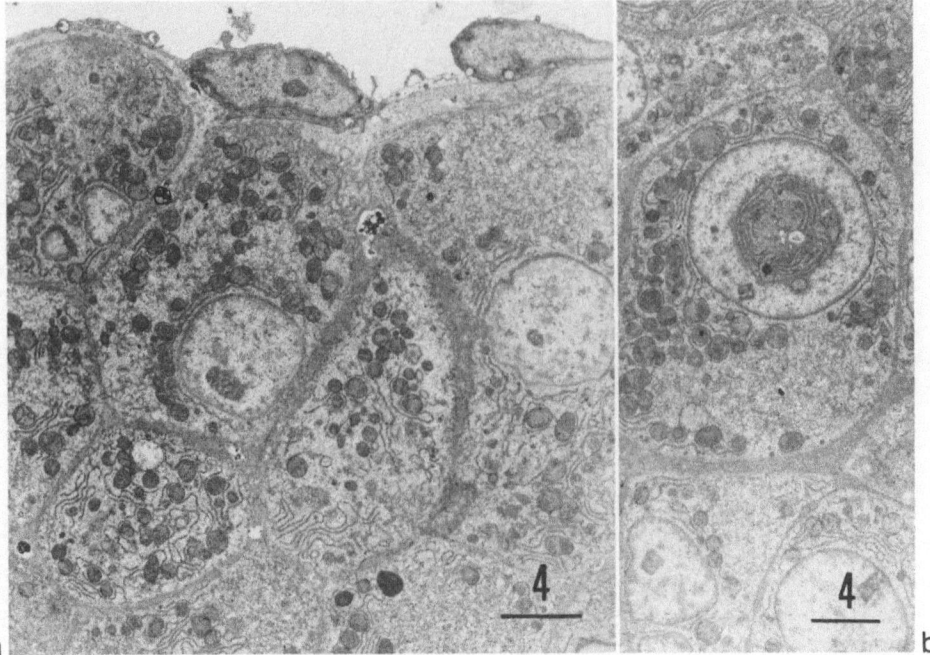

Fig. 3.2a–b. Trabecular HCC, well-differentiated. **a** Bile canaliculi are seen between tumor cells. **b** Pseudoinclusion is observed in the nucleus

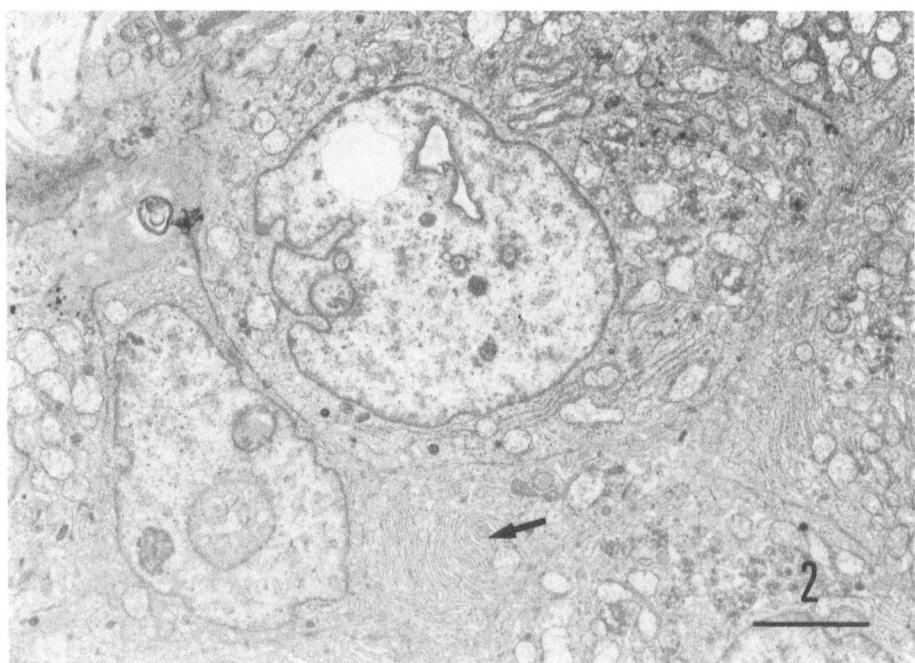

Fig. 3.3. Trabecular HCC, moderately differentiated. The nucleus/cytoplasm ratio is increased and nuclear irregularity is dominant. The rER shows a lamellar structure (*arrow*)

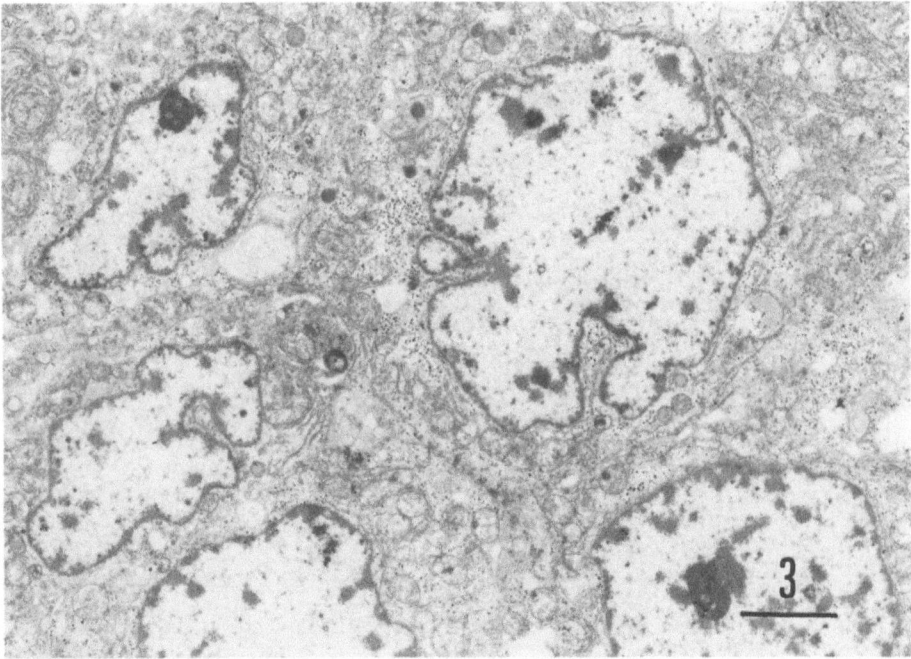

Fig. 3.4. Trabecular HCC, moderately differentiated. Although nuclear irregularity is prominent, intracytoplasmic organelles are well developed

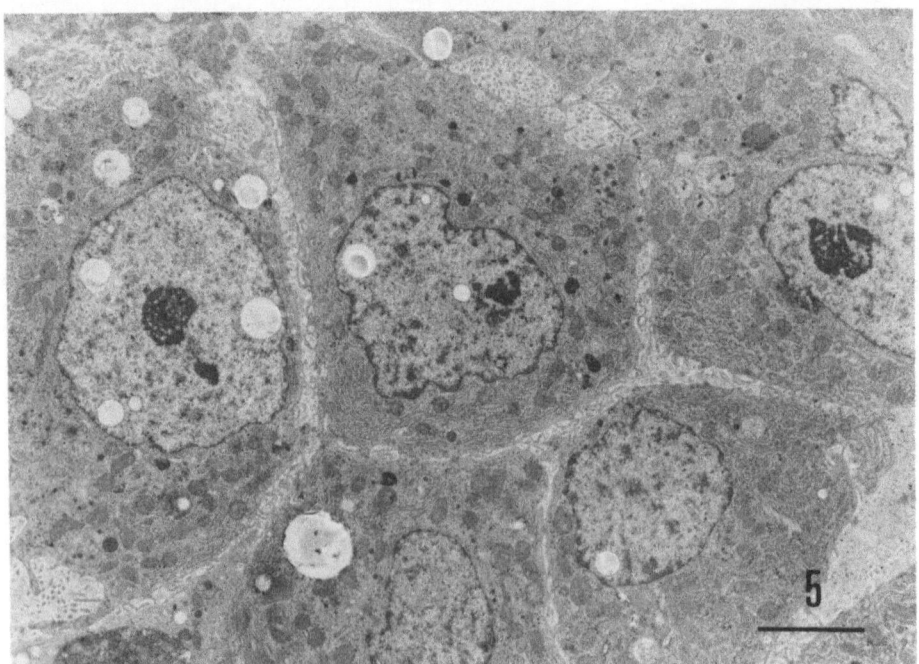

Fig. 3.5. Trabecular HCC, moderately differentiated. Cellular atypism is not dominant, but the tumor cells show poor mutual adhesion

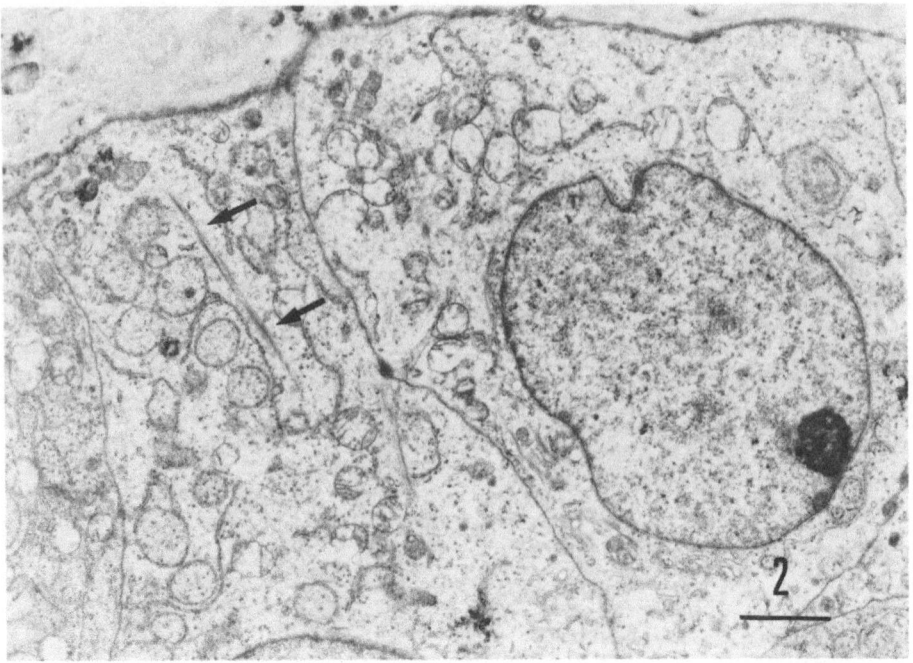

Fig. 3.6. Trabecular HCC, moderately differentiated. Filament-like structures (*arrows*) in the cytoplasm

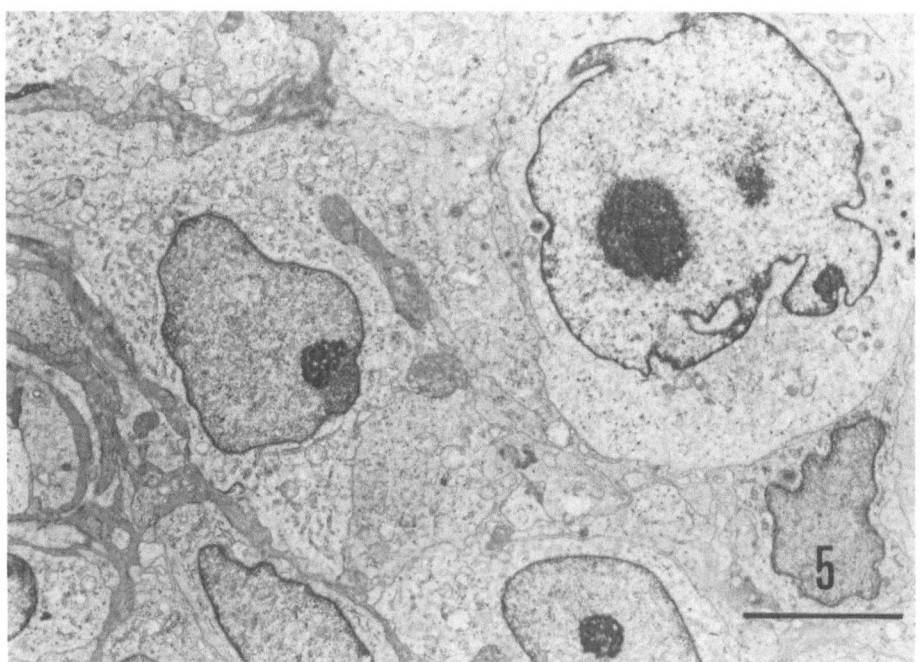

Fig. 3.7. Trabecular HCC, poorly differentiated. Nuclear irregularity is increased and nucleoli are prominent

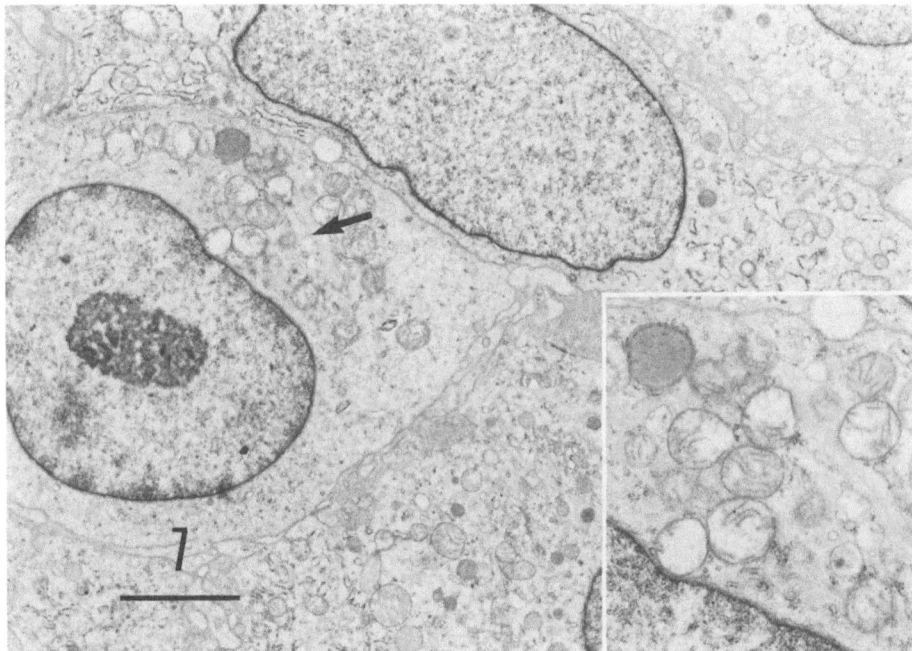

Fig. 3.8. Trabecular HCC, poorly differentiated. Filament-like structure (*arrow*) in cytoplasm. *Inset*: detail of filament-like structure

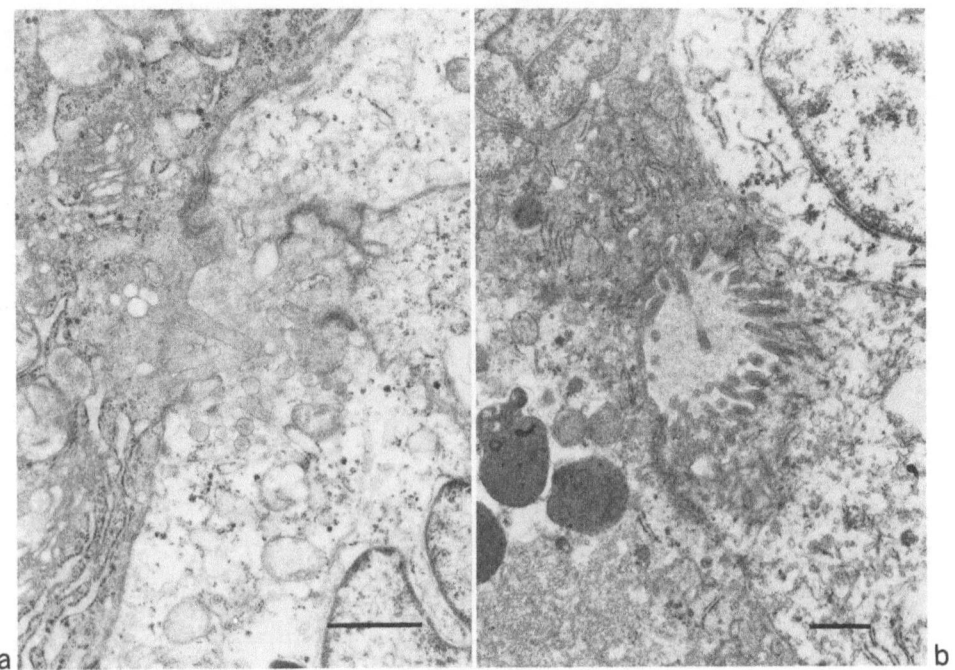

Fig. 3.9a, b. Bile canaliculi seen between well-differentiated HCC cells

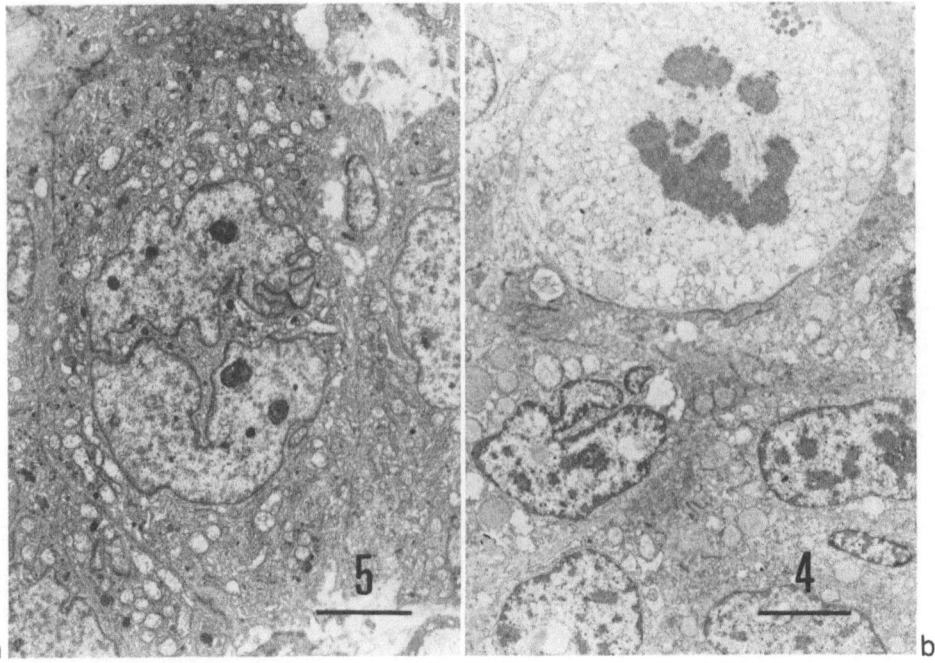

Fig. 3.10a, b. Pleomorphic HCC cells. **a** Binucleated giant cell. **b** Mitosis in HCC cell

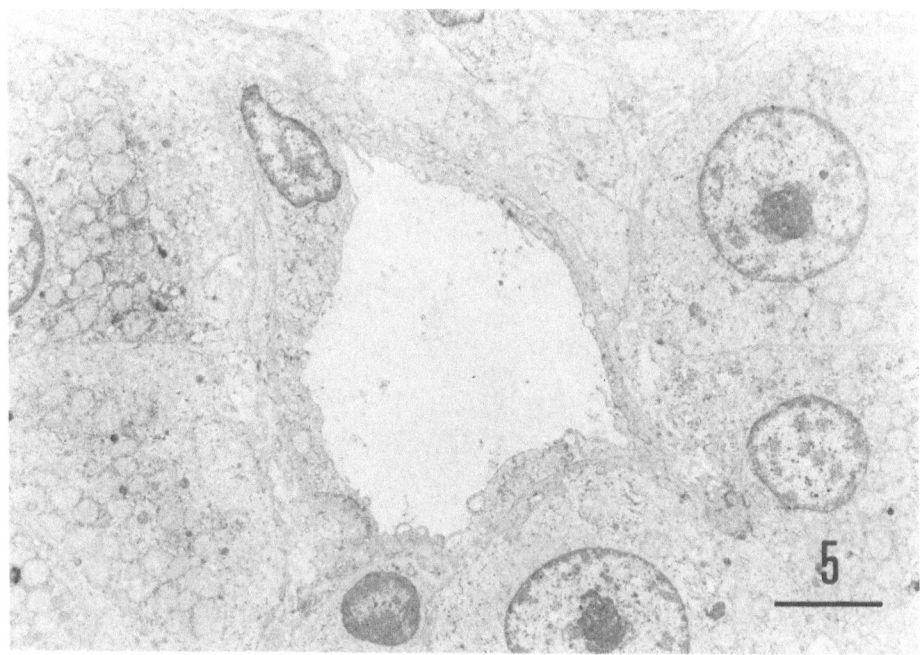

Fig. 3.11. Blood space in HCC. Endothelial cells lack pore formation

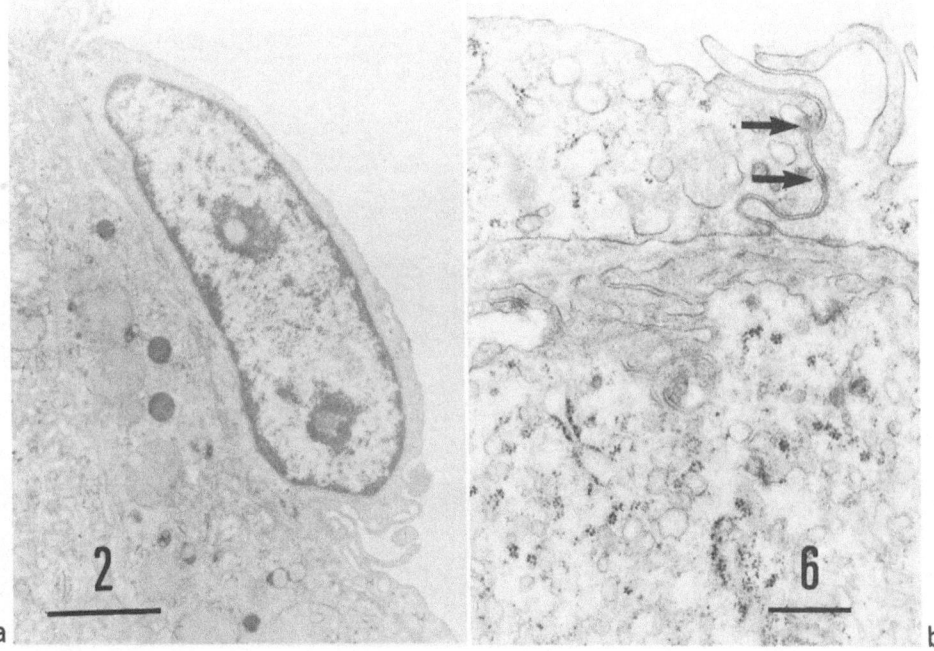

Fig. 3.12. **a** Well-developed marginal folds in endothelial cell of blood space. **b** Junctional complexes between endothelial cells (*arrows*)

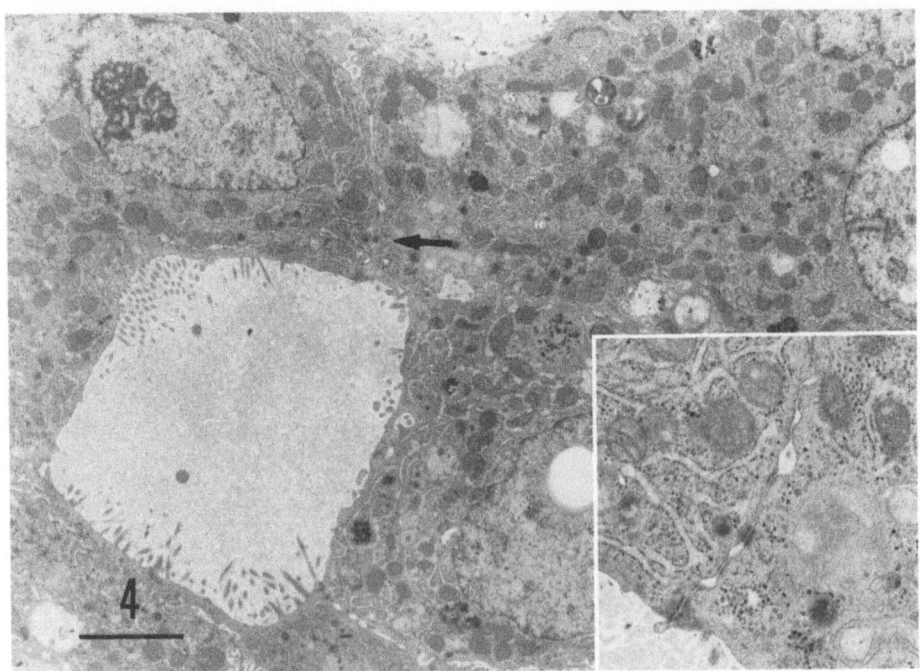

Fig. 3.13. Pseudoglandular HCC. Microvilli are well developed in the luminal border. A juctional complex (*arrow*) is observed between the tumor cells. *Inset*: junctional complex

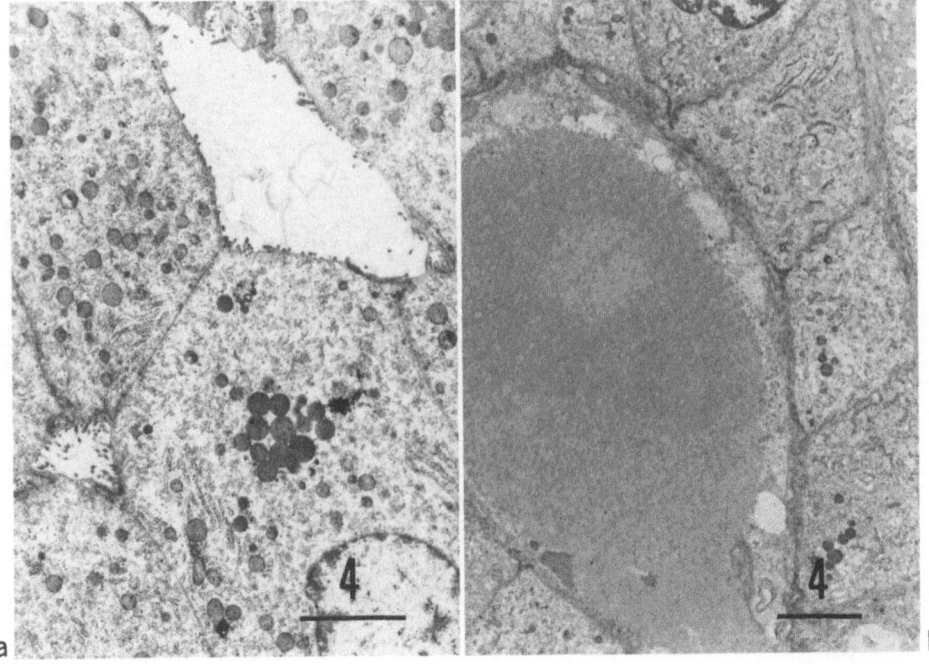

Fig. 3.14a, b. Pseudoglandular HCC. **a** Glandular structure with microvilli. **b** Lumen without microvilli

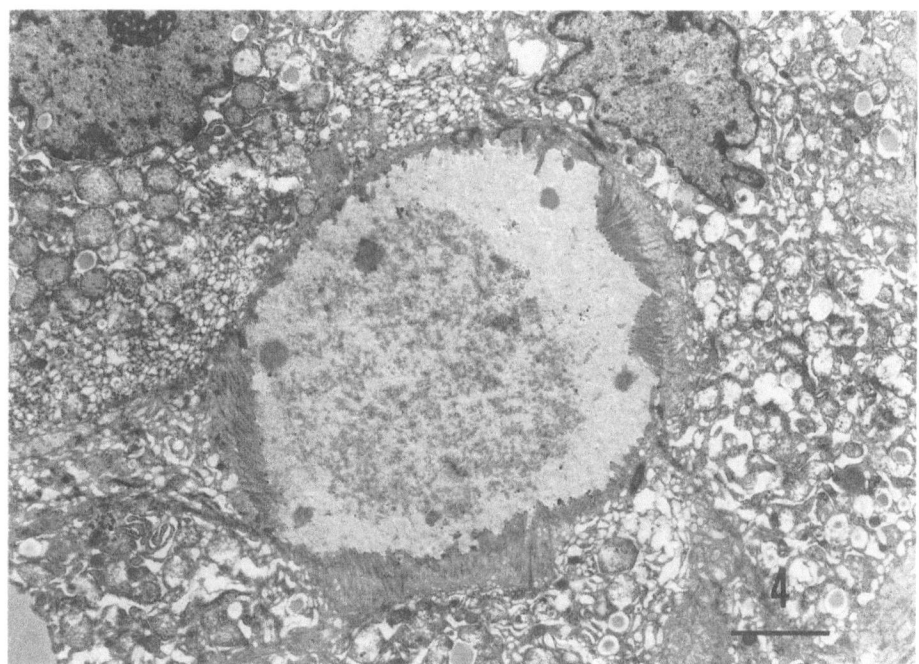

Fig. 3.15. Pseudoglandular HCC with well-developed microvilli in the lumen

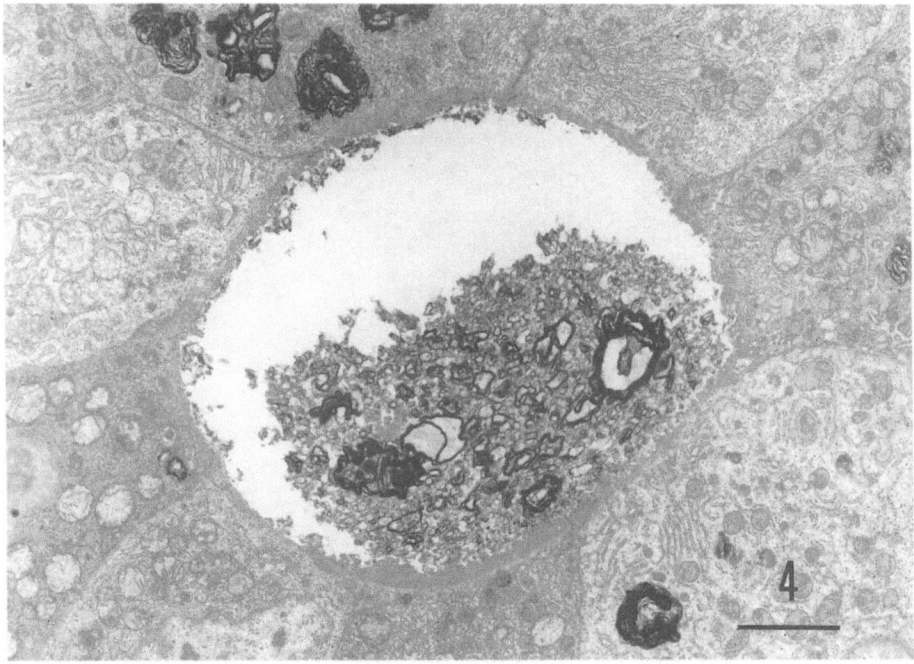

Fig. 3.16. Pseudoglandular HCC containing degenerative materials in the lumen

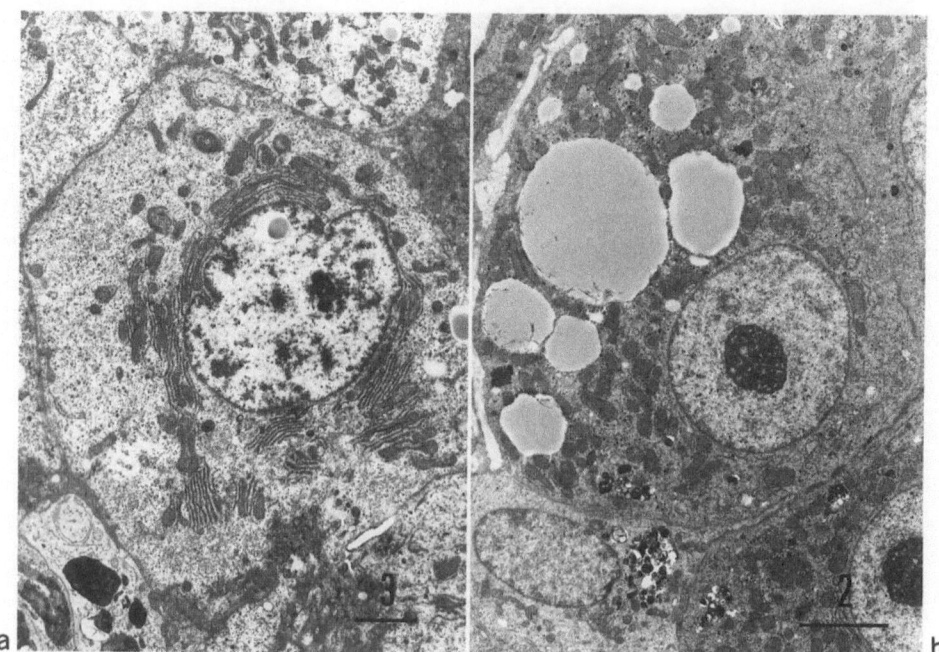

Fig. 3.17a, b. Clear cell HCC. **a** Abundant glycogen granules are observed. **b** The HCC cell contains varying sized fat droplets

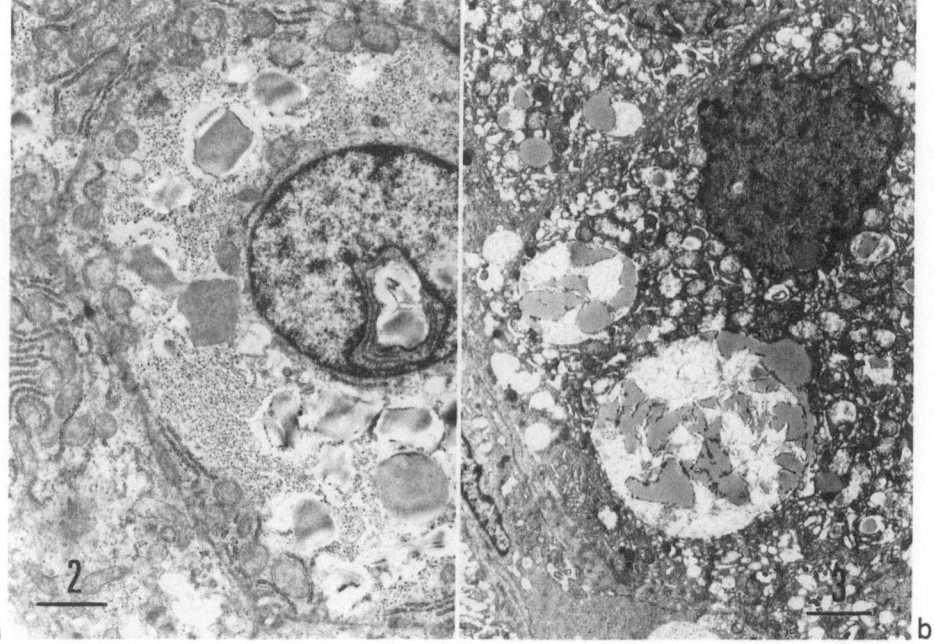

Fig. 3.18a, b. Clear cell HCC. **a** The HCC cells contain fat droplets and glycogen granules of varying size. **b** Fat droplets in HCC cells tend to fuse with each other

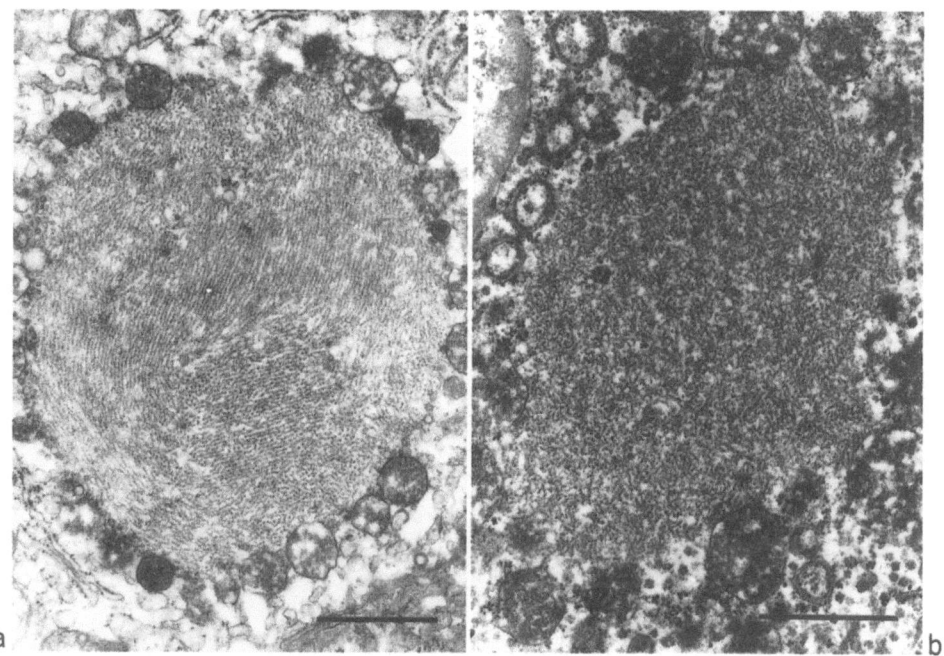

Fig. 3.19a, b. Hyaline inclusions (Mallory bodies) in HCC cells. Hyalins are seen as an accumulation of fibrillar structure. **a** Yokoo's type I hyalin. **b** Yokoo's type II hyalin. Both are surrounded by peroxisomes

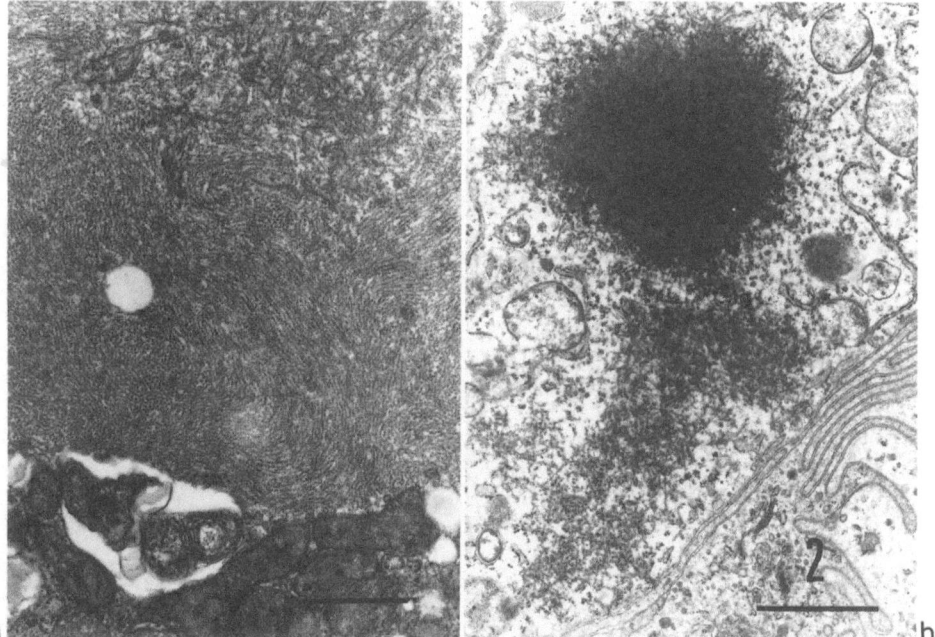

Fig. 3.20a, b. Mallory bodies in HCC cells. **a** Yokoo's type I + II hyalins. **b** Yokoo's type II + III hyalins

Chapter 4
Histological Growth Patterns of Hepatocellular Carcinoma

Macroscopically, HCC grows in either an infiltrative or an expansive pattern. The growth patterns at the tumor-nontumor boundary, however, can be histologically divided into two basic categories, sinusoidal and replacing. Occasionally, a lesion is encountered that pushes normal hepatic cells ahead of it as it grows—although it is primarily of the replacing type—because of the predominance of expansive growth. In such lesions, a pseudocapsule of reticulin fibers is formed, concentrated along the boundary (pseudocapsular growth). These lesions are classified separately and designated pseudocapsular.

Sinusoidal Growth Pattern

In the sinusoidal growth pattern (Figs. 4.1–12), tumor cells grow in an infiltrating fashion in the sinusoids at the boundary, compressing liver cell cords and hepatocytes. On silver impregnation, reticulin fibers are seen to be condensed in the areas where liver cells have disappeared, with irregular destruction of the reticulin framework. The tumor cells tend to be free with little mutual contact, and extrahepatic metastasis is most frequent in this type [100, 101]. Grossly, HCC displaying the sinusoidal growth pattern is mainly of the infiltrative type. No surgical cases are of the sinusoidal type. Because HCC of the sinusoidal type does not form a capsule, it is difficult to detect early using imaging techniques such as computed tomography and/or ultrasonography. Extrahepatic metastasis in HCC of the sinusoidal type occurs earlier and more frequently than in other kinds of HCC. Surgery is rarely indicated in the sinusoidal type.

Replacing Growth Pattern

In the replacing growth pattern (Figs. 4.13–28), tumor cells are seen replacing hepatocytes along the liver cell cords. This is a basic growth pattern in HCC. There is some increase of reticulin fibers at the boundary, but the basic reticulin framework is preserved. In the area where HCC cells are arranged along the liver cell cords, the sinusoids communicate with blood spaces of cancerous tissue.

Electron-microscopic examination of the replacing type of HCC in the region of the tumor-nontumor boundary reveals the cancer cells to be proliferating along the liver cell cord, as if they were replacing liver cells. The cell membranes of both hepatic and cancer cells are recognizable at the boundary. The hepatic cells are deformed and irregular, cytoplasmic processes of cancer cells project into the hepatic cells, and lipofuscin granules are increased in hepatic cells near the cancer cells. All these findings suggest that cancer cells in the hepatic cords compress the hepatic cells. Where cancer cells are arranged along the hepatic cords, the sinusoids communicate with the blood spaces of the cancerous tissue, and Disse's spaces with the subendothelial space of cancerous tissue [102, 103]. In accordance with these findings, continuity of the hepatic cell cord and cancer cell plate is demonstrated in the reticulin fibers, which are not heavily destroyed.

The continuity of the sinusoids and blood spaces can also be demonstrated by means of silver impregnation in a 1-μm section stained with Giemsa. In such a region, the endothelial cells are enlarged and there is a conglomeration of immature hepatic cells, with few intracellular organelles, near the cancer cells. The cancer tissue at the front of the replacing growth may be nourished by blood from the portal vein. In HCC growing in a replacing fashion, poorly differentiated endothelial cells in the periboundary of the tumor tissue constitute the stroma of tumor nests. They resemble sinusoidal endothelial cells but have fewer cytoplasmic organelles. In such areas, the cancer cells are arranged relatively close to each other with desmosomes and interdigitations. The transition between sinusoidal endothelial cells and endothelial cells in the cancer nest can hardly be observed.

Pseudocapsular Growth Pattern

We occasionally encounter a tumor which, although primarily of the replacing growth type, compresses noncancerous tissue in an expansive fashion. Reticulin fibers concentrate along the boundary, and a pseudocapsule is formed. Ultrastructurally, the endothelial cells form nests and, besides Disse's spaces containing collagen, intercellular collagen is evident in the endothelium. This feature indicates that hepatic cells are obliterated following degeneration, leaving the sinusoids in layers. Such changes correspond to the changes in the early stage described by Okabe [39], who stated that obliteration of the reticulin fibers, collagenization, and occasional hyalinization occur with progression of HCC, diminishing the importance of the capsule. Metastasis is most infrequent in the pseudocapsular growth type (Figs. 4.29–44).

HCC in which surgical excision is indicated is mostly of the pseudocapsular type. Among 92 patients who have undergone surgery in our institute, about 90% had HCC of this type. Despite the pseudocapsular growth pattern, extracapsular tumor growth was found in about 44% of the cases, and all the extracapsular tumor foci had grown in a replacing manner. Therefore, pseudocapsular growth should be considered a category of replacing growth.

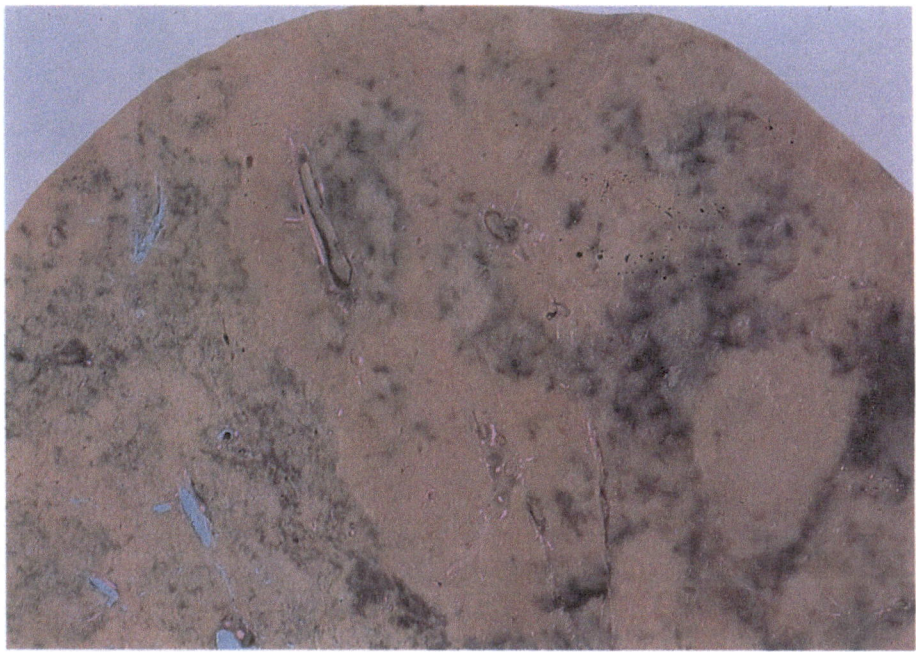

Fig. 4.1. Infiltrative HCC. The tumor-nontumor boundary is obscure. Histologically, the tumor shows a sinusoidal growth pattern. Colored contrast media were injected into the blood vessels: *red*, artery; *blue*, portal vein

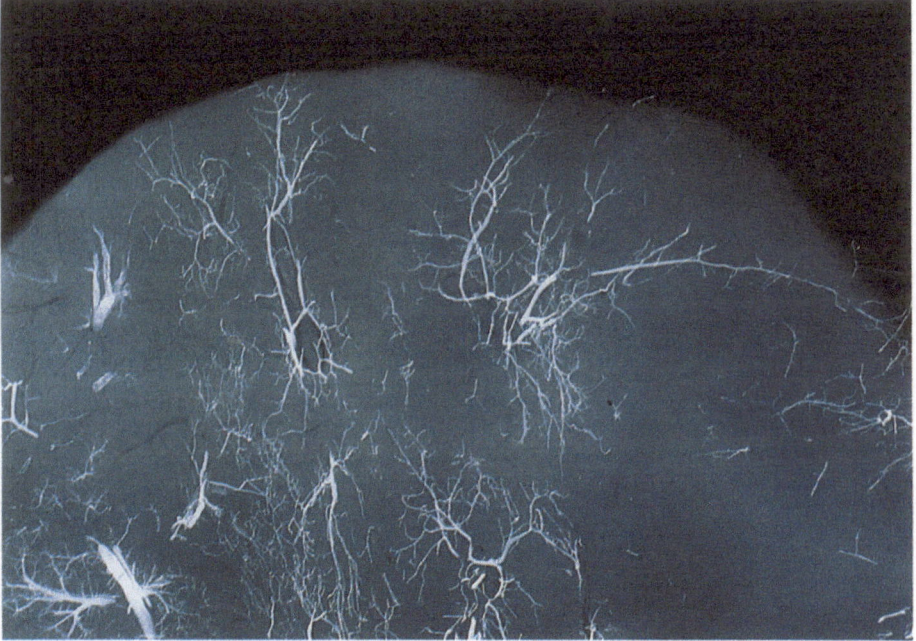

Fig. 4.2. Same case. Soft X-ray finding. The portal veins were not imaged due to a massive tumor thrombus

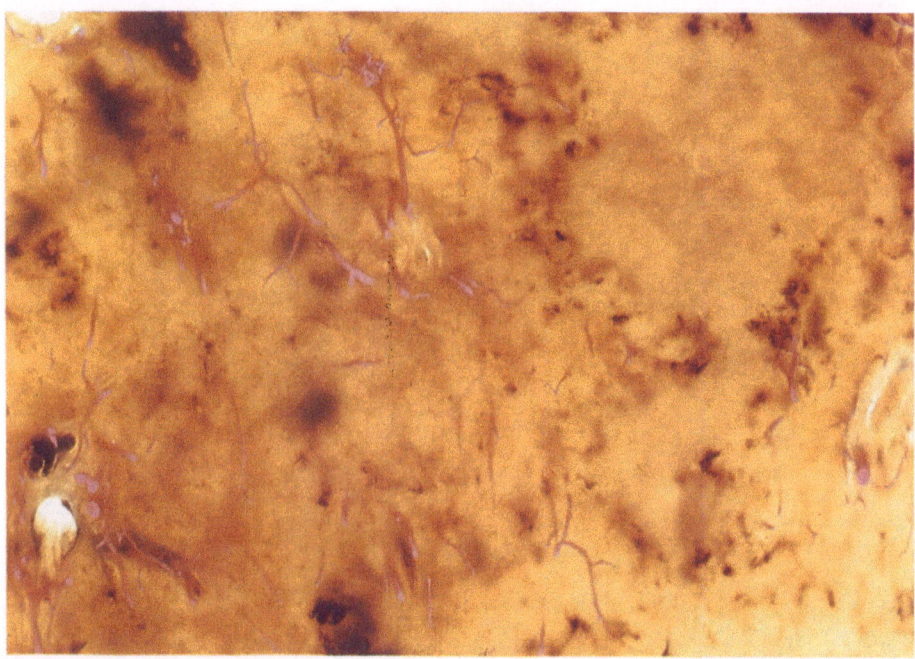

Fig. 4.3. Same case. The arteries show narrowing and interruption in the cancerous areas with fibrosis. Colored contrast medium could not be injected into the portal vein due to tumor thrombus. Transparent preparation

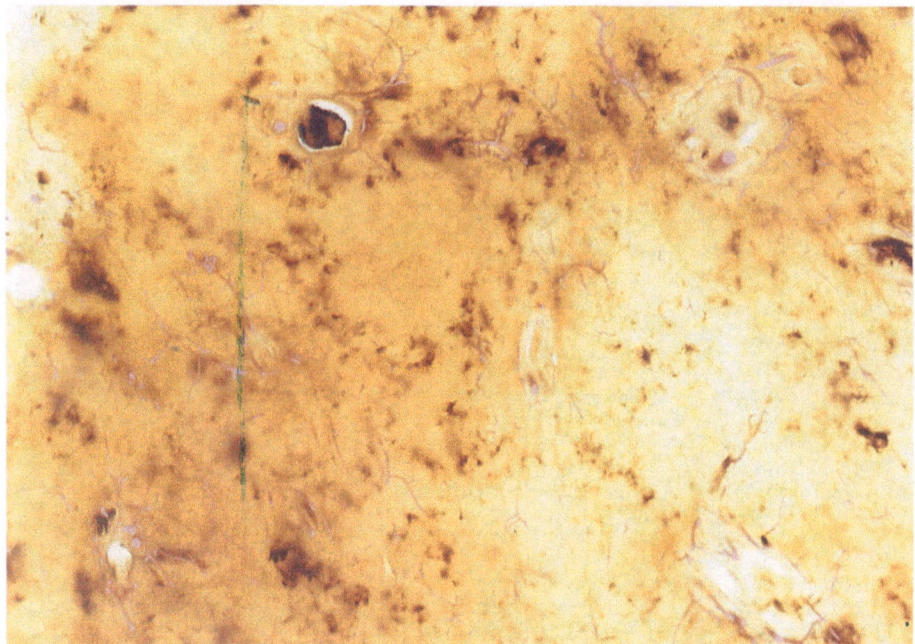

Fig. 4.4. Same case. The center of the cancerous area shows fibrosis and hyalinization

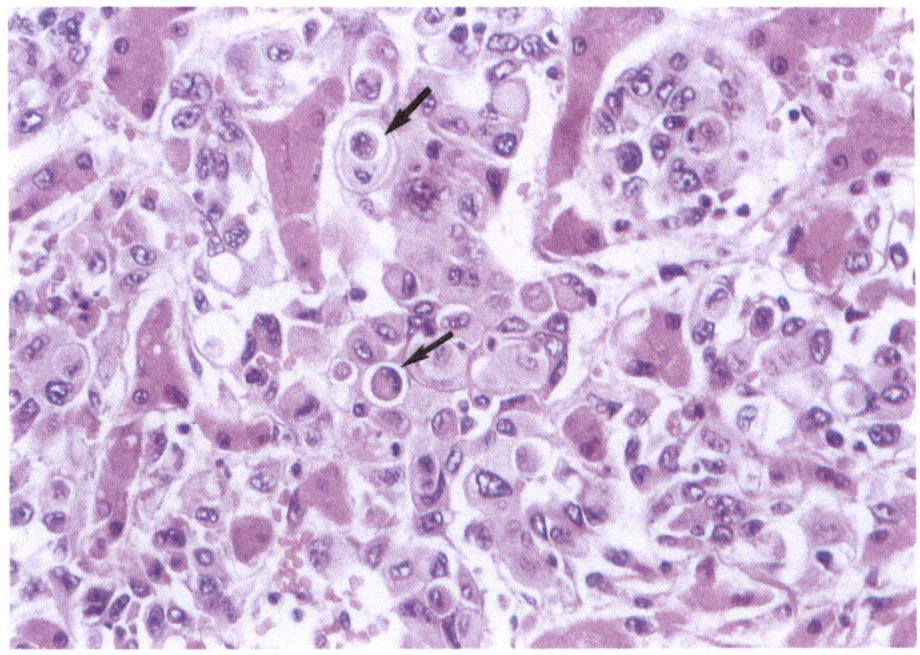

Fig. 4.5. Sinusoidal growth. The cancer cells lack a mutual contact (free-cell type) and are pleomorphic. They are growing in the sinusoids, some cancer cells show cannibalism (*arrows*). HE, × 400

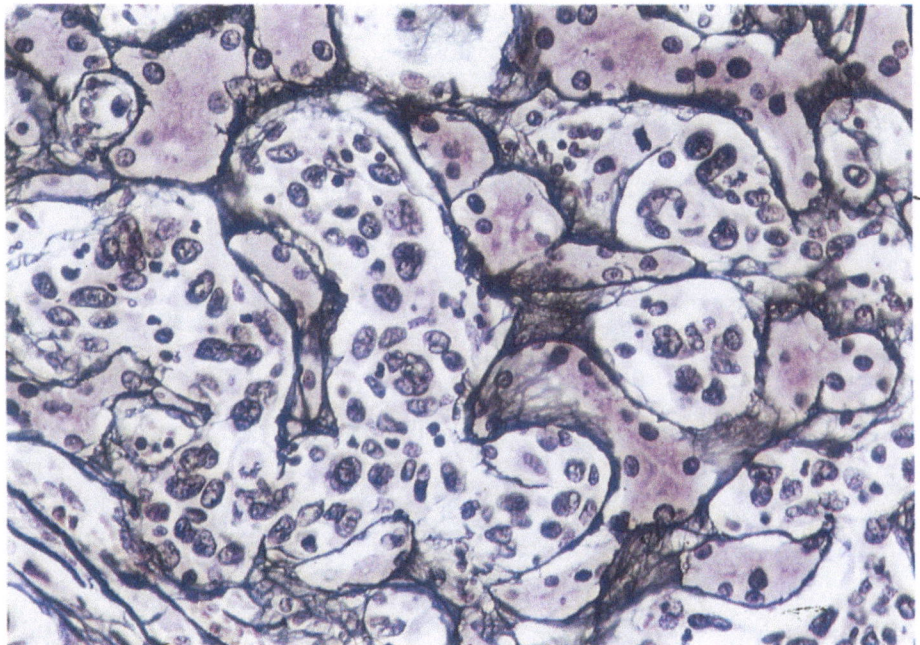

Fig. 4.6. Same case. The reticulin framework of the liver cell cords is markedly distorted. Reticulin, × 400

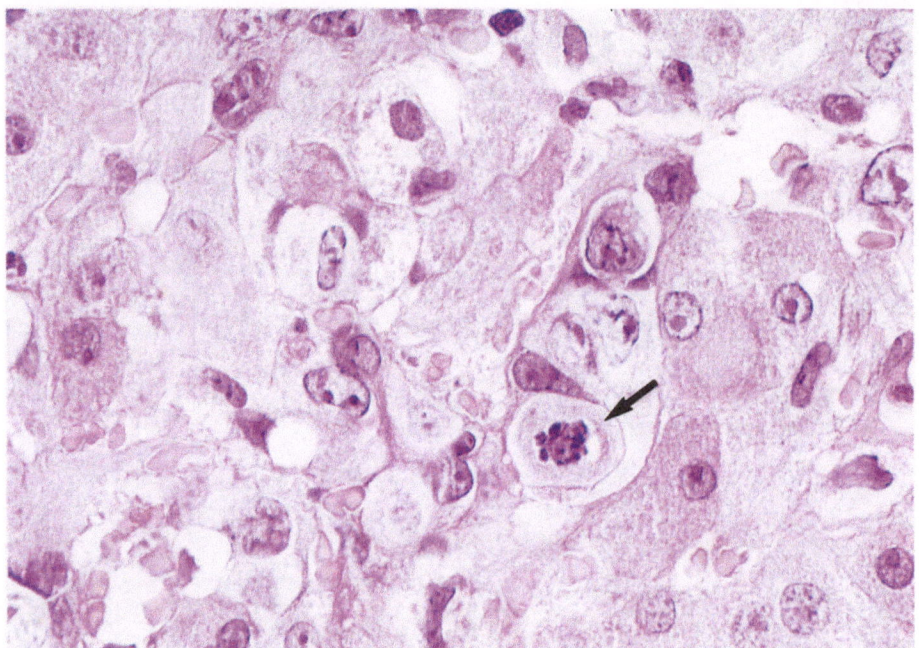

Fig. 4.7. Sinusoidal growth. Free-cell type cancer cells (*arrow*) are growing in the sinusoids. Epon-embedded 1-μm section, HE, $\times$ 600

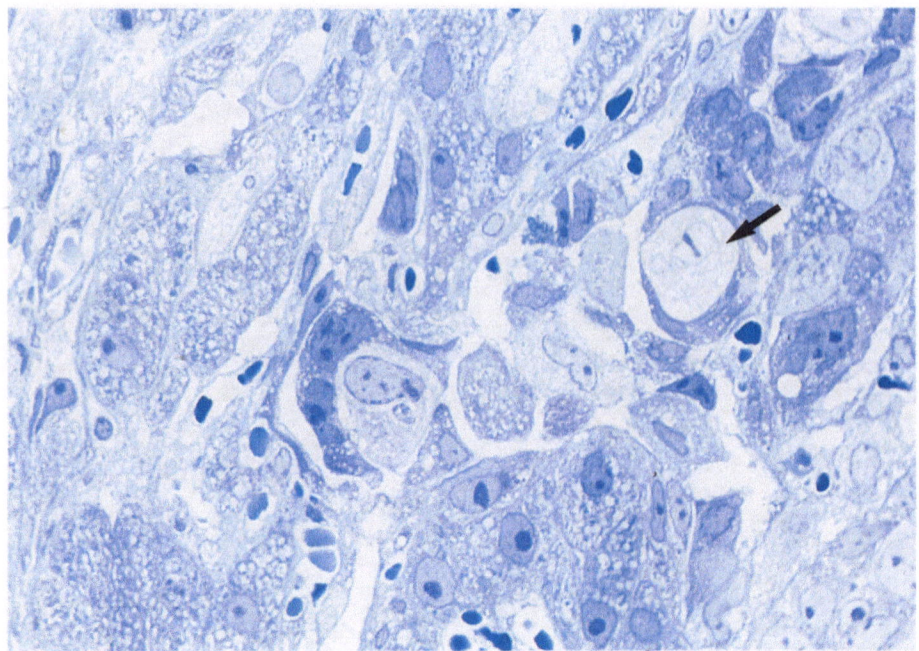

Fig. 4.8. Same case. Cancer cells growing in the sinusoids are pleomorphic (*arrow*). Epon-embedded 1-μm section, Giemsa, $\times$ 600

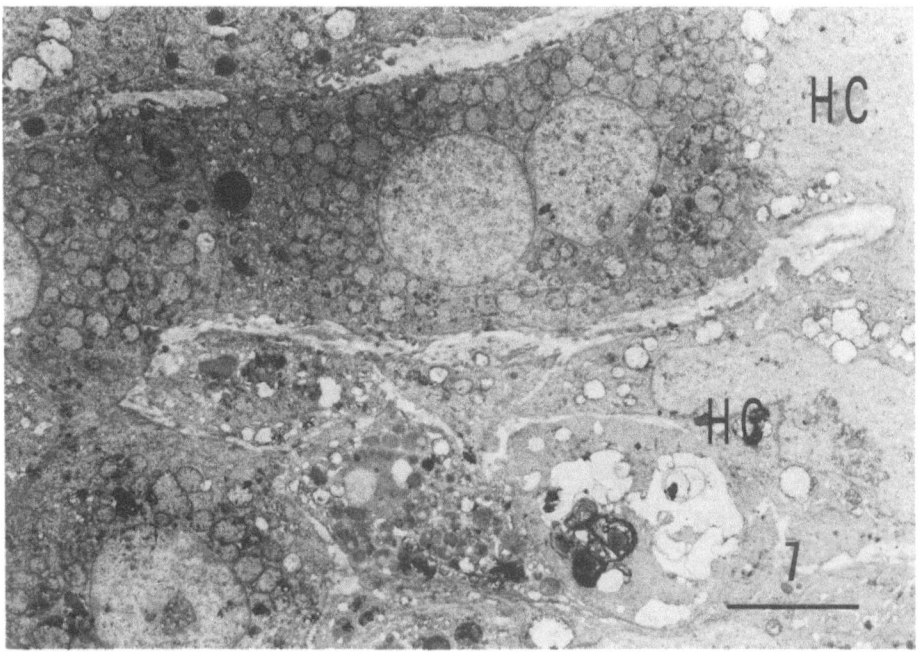

Fig. 4.9. Sinusoidal growth. One cancer cell (*upper HC*) is directly attached to the hepatocyte and another (*lower HC*) is located in the sinusoid

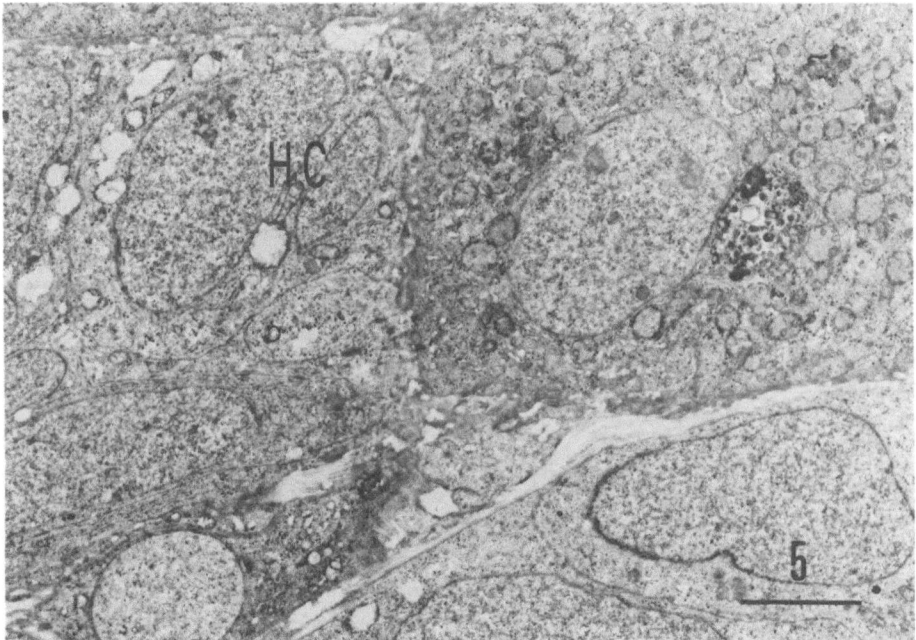

Fig. 4.10. Sinusoidal growth. Cancer cell (*HC*) in the sinusoid

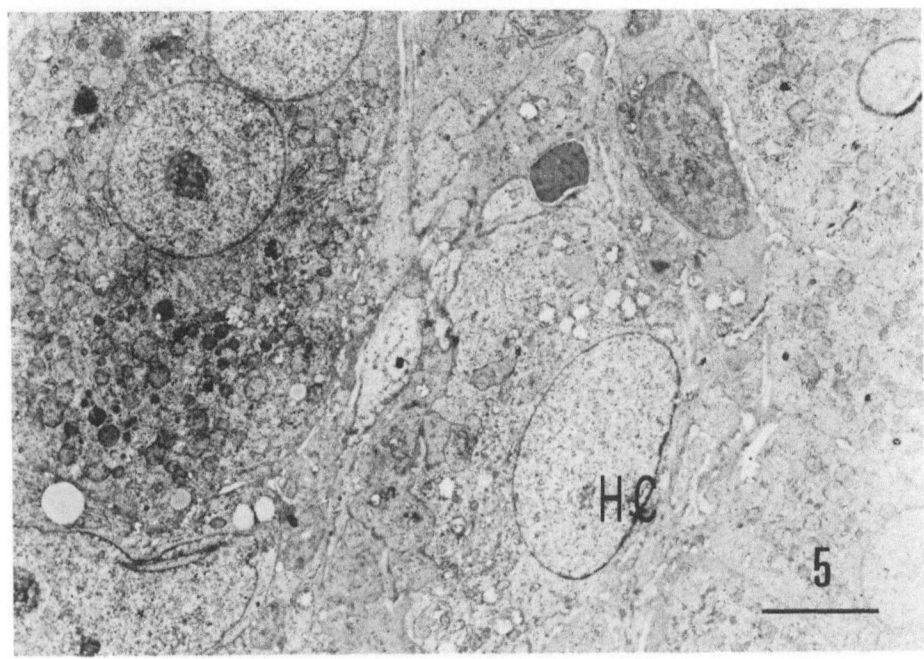

Fig. 4.11. Sinusoidal growth. Cancer cell (*HC*) in the sinusoid

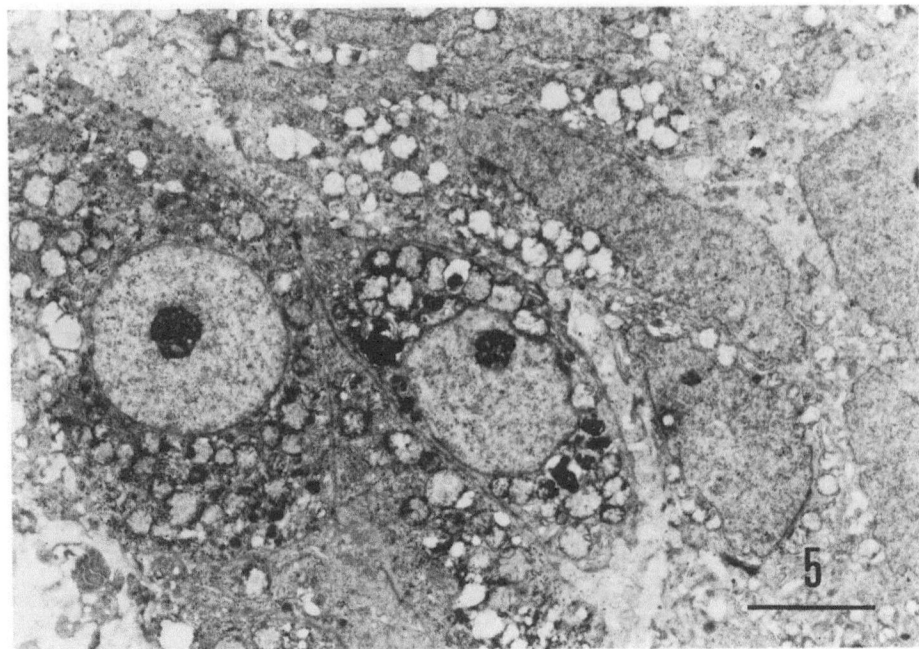

Fig. 4.12. Sinusoidal growth. The cancer cells in the sinusoid lack a mutual contact

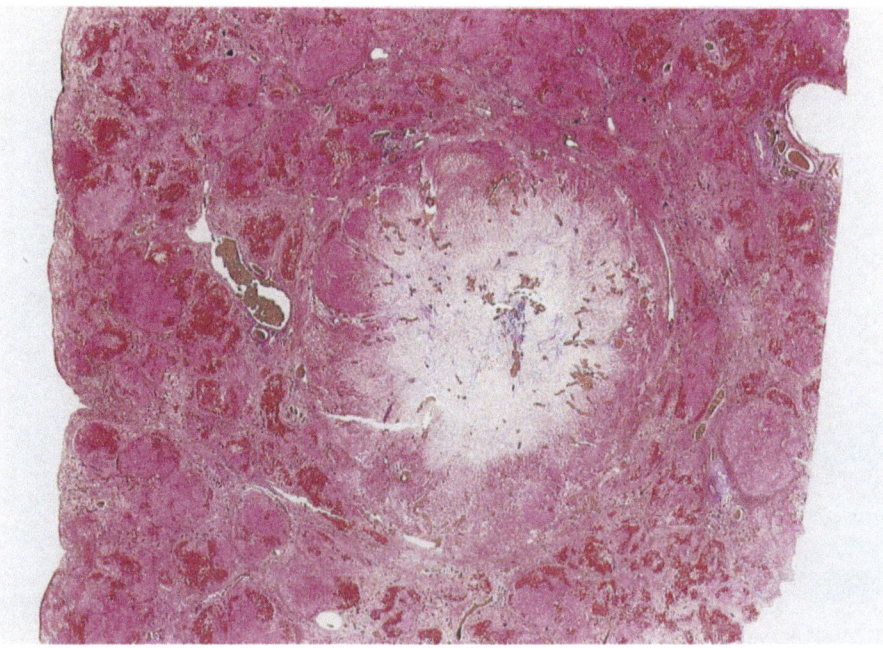

Fig. 4.13. Replacing growth. The tumor nodule, 1 cm in diameter, shows expanding growth but lacks a fibrous capsule. HE, × 1

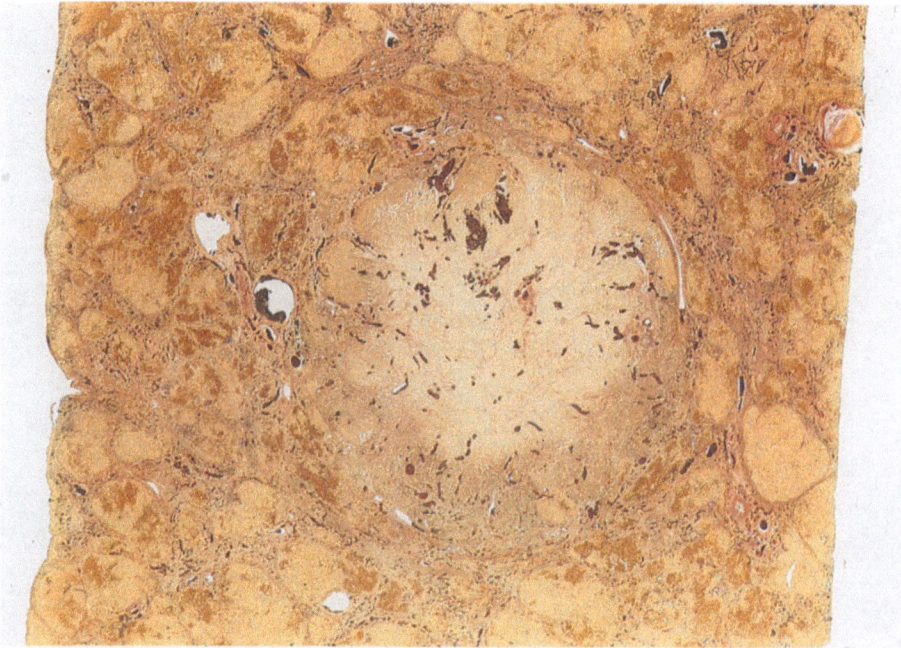

Fig. 4.14. Same tumor. Elastica Van Gieson

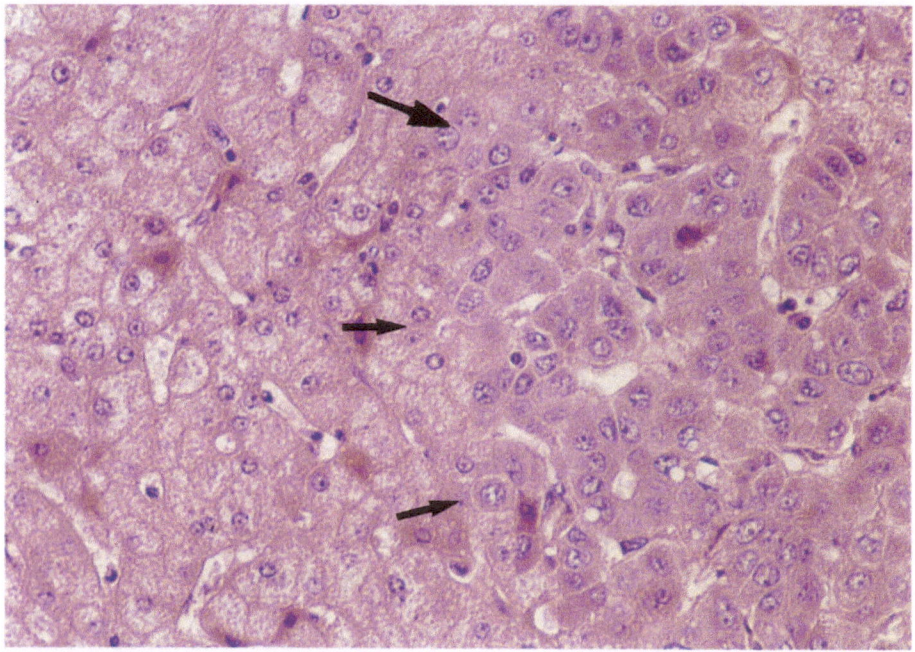

Fig. 4.15. Replacing growth. The cancer cells grow as they replace the hepatocytes at the tumor-nontumor boundary (*arrows*). HE, × 400

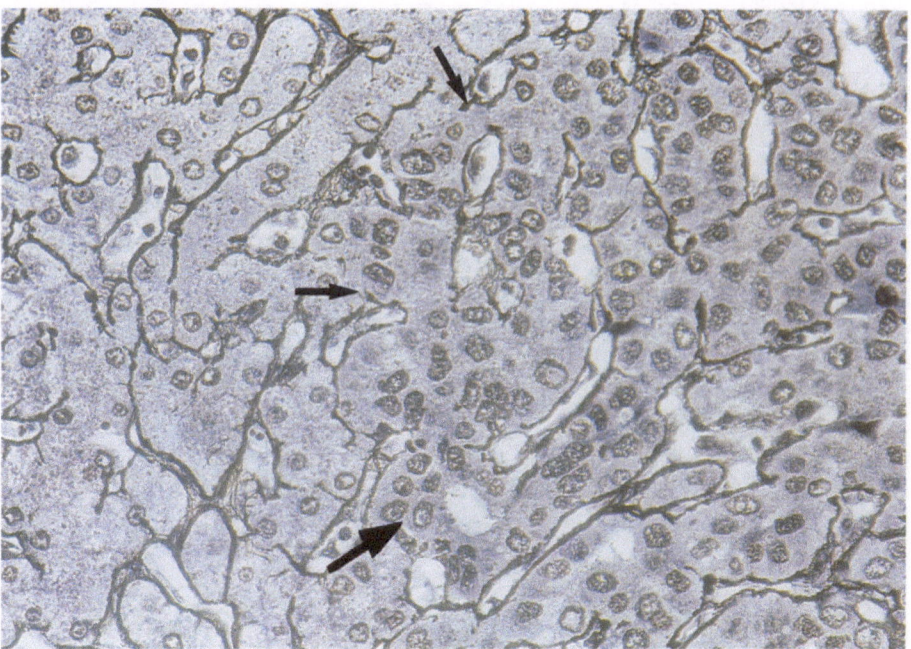

Fig. 4.16. Replacing growth. The reticulin framework at the tumor-nontumor boundary is preserved, and the sinusoids appear to be in the process of becoming blood spaces in cancerous tissue (*arrows*). Reticulin, × 400

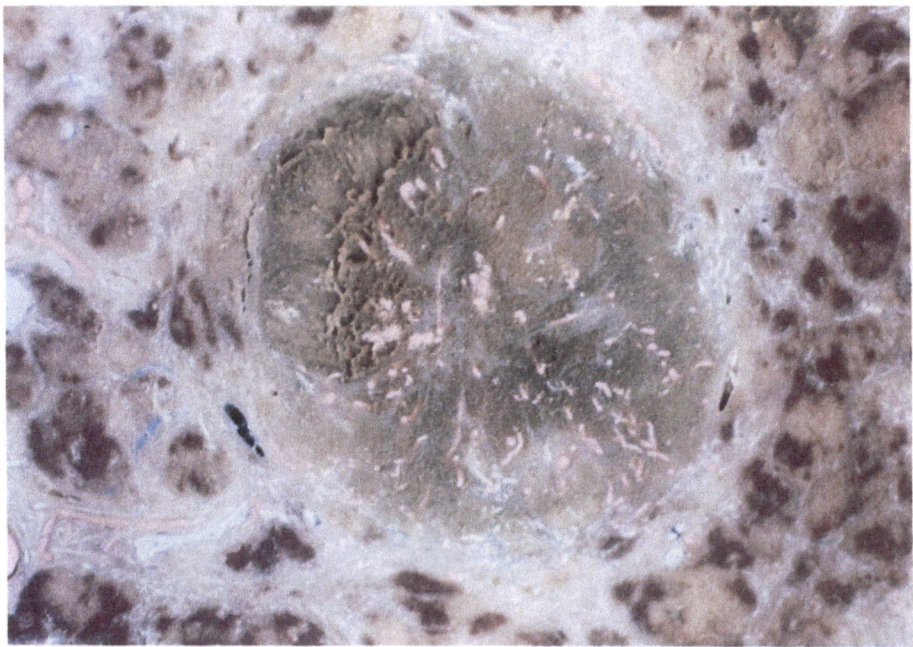

Fig. 4.17. Small liver cancer showing replacing growth. Although irregular fibrosis is observed around the tumor nodule, capsule formation is not distinct. The tumor mostly receives arteries, but portal veins are also observed: *red*, artery; *blue*, portal vein

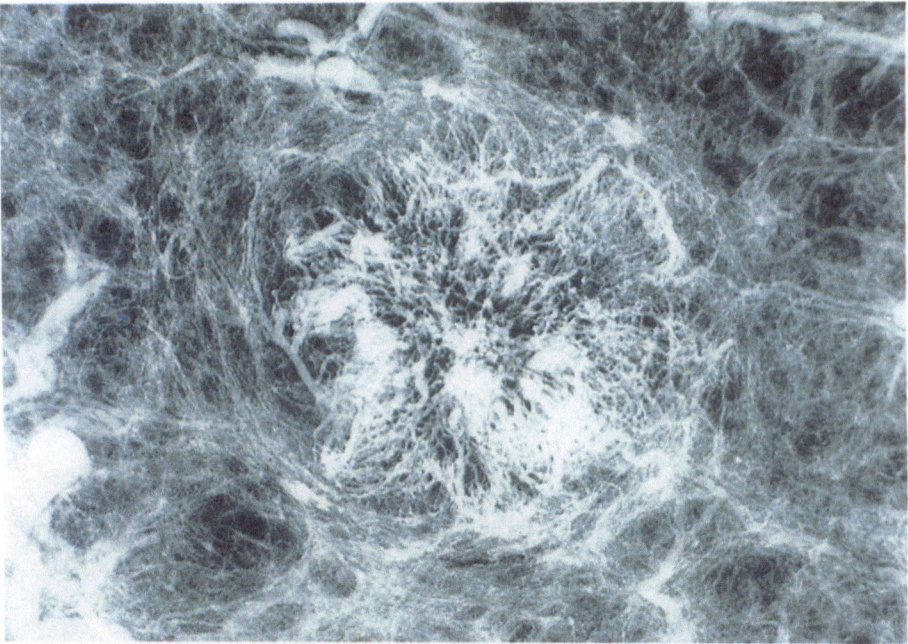

Fig. 4.18. Same tumor. Soft X-ray finding. The tumor is markedly hypervascular

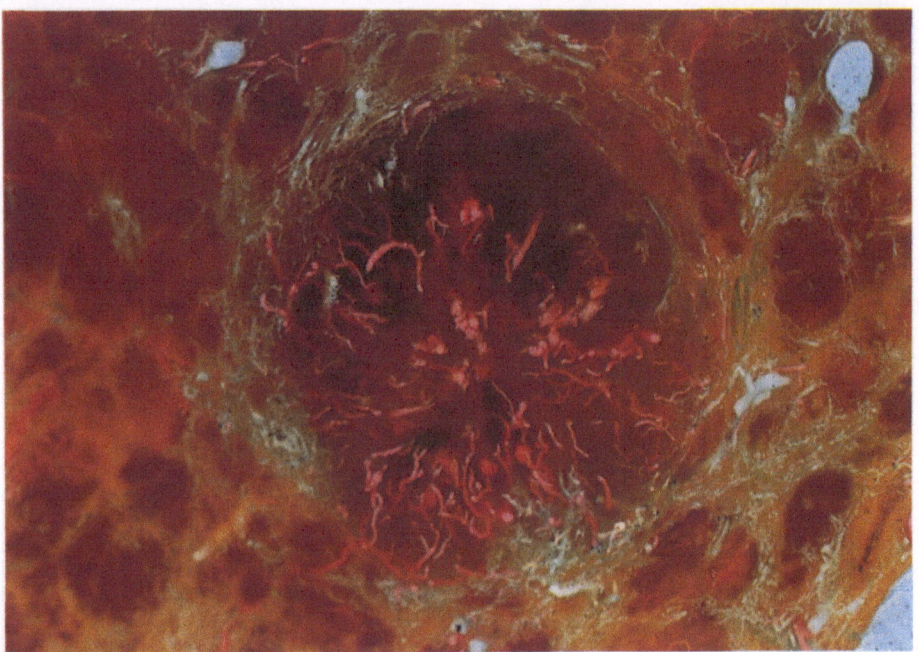

Fig. 4.19. Same tumor. The portal vein branches intermingle with the arterial branches at the boundary in the hypervascular tumor. Transparent preparation

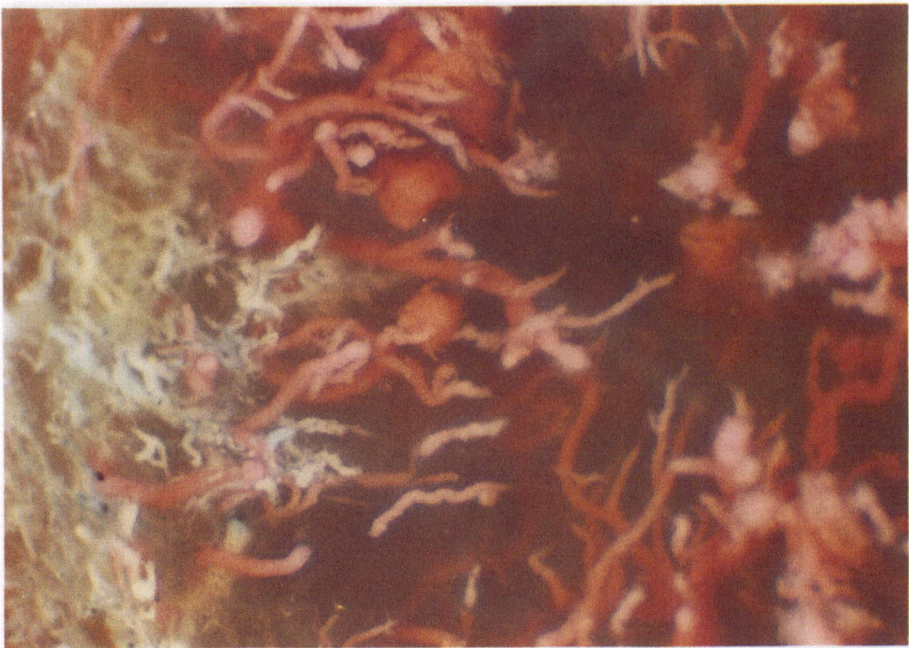

Fig. 4.20. Close-up view of the same tumor. Intermingling of the portal vein branches and arterial branches at the tumor-nontumor boundary.

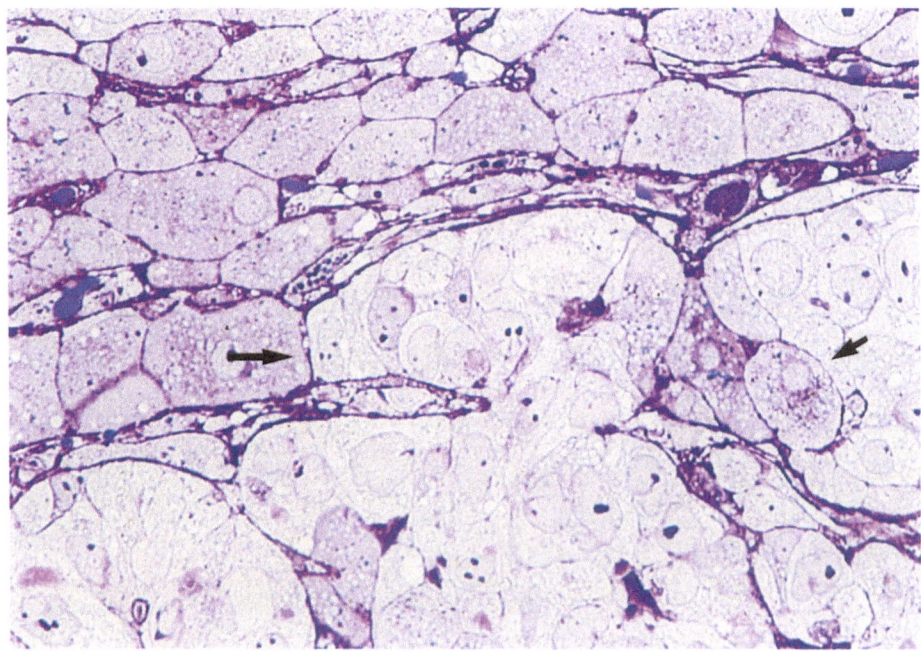

Fig. 4.21. Replacing growth. The cancer cells attach directly to the hepatocytes (*long arrow*) and a hepatocyte is retained in the cancer nest (*short arrow*). Epon-embedded 1-μm section, Giemsa, × 600

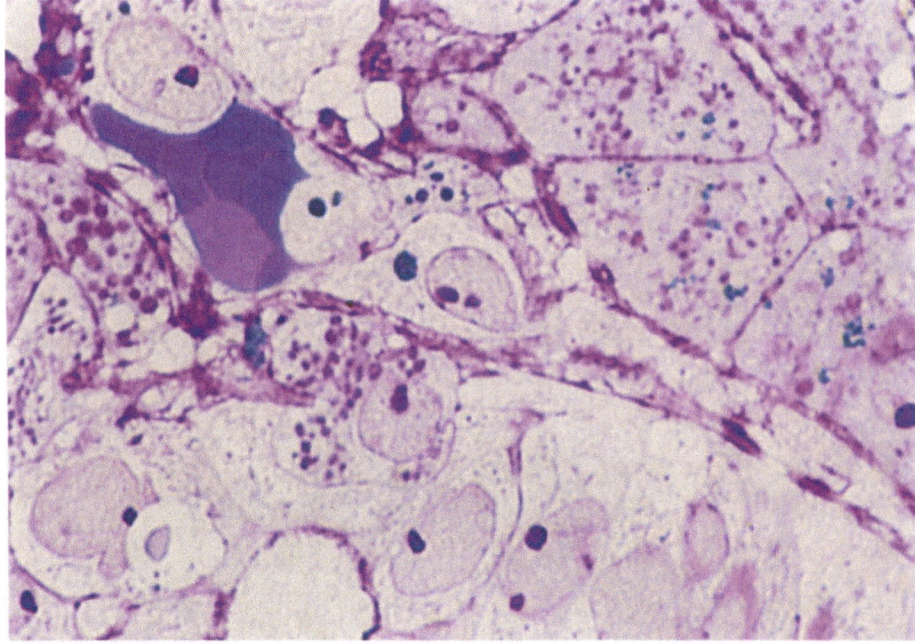

Fig. 4.22. Replacing growth. A sinusoid is seen between the cancerous tissue (*lower half*) and the noncancerous tissue (*upper half*). The endothelial cells of the sinusoid are markedly swollen. Epon-embedded 1-μm section, Giemsa, × 1000

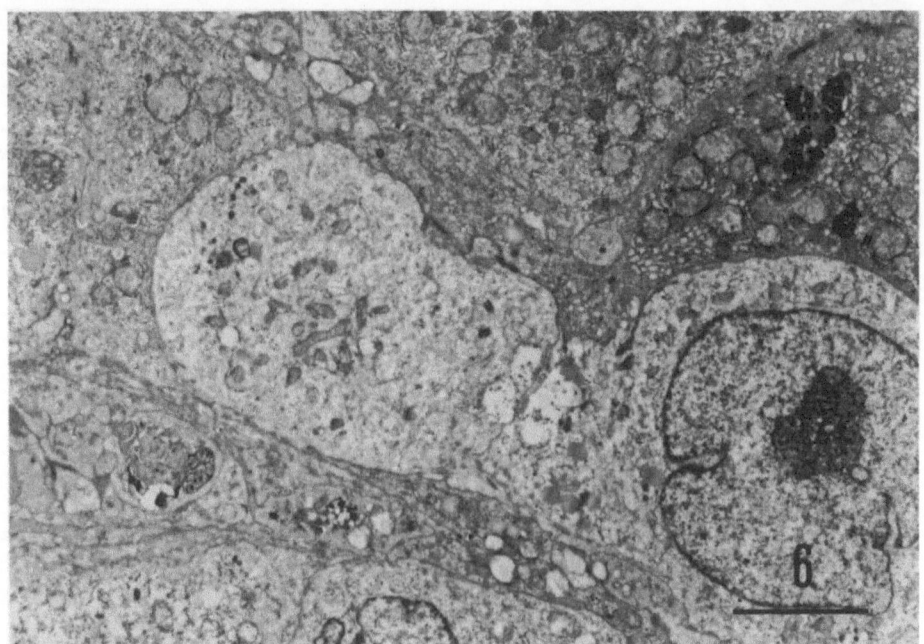

Fig. 4.23. Replacing growth. The cancer cell is replacing the hepatocyte

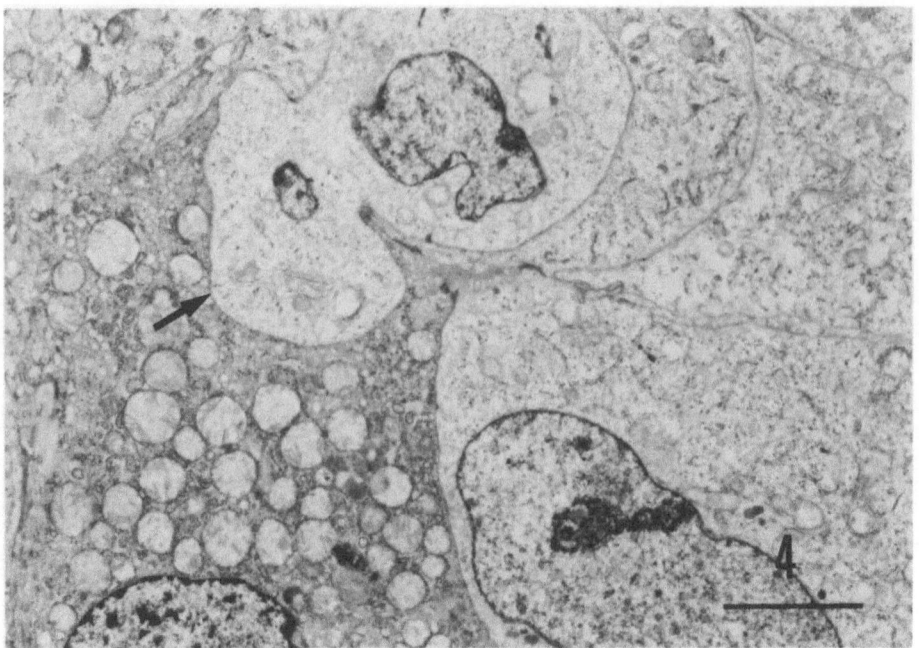

Fig. 4.24. Replacing growth. Budding of the cytoplasm of the cancer cell into the hepatocyte (*arrow*)

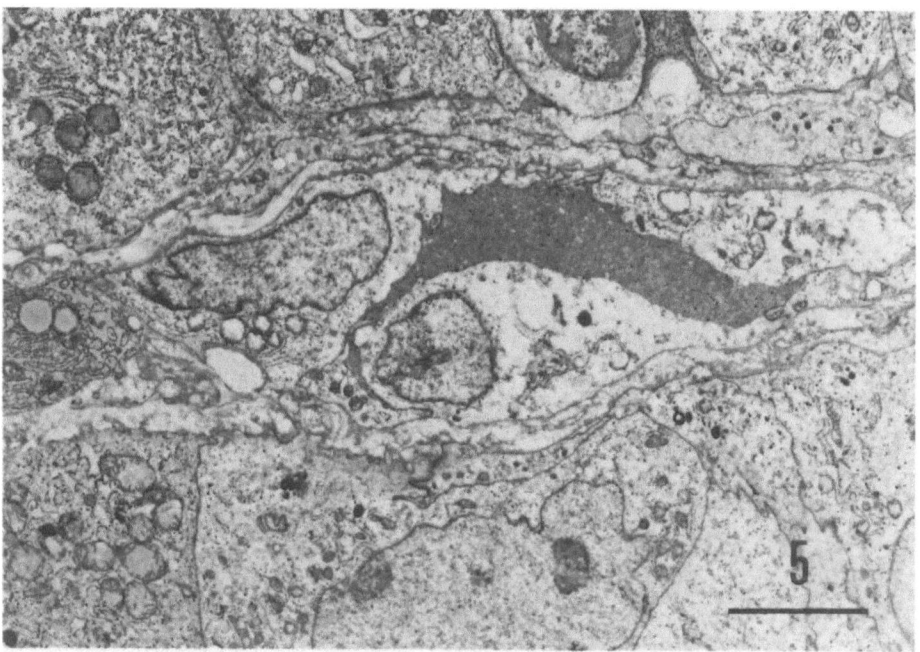

Fig. 4.25. Replacing growth. Blood space (sinusoid) seen between the hepatocytes (*upper half*) and cancer cells (*lower half*)

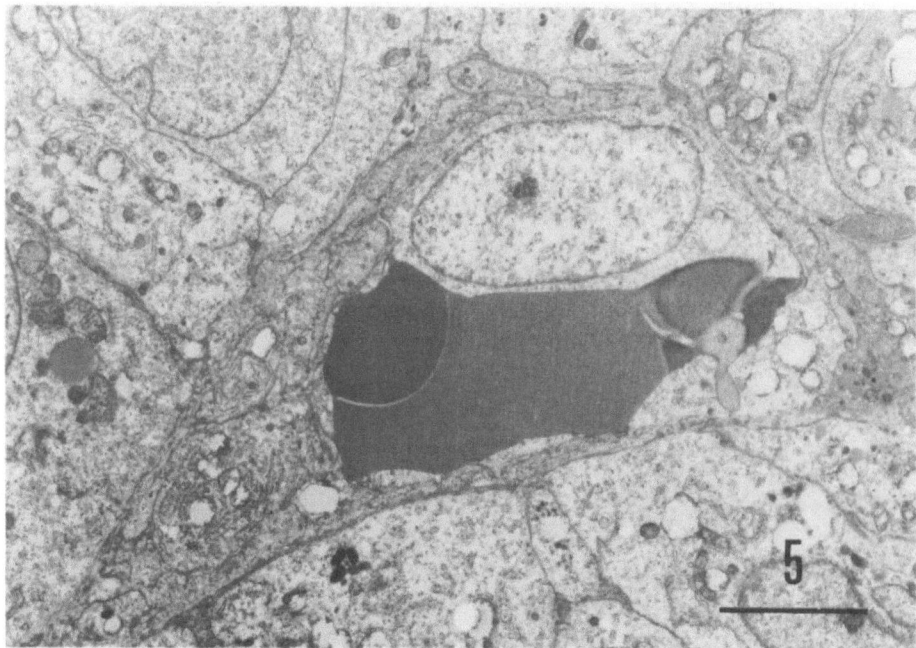

Fig. 4.26. Replacing growth. Markedly swollen endothelial cells of the blood space in cancerous tissue

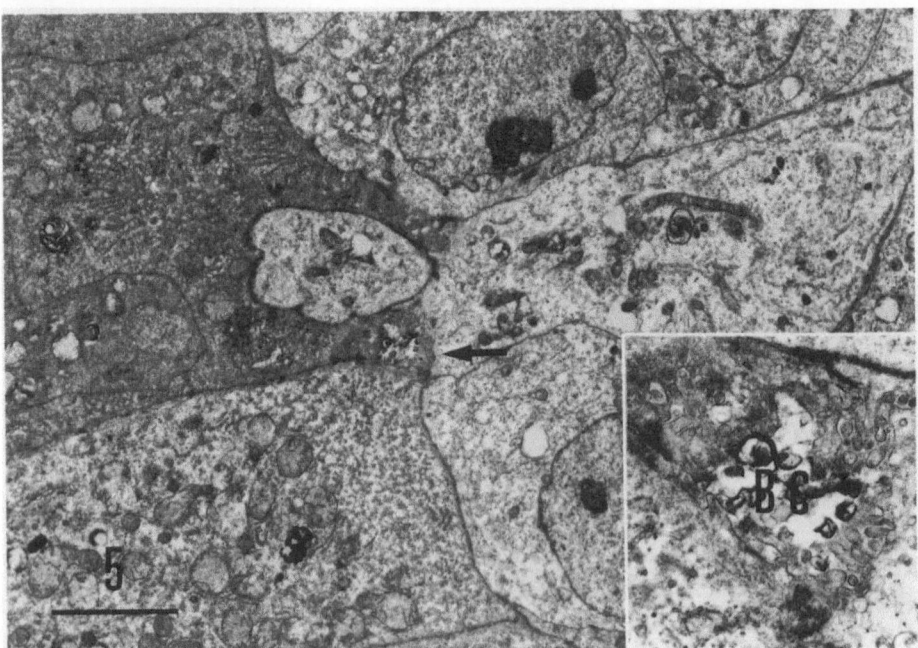

Fig. 4.27. Replacing growth. Bile-canaliculi-like structure (*arrow*) between the hepatocytes and cancer cells. *Inset*: high-power view of bile-canaliculi-like structure

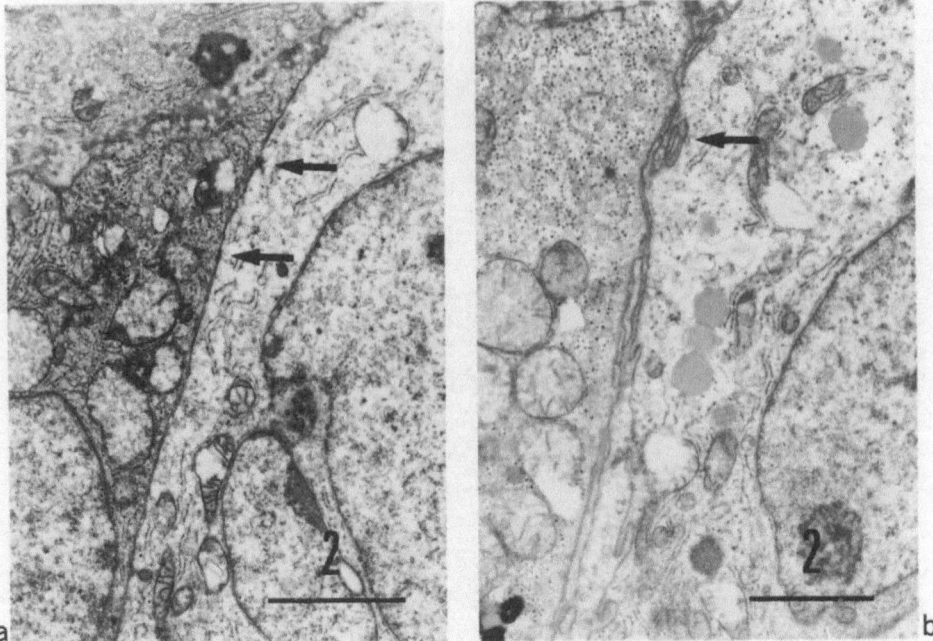

Fig. 4.28a, b. Replacing growth. Desmosomes (*arrows*) (**a**) and interdigitation (*arrow*) (**b**) between the hepatocyte and the cancer cell

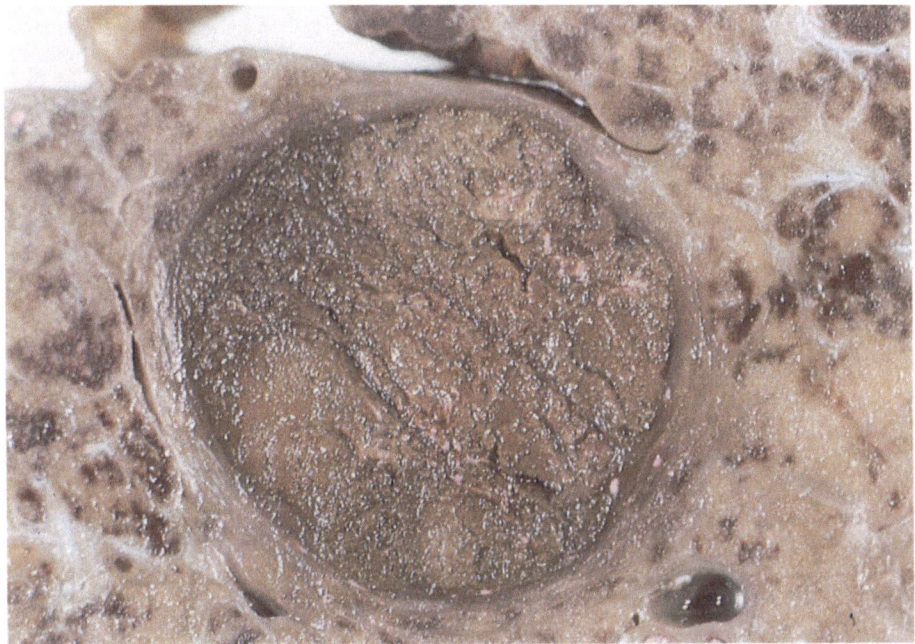

Fig. 4.29. Pseudocapsular growth. The expansive type tumor is enclosed by a thin fibrous capsule

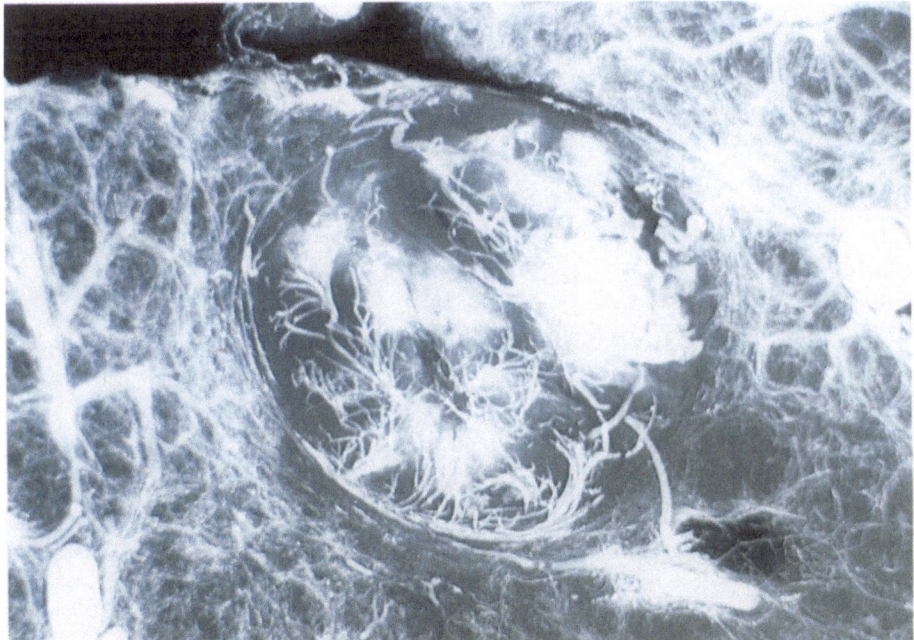

Fig. 4.30. Same tumor. Soft X-ray finding. The tumor is hypervascular

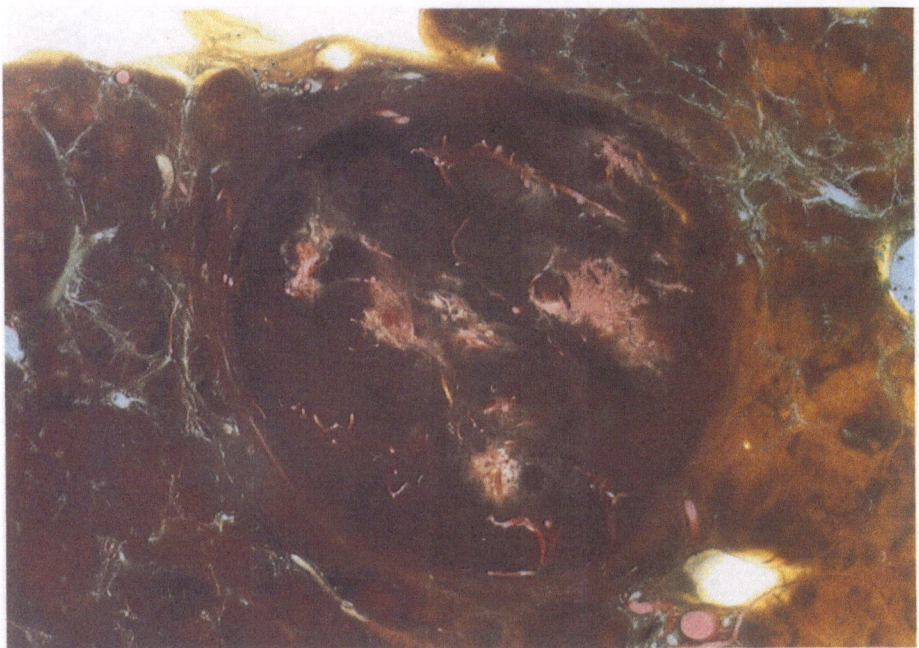

Fig. 4.31. Same tumor. The angioarchitecture of the tumor nodule consists solely of arterial vessels. Transparent preparation: *red*, artery; *blue*, portal vein

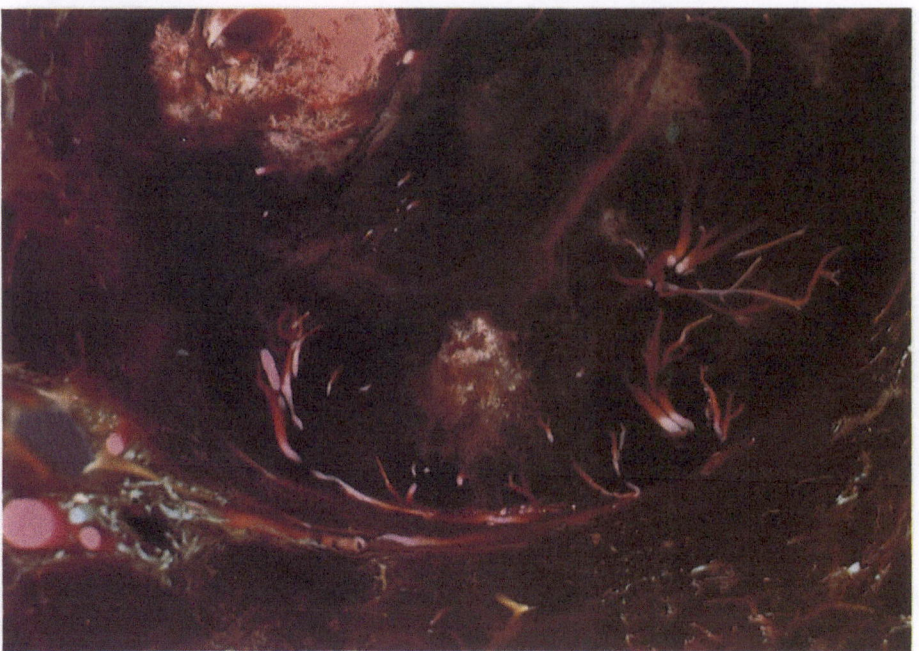

Fig. 4.32. Detail of a different section of the same tumor. The arterial tumor vessels originate from the arteries running along the capsule

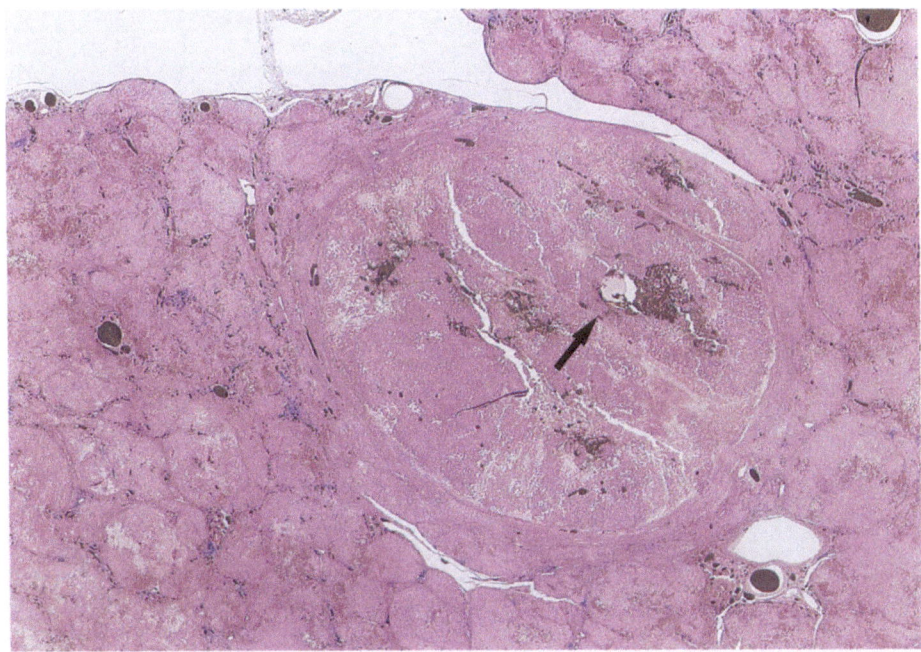

Fig. 4.33. Pseudocapsular growth. The tumor nodule is enclosed by a thin fibrous capsule, and a thin fibrous septum (*arrow*) is seen in the tumor. HE, × 1

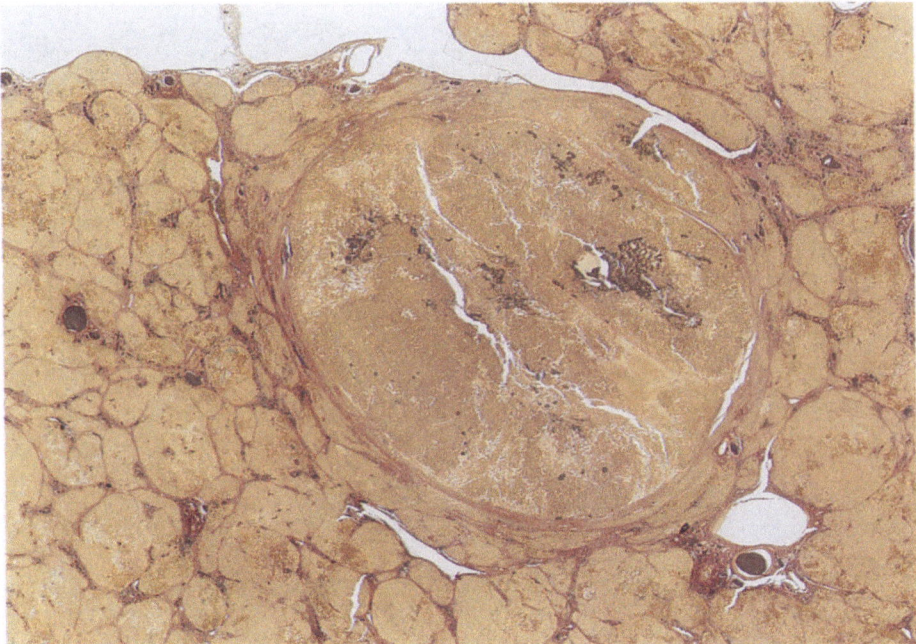

Fig. 4.34. Same tumor. Elastica Van Gieson

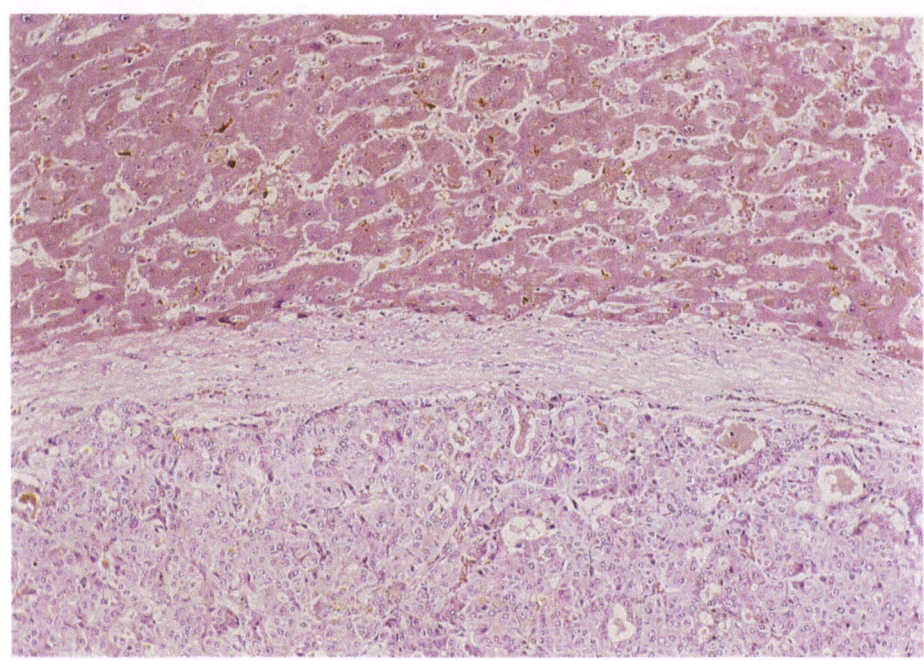

Fig. 4.35. Pseudocapsular growth. Fibrous capsule at the tumor-nontumor boundary. HE, × 100

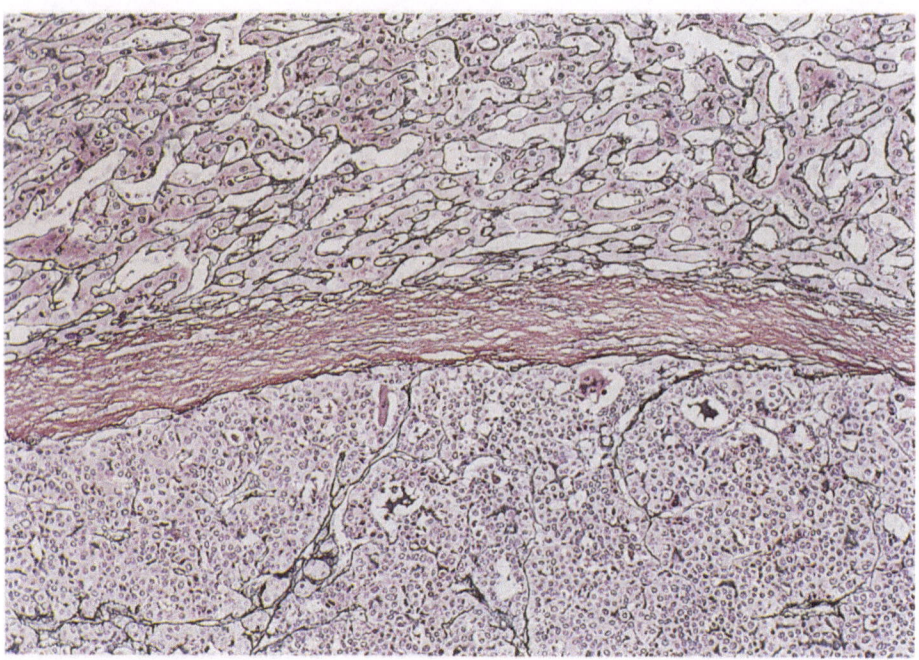

Fig. 4.36. Same tumor. It is suggested that capsule formation results from the aggregation of reticulin fibers. Reticulin, × 100

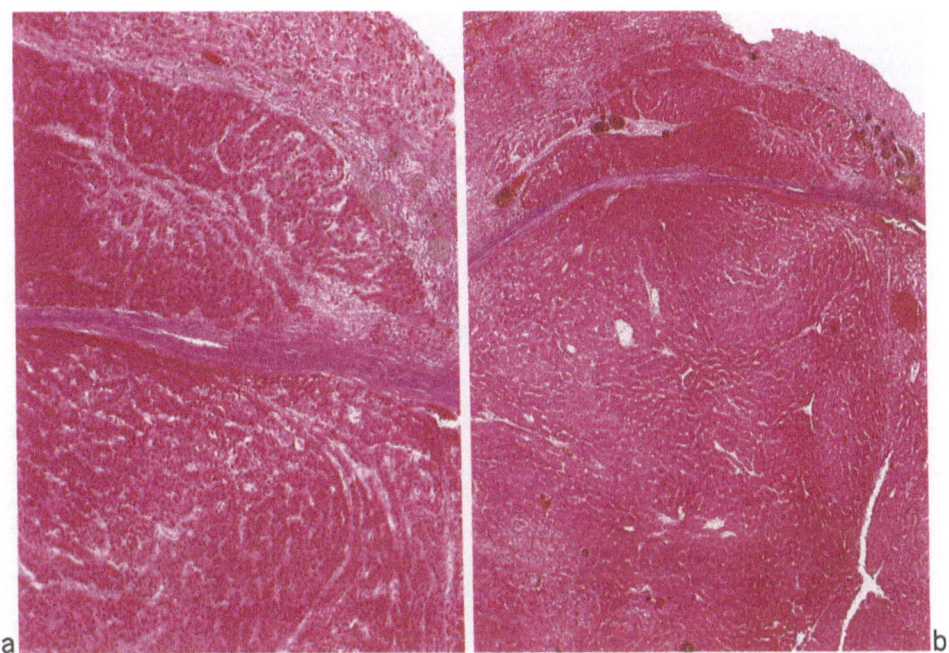

Fig. 4.37a, b. Extracapsular tumor growth. Budding of the tumor beyond the capsule. Azan-Mallory; **a** × 50, **b** × 20

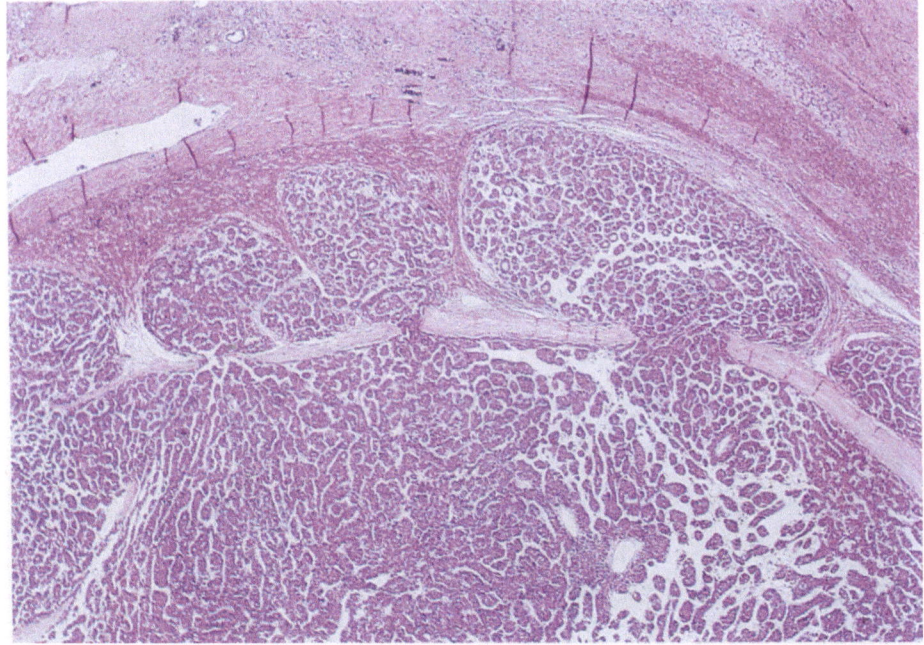

Fig. 4.38. Extracapsular tumor growth. A new, still incomplete capsule is forming at the boundary of the extracapsular tumor, and the old capsule seems to be remaining in the tumor as a fibrous septum. HE, × 50

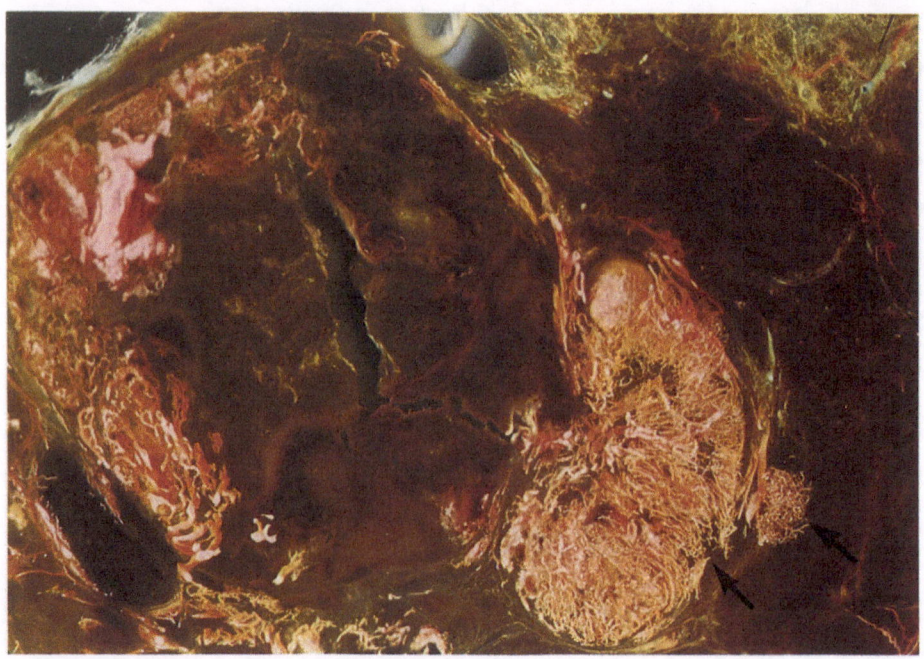

Fig. 4.39. Extracapsular tumor growth. The tumors growing beyond the capsule are markedly hypervascular (*arrows*). Transparent preparation

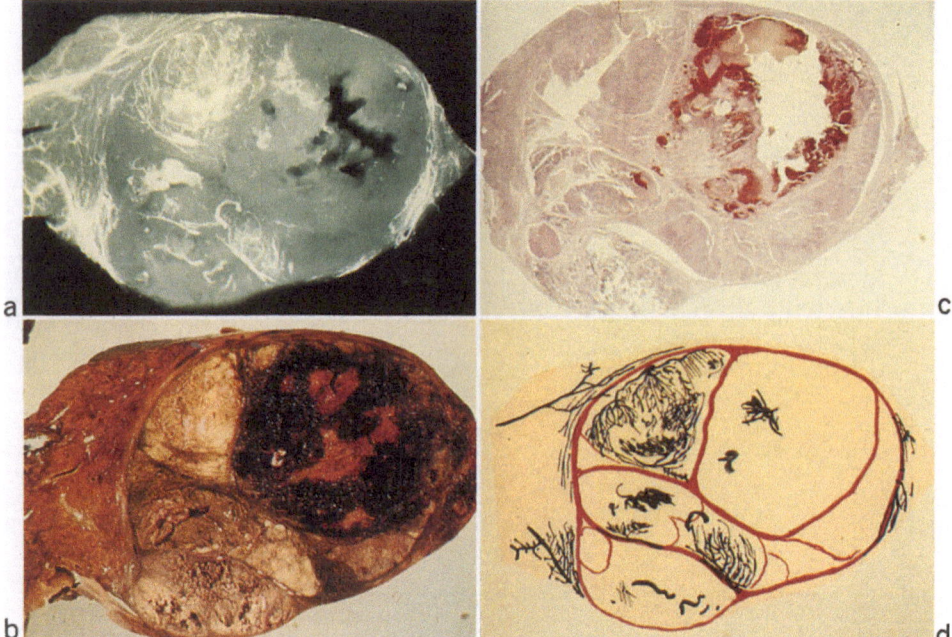

Fig. 4.40a–d. Encapsulated tumor. The tumor is divided by fibrous septa, and each part of the tumor shows independent vasculature. **a** Soft X-ray finding; **b** Gross features; **c** HE stain; **d** Schema of the vasculature

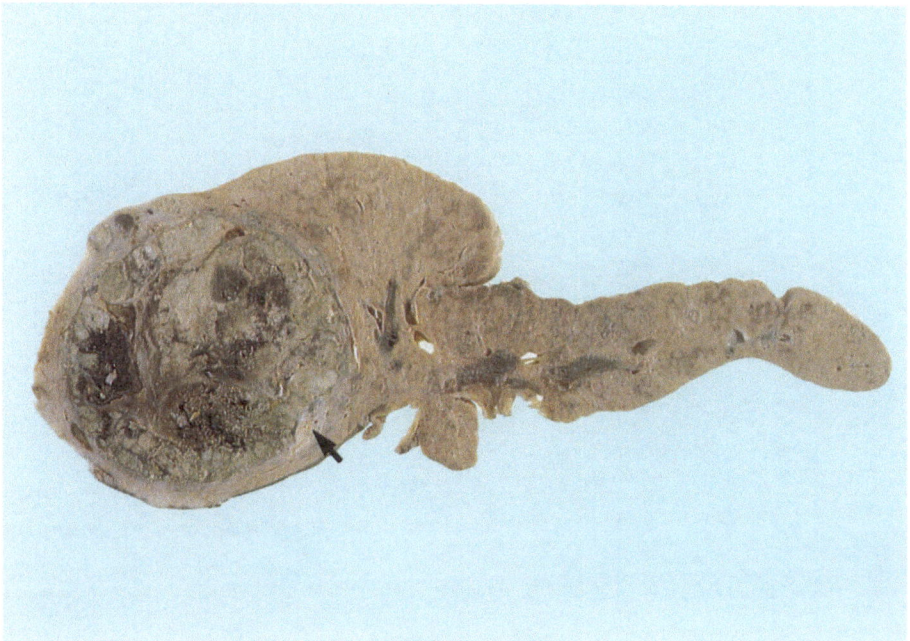

Fig. 4.41. Encapsulated tumor with sinusoidal growth in part (*arrow*)

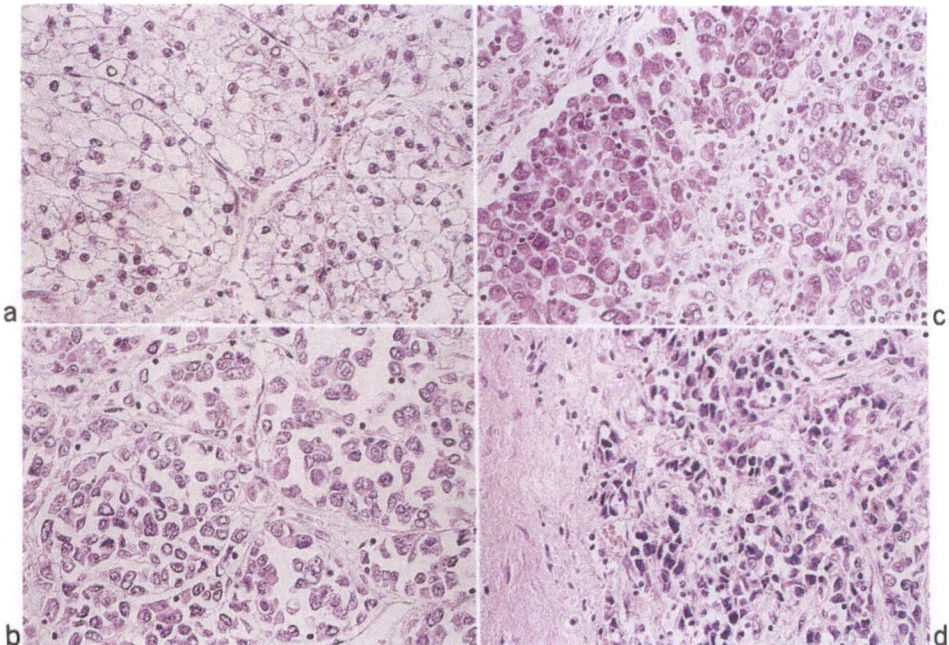

Fig. 4.42a–d. Same case. **a** Trabecular HCC seen in most of the tumor. **b** Free-cell HCC seen in the part showing a sinusoidal growth pattern. **c** Metastasis in the periaortic lymph node. **d** Metastasis in the spleen. The metastates are of the free-cell type. HE; **a–c** × 200, **d** × 100

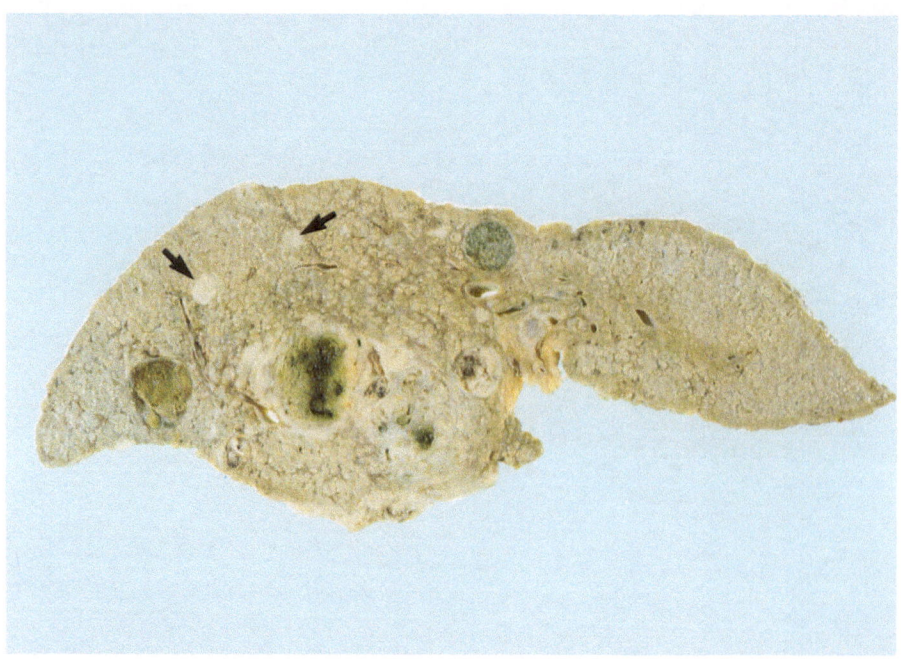

Fig. 4.43. Coexistence of tumors with different growth patterns. There are infiltrative tumor nodules (*arrows*) and encapsulated tumor nodules

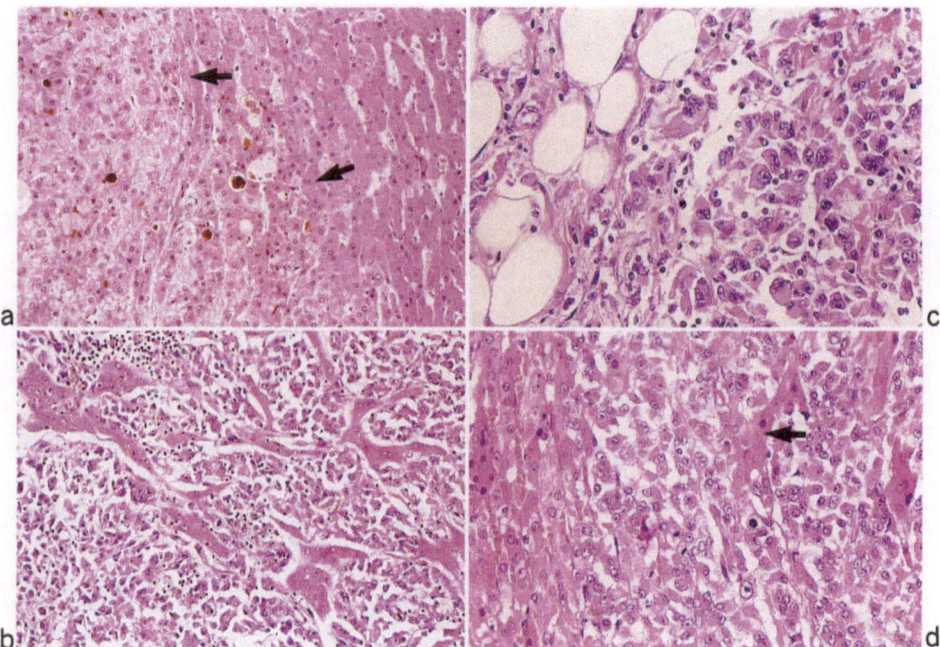

Fig. 4.44a–d. Same case. **a** Trabecular HCC showing a replacing growth (*arrows*) seen in a greenish tumor nodule. **b** Marked sinusoidal growth of free-cell cancer cells seen in an infiltrative tumor nodule. Free-cell cancer cells metastasized in the mesenteric lymph node (**c**) and in the adrenal gland. *Arrow* shows atrophied adrenal cells (**d**). HE; **a, b** × 50, **c, d** × 100

Chapter 5
Angioarchitecture of Hepatocellular Carcinoma

Bierman et al. [104] employed for the first time a catheter technique for selective celiac arteriography and described the assessment of tumor angioarchitecture based on pictorial delineation in three cases of HCC and one case of cholangio-carcinoma. The technique was modified by Seldinger [105] and Odman [106], who utilized ·percutaneous catheterization. These techniques stimulated remarkable developments in arteriography for HCC. With further progress, the arteriographic features of HCC have been studied more closely. As in the gross classification, HCC was divided into nodular, massive, and diffuse types on the basis of arteriography by Boijsen and Abrams [107]. Since then, the arteriographic features of HCC have been examined by a number of researchers [108–110]. It has been disclosed that changes in the arterial system, such as arteriovenous shunt and tumor stains, are clinically significant [111–113].

Transarterial embolization therapy has produced good results as a conservative treatment for advanced HCC and depends principally on obstruction of the arteries communicating with cancer foci. This causes necrosis of tumor cells, leading to prevention of tumor growth [114–116]. This therapy has also been widely employed preoperatively to improve the postoperative course. A comparative study of angiograms taken while the patient is alive with postmortem angiograms is indispensable for more accurate assessment of the angioarchitecture of HCC. As seen in postmortem angiograms and transparent preparations, the angioarchitecture visualized by angiography is so complicated because the individual angioarchitectures of the primary foci, tumor thrombi, and intrahepatic tumor spreads are combined en bloc [117–120].

Angioarchitecture of Cancer Nodules

The angioarchitecture of cancer nodules varies widely depending on the tumor growth pattern; For detailed discussion of histological growth patterns, see Chap. 4. Here we will describe the basic angioarchitecture in HCC of the multinodular expansive type. The angioarchitecture of multinodular HCC varies widely depending on the presence or absence of liver cirrhosis, the presence or absence of a capsule, and the thickness of the capsule when present. As the influence of liver cirrhosis on the angioarchitectural pattern is the most striking, the angioarchitecture of multinodular HCC is illustrated in one case each of HCC with and without associated liver cirrhosis.

HCC without associated liver cirrhosis

In HCC without liver cirrhosis (Figs. 5.1–8), the surface of the liver is smooth and undulates gently, depending on the size of the superficial nodules, which varies. The frontal plane presents numerous nodules of various size which are clearly demarcated from the surrounding hepatic parenchyma. In the transparent preparation, the angioarchitecture in the cancer nodules exclusively comprises arterial tumor vessels. The tumor vessels branch, forming a tree-like pattern within the tumor nodule, and injected colored gelatin is observed in a diffuse pattern in the peripheral area, suggesting that the tumor vessels empty into blood spaces in the HCC.

The ramification of the tumor vessels varies in extent in different parts. The vessels branch finely at the site where proliferation of cancer cells is active, while accumulation of colored gelatin in necrotic foci is indicative of the formation of a blood lake; sparse branching is observed at sites of abundant fibrous stroma. Individual vessels differ in appearance. Some are collapsed and others are bent, with irregularity of the lumen.

HCC with associated liver cirrhosis

In HCC with liver cirrhosis (Figs. 5.9–16), the surface of the liver is granular. A superficial tumor produces a smooth and lustrous hemispheric protrusion from the surface. Abnormal dilatation, proliferation, and distribution of blood vessels is observed beyond the hepatic capsule. In the frontal plane, there are several cancer nodules covered with a thick fibrous capsule clearly demarcating the tumor from noncancerous tissue. The angioarchitecture consists solely of arterial tumor vessels branching in a tree-like pattern. Tumor nodules encased in a thick capsule appear to be hypovascular on a soft X-ray film. In transparent preparations, fine arterial tumor vessels can be observed in some of the tumor nodules with a thick capsule.

Angioarchitecture of the capsule of HCC nodules

Tumor nodules of the expansive type are enclosed by a pseudocapsule of reticulin fibers or, in long-standing nodules, by a thick fibrous capsule resulting from collagenization of the pseudocapsule. The capsule develops in the condensed reticulin framework of heptaic parenchyma following the atrophic changes that result from compression due to tumor growth.

HCC generally presents hypervascular cancer nodules in arteriograms, but expansive cancer nodules are often hypo-or avascular at autopsy. This indicates that the pictorial delineation by angiography involves capsular blood vessels, leading to an apparent hypervascularity (Figs. 5.3–12).

In the capsule, large arterial branches which have been replaced and translocated are dilated, and numerous regenerated arterial branches form irregular nests. The portal veins are also markedly pushed and flattened. There is, however, no evidence of penetration of such capsular blood vessels into the cancer nodule (Figs. 5.3–6).

Extension of cancer nodules and angioarchitecture

Expansive tumor nodules yield daughter nodules in their close vicinity and, as described above, coalesce with the daughter nodules and grow in an expansive manner into larger nodules. The angioarchitecture of the daughter nodules is independent of that of the primary nodule. This is because the arterial tumor vessels of the daughter nodules arise from arterial branches entirely different to those from which the arterial tumor vessels communicating with the primary nodule arise. In addition, a fibrous capsule intervenes between the primary and daughter nodules. Fresh cancer nodules are rich in tumor vessels (hypervascular), while longstanding cancer nodules have few tumor vessels (hypo- or avascular) (Figs. 5.13–16).

Angioarchitecture of Tumor Thrombus of the Portal Vein

The detailed angioarchitecture of a tumor thrombus of the portal vein is discussed separately in Chap. 6. In general, a tumor thrombus of the proliferative type is hypervascular. The arterial tumor vessels are not evident in a tumor thrombus of HCC of the free-cell type.

Angioarchitecture of Periportal Tumor Spreads

Intrahepatic tumor spreads that surround a tumor thrombus of the portal vein receive branches of the arterial tumor vessels which originate in dilated periportal arteries.

Angioarchitecture of Intrahepatic Metastasis

Intrahepatic metastatic foci via the portal vein receive the arterial tumor vessels branching from the interlobular artery.

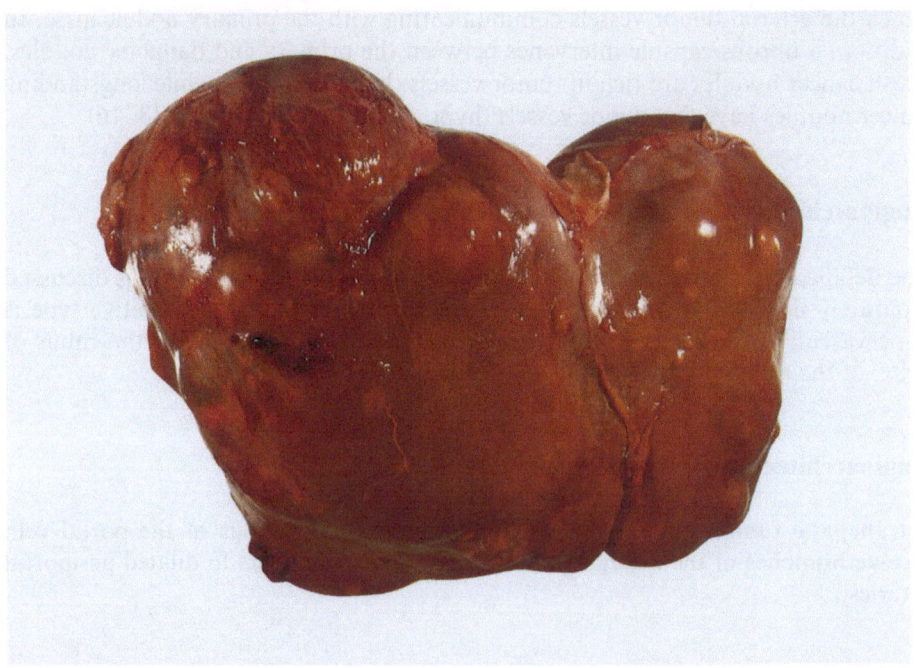

Fig. 5.1. Expansive HCC, multinodular, without liver cirrhosis. Tumor nodules of varying size can be recognized on the liver surface

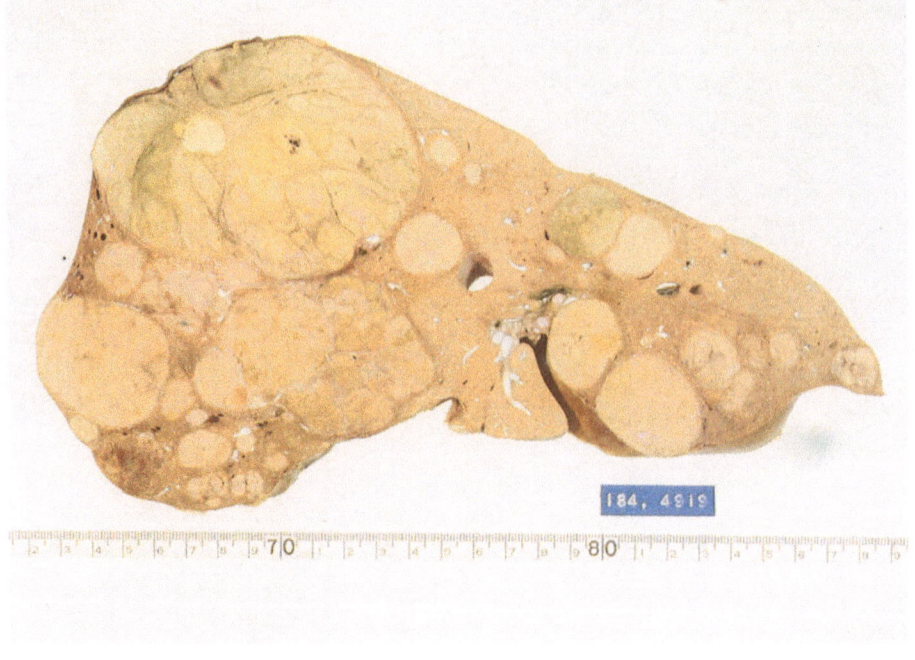

Fig. 5.2. Cut surface of the same case. Well-demarcated tumors of varying size are distributed throughout the liver

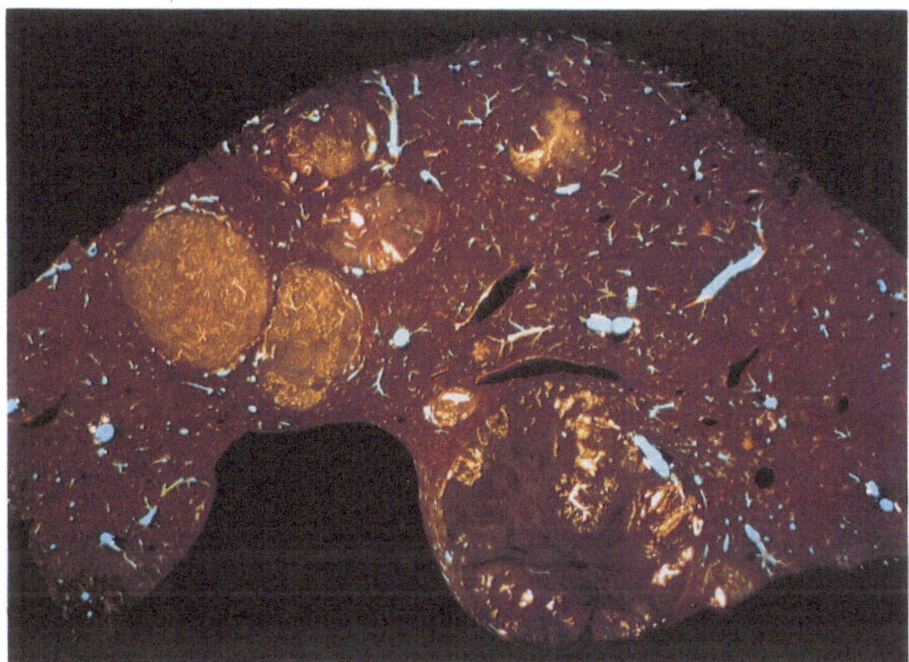

Fig. 5.3. Angioarchitecture of the same case. The angioarchitecture of the tumor nodules, which are hypervascular, consists solely of arterial tumor vessels. Transparent preparation: *red*, artery; *blue*, portal vein

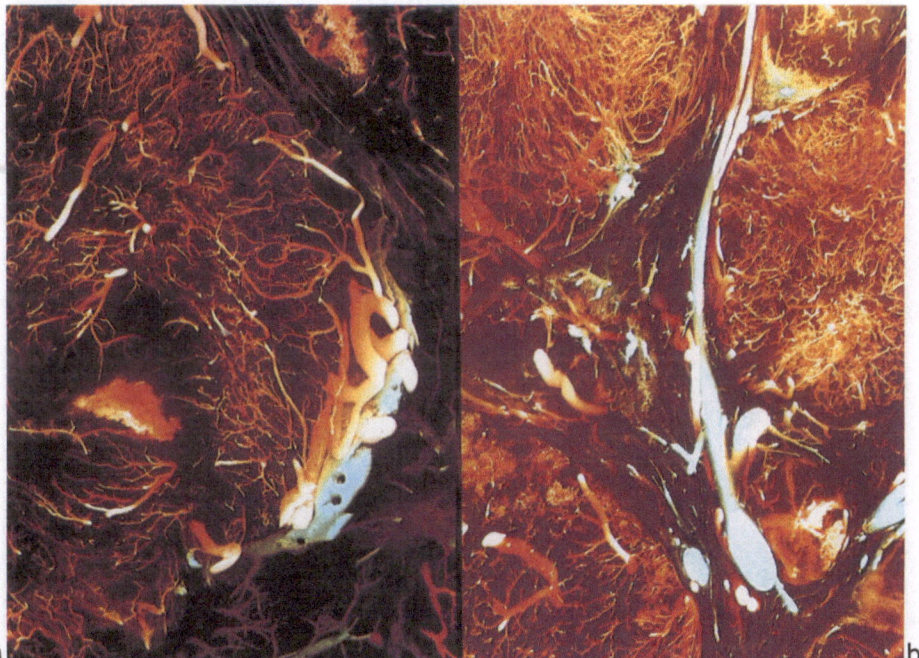

Fig. 5.4a, b. Angioarchitecture of tumor nodules in the same case. The nodules are markedly hypervascular and their angioarchitecture consists of the arterial tumor vessels. Portal veins are observed only in the boundary. Transparent preparation: *red*, artery; *blue*, portal vein

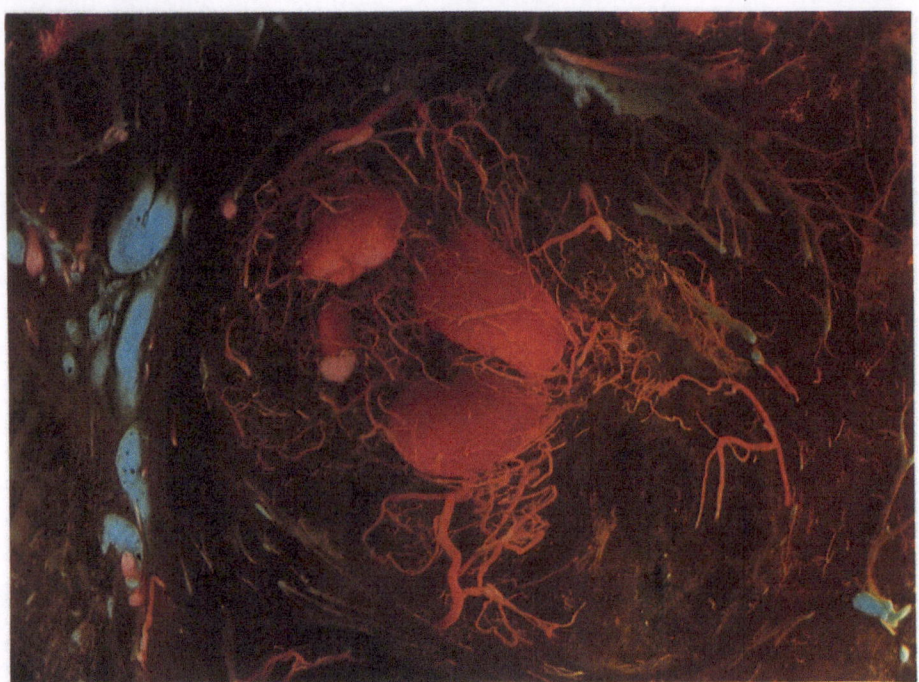

Fig. 5.5. Same case. Aneurysmal change of the arterial tumor vessels

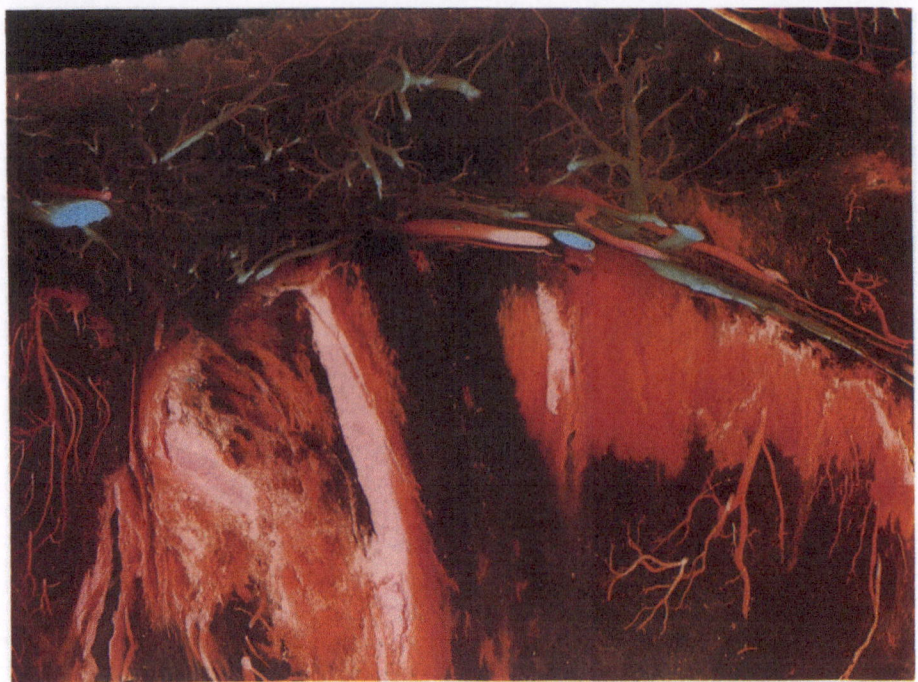

Fig. 5.6. Same case. Red dye injected via the artery flows into the tumor from dilated pericapsular arteries damaged by tumor invasion. Transparent preparation

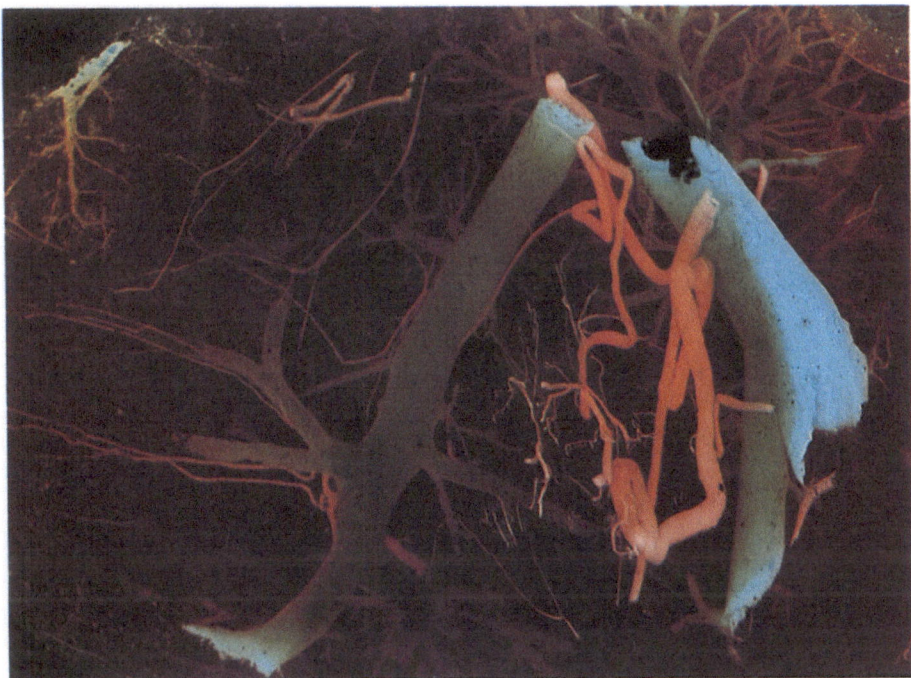

Fig. 5.7. Dilated arteries and portal veins in the capsule of an expansive-type tumor nodule. Transparent preparation

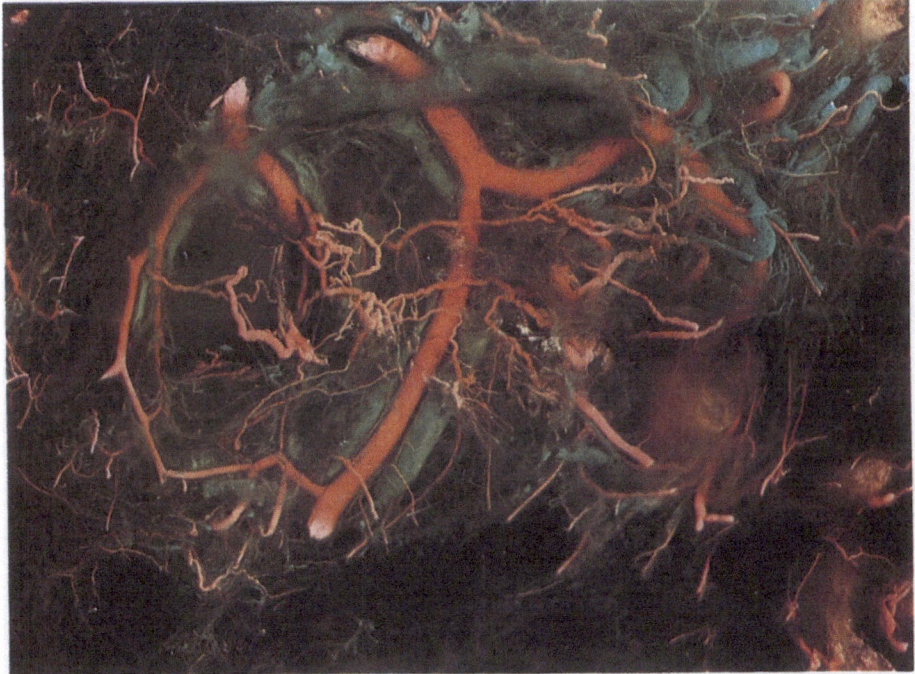

Fig. 5.8. The presence of numerous arteries along the tumor capsule, in addition to the arterial tumor vessels, seems to contribute to the hypervascularity of the tumor on angiography. Transparent preparation

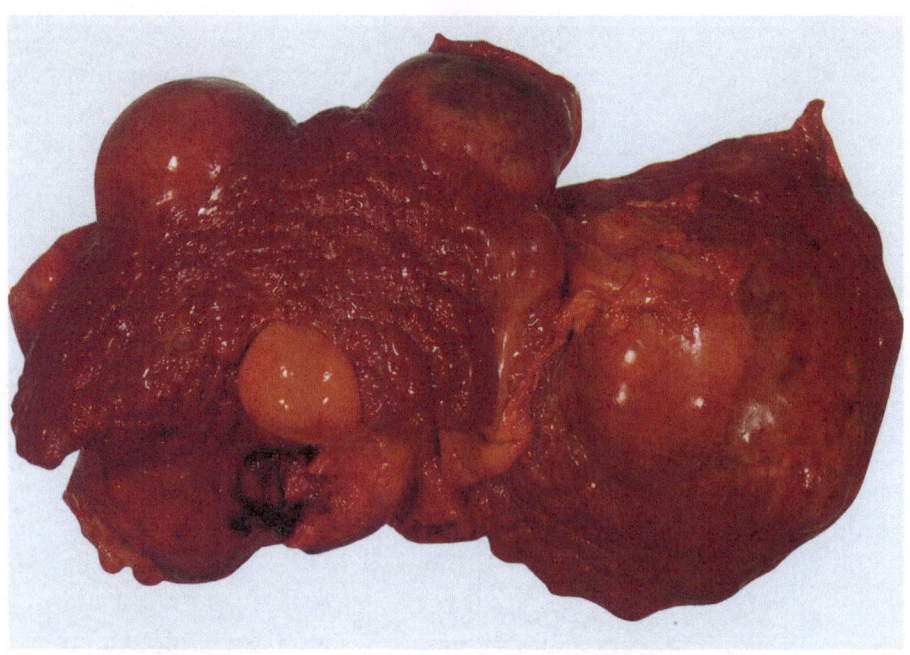

Fig. 5.9. Expansive HCC, multinodular, with liver cirrhosis

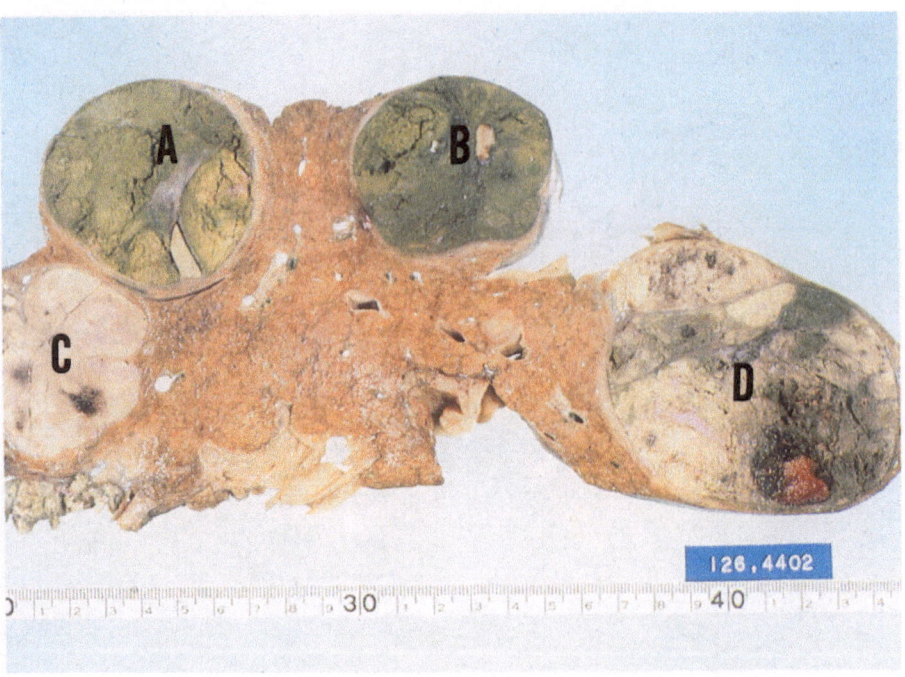

Fig. 5.10. Cut surface of the same case. Four well-demarcated tumors show different gross features. **A, B** Well-encapsulated tumors showing a greenish color. **C** Whitish-gray nonencapsulated tumor. **D** Tumor with thin fibrous septa

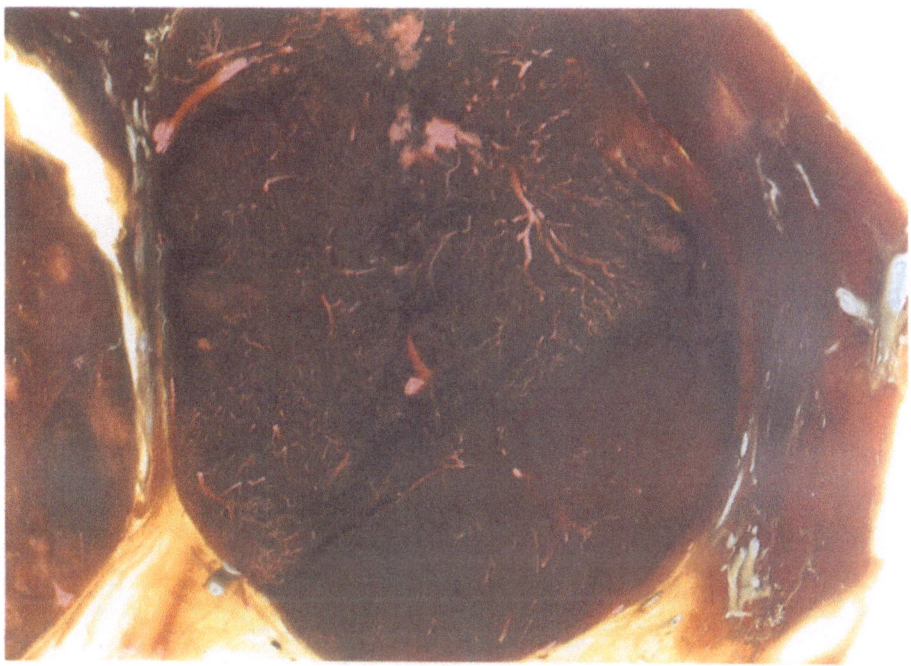

Fig. 5.11. Same case. The encapsulated tumor has a hypervascular and a hypovascular portion. It is suggested that this tumor receives different arterial branches from outside the tumor. Transparent preparation

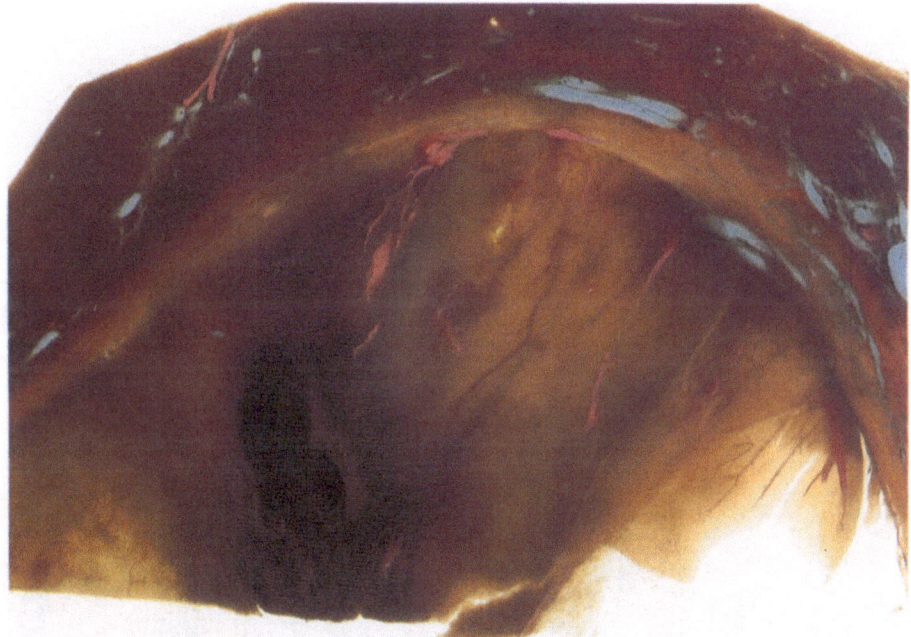

Fig. 5.12. Same case. Fine arterial tumor vessels branching from the pericapsular artery. Transparent preparation

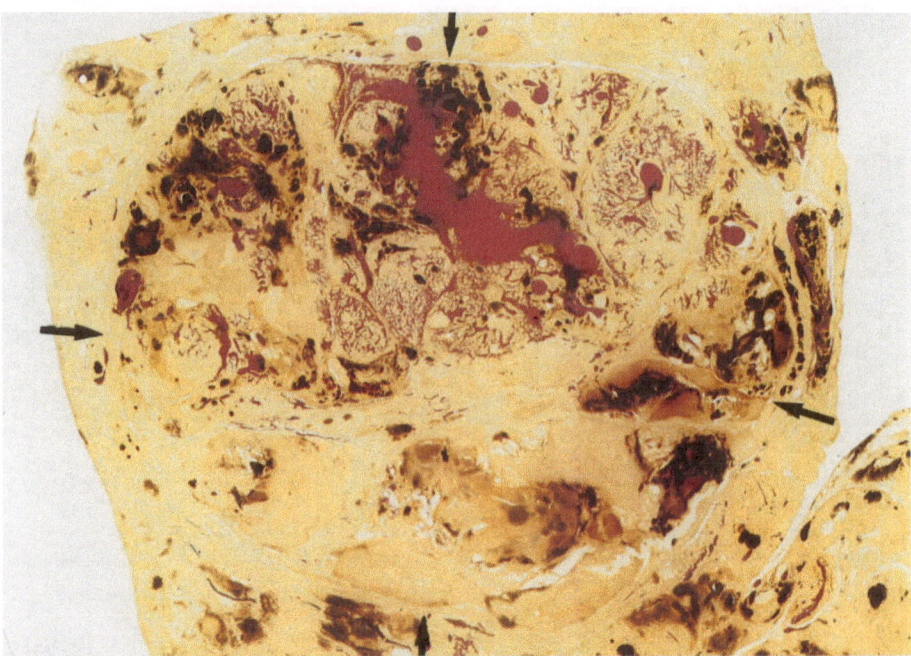

Fig. 5.13. Angioarchitecture of an encapsulated tumor. The fibrous capsule is avascular (*arrows*). The different parts of the tumor, separated by fibrous septa, show different vasculature. Transparent preparation

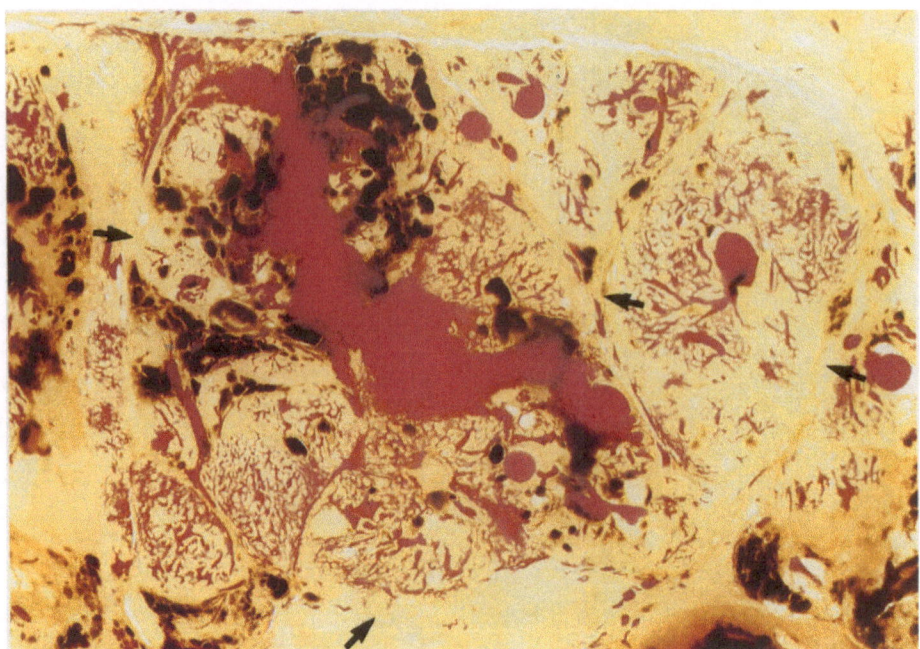

Fig. 5.14. Detail of the same tumor. Different vasculature in each of the parts separated by fibrous septa (*arrows*). Transparent preparation

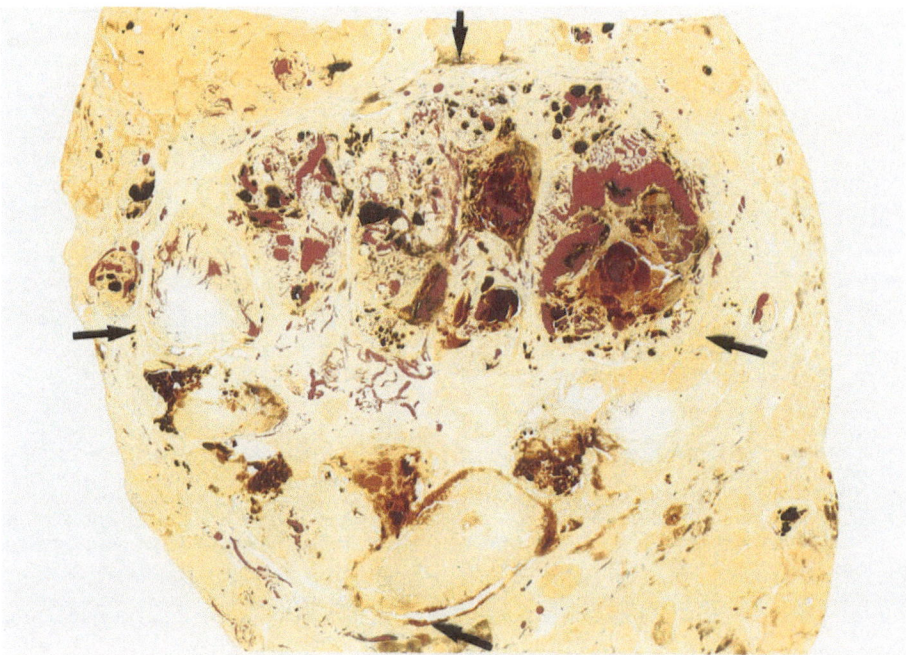

Fig. 5.15. Different vasculature is seen in each of the parts, separated by fibrous septa, of this tumor enclosed by a thick fibrous capsule (*arrows*). Transparent preparation

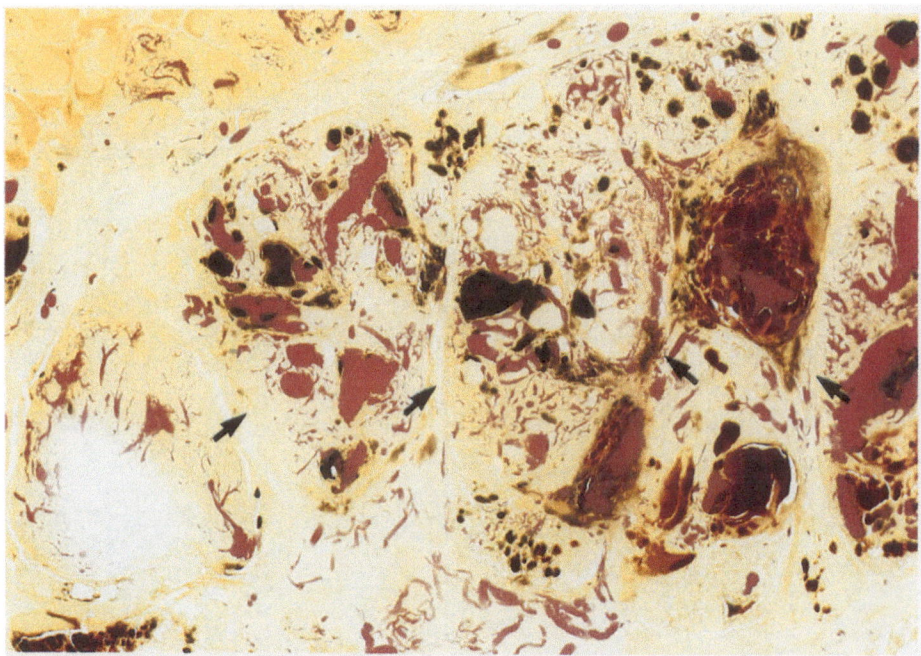

Fig. 5.16. Close-up view of the hypervascular part of the same tumor. Transparent preparation. *Arrows* show fibrous septa

Chapter 6
Tumor Thrombus of the Hepatic and Portal Veins

Hepatocellular carcinoma commonly involves the portal and/or hepatic veins, causing a tumor thrombus. The incidence of tumor thrombus of the portal vein, in particular, is extremely high among patients with HCC. Rarely, HCC is characterized only by a prominent tumor thrombus of the portal and/or hepatic veins with no recognizable main tumor mass.

Tumor Thrombus of the Portal Vein

Histological findings
The tumor thrombus frequently takes the form of a thin, elongated trabecular structure along the vessel which has been called "finger-like column" (Figs. 2.7, 6.2a). Tumor thrombi of the portal vein may be classified into four types [121]—proliferative (Fig. 6.2a), necrotic (Fig 6.2b), mixed proliferative and necrotic, and organized (Fig. 6.2c, d)—but the tumor thrombi in a single portal vein may not all be of one particular type. In many cases, the histological findings vary. In portal vein branches (fifth and sixth branches), the proliferative type is most common, occurring in 64.7% of cases, followed by the mixed proliferative and necrotic type in 28%, and the necrotic type in 18.7%.

The proliferative type tumor thrombus can be subdivided into three types as follows [122]. *Type I*: the tumor thrombus consists of a well-differentiated tumor, receives the arterial blood vessels from the dilated periportal arteries, and is covered by a single layer of endothelial cells (Fig. 6.3c, d). *Type II*: the tumor thrombus consists of a poorly differentiated tumor, with no trabecular structure, and the tumor cells are frequently of the free-cell type (Fig. 6.4a, b). *Type III*: mixture of types I and II.

Shunt formation between artery and portal vein
Retrograde portal circulation through a shunt between the artery and portal vein results more frequently from HCC than from liver cirrhosis. The affected portal vein is delineated by celiac angiography earlier than usual because of the artery-portal vein (A-P) shunt through the tumor thrombus [123]. A large tumor thrombus that has grown within the portal vein has a predisposition to form an A-P shunt because virtually its entire vascular framework is comprised by the arterial tumor vessels. A-P shunts can be divided into three types as follows.

Type 1. The blood flows from the arterial branches covering the portal vein into the arterial tumor vessels of the tumor thrombus and thence into the blood space of the tumor thrombus, which drains into the portal lumen (Fig. 6.5).

Type 2. The dilated branches of the hepatic artery, located around the portal vein, are directly destroyed by the rapidly expanding tumor thrombus. Thus, arterial blood of the interlobular artery drains directly into the portal vein (Fig. 6.6).

Type 3. This is a relatively large shunt between the interlobular artery and the portal vein caused by a large thrombus in the latter. When tumor invasion extends to the periportal collateral circulation involving the interlobular artery, necrosis and destruction of the branches of the hepatic artery result in communication of the hepatic artery with the portal vein (Figs. 6.7, 8).

Vascular architecture
Besides the tumor masses, a tumor thrombus of the portal vein contributes greatly to the formation of the complicated vasculature in HCC. Dilatation with increased branching is evident in the branches of the artery around the portal vein that has a tumor thrombus. From such arterial branches, the arterial tumor vessels extend into the tumor thrombus, indicating that it is also nourished by these vessels (Figs. 6.9–13, 16). In some poorly differentiated types of HCC, the cancer fails to form a tumor nest because the cancer cells lack adhesiveness with each other. In such cases, the tumor thrombus occasionally appears not to be provided with the arterial tumor vessels.

Organization
Recent progress in the therapy of HCC has been striking. Intra-arterial injection of anticancer agents (one-shot injection therapy and infusion therapy) and arterial embolization therapy have enhanced the 1 year survival rate of patients with HCC; consequently, organization of the tumor thrombus has become frequent. The manner of organization may be divided into three types as follows. *Type I*: the organization begins with the tumor tissues adjacent to the arterial tumor vessels, which originate in the arteries around the portal vein (Figs. 6.17, 18). *Type II*: the organization starts around the central necrotic focus in a tumor thrombus which is poorly supplied by the blood circulation (Figs. 6.17, 18). *Type III*: The organization begins with fibrotic changes in a subendothelial space of trabecular tumor nests (Figs. 6.21, 22).

Intrahepatic tumor spread
Although distant metastasis is relatively infrequent in HCC, intrahepatic metastasis through a tumor thrombus of the portal vein occurs in the early stage, resulting in diffuse infiltrates. Intrahepatic infiltrates and metastases have been observed to form around branches of the portal vein (Fig. 6.14a, b). Such foci are connected with the dilated branches of the hepatic artery and constitute a periductal capillary plexus around the portal vein with the arterial tumor vessels, which nourish the foci (Fig. 6.14c). When there is associated liver cirrhosis, the tumor extends as it replaces cirrhotic lobules, and so the vascular framework in the intrahepatic metastasis assumes a "glomoid structure," comprising the arterial tumor vessels, in postmortem angiograms or transparent preparations. The vascular architecture in an isolated intrahepatic metastatic focus is comprised solely of the arterial tumor vessels (Fig. 6.16).

Tumor Thrombus of the Hepatic Vein

Compared with a tumor thrombus in a branch of the portal vein, it is difficult to identify a thrombus in the hepatic vein (Figs. 6.23, 24), because the peripheral branches of the hepatic vein are destroyed at an earlier stage. Since only tumor thrombi occurring in the relatively large venous branches in the hepatic hilus are identified, the reported incidence is far lower than the actual figure. Thrombi that form in the hepatic vein are also connected by the arterial tumor vessels with the branches of the artery located around the hepatic vein.

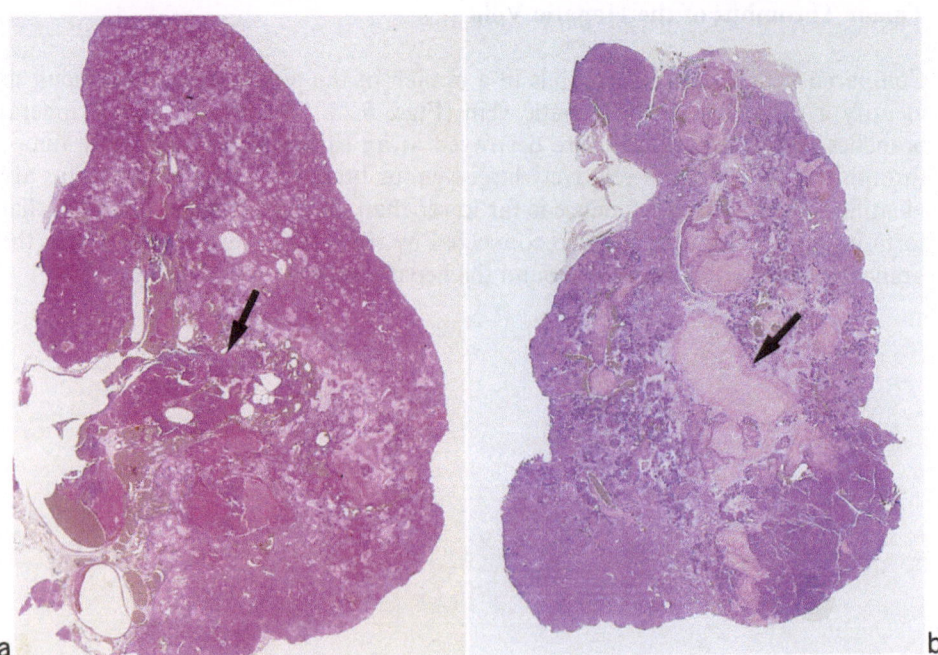

Fig. 6.1a, b. Tumor thrombus of the portal vein (*arrows*). **a** Proliferative type; **b** Necrotic type. HE, × 1

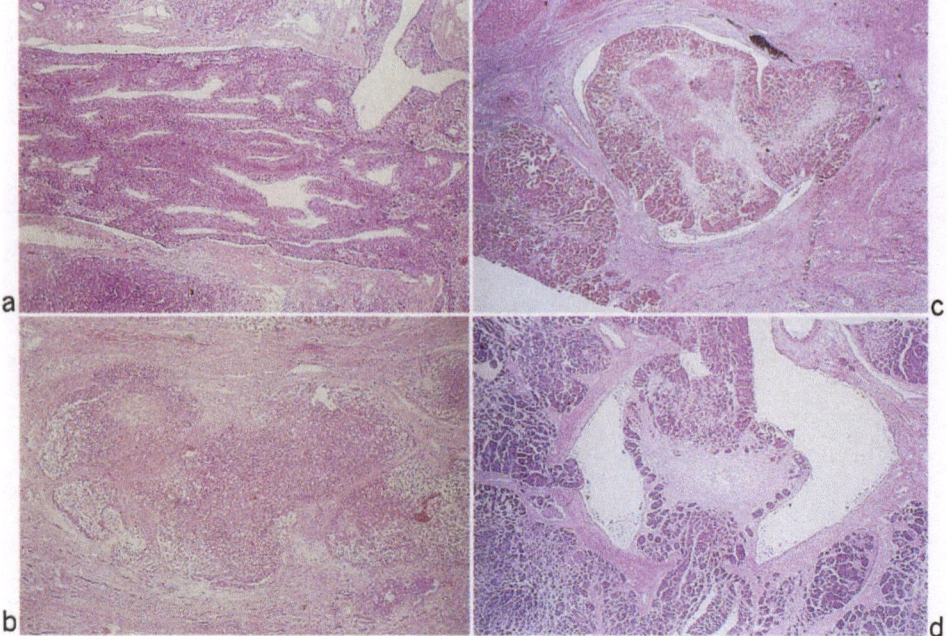

Fig. 6.2a–d. Histological findings of tumor thrombus of the portal vein. **a** Proliferative type; **b** Necrotic type; **c, d** Organized type. HE, × 20

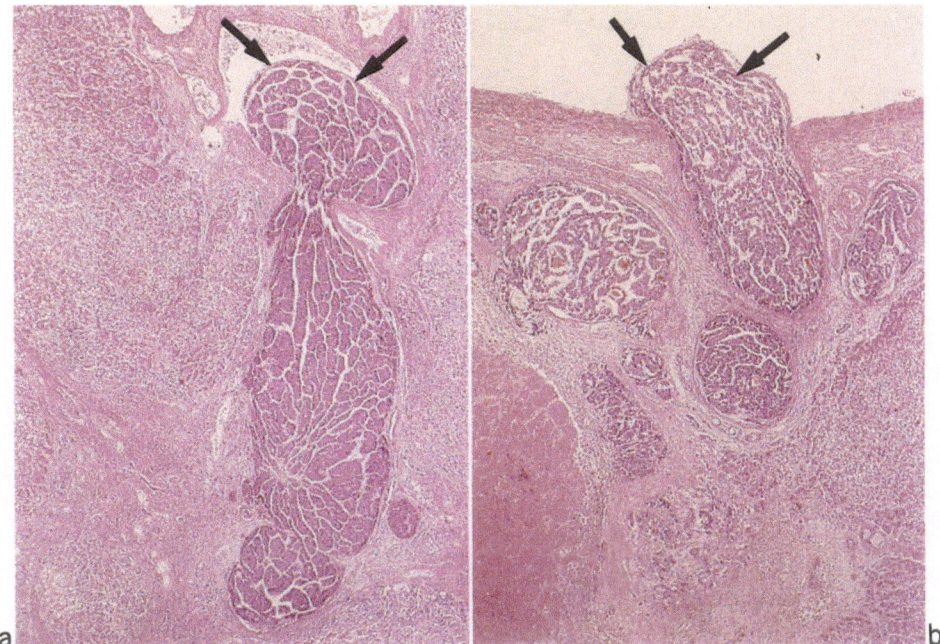

Fig. 6.3a, b. Proliferative tumor thrombus of well-differentiated type (type I) of the portal vein. Tumor thrombi showing a trabecular pattern completely obstruct the portal vein and are covered by a single layer of endothelial cells (*arrows*). HE, × 20

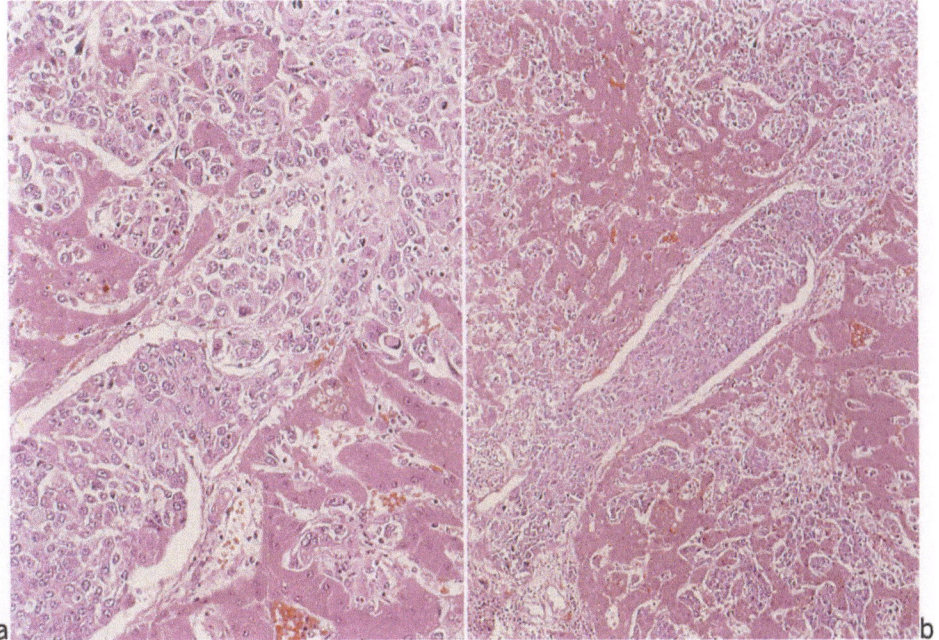

Fig. 6.4a, b. Proliferative tumor thrombus of poorly differentiated type (type II) of the portal vein. The tumor thrombi consist of tumor cells of the free-cell type, and extravascular tumor cells proliferate in the sinusoids. HE; **a** × 100, **b** × 50

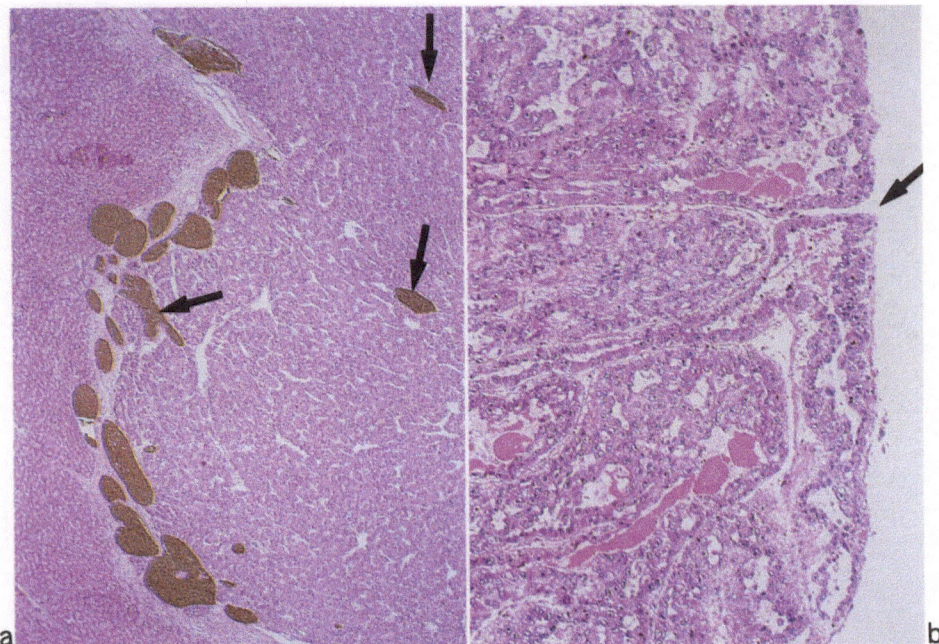

Fig. 6.5a, b. Artery-portal vein shunt, type I. **a** Arterial tumor vessels (*arrows*) in the tumor thrombus originate from the dilated periportal arteries. **b** The blood space of the tumor thrombus drains into the lumen of the portal vein (*arrow*). HE; **a** × 20, **b** × 50

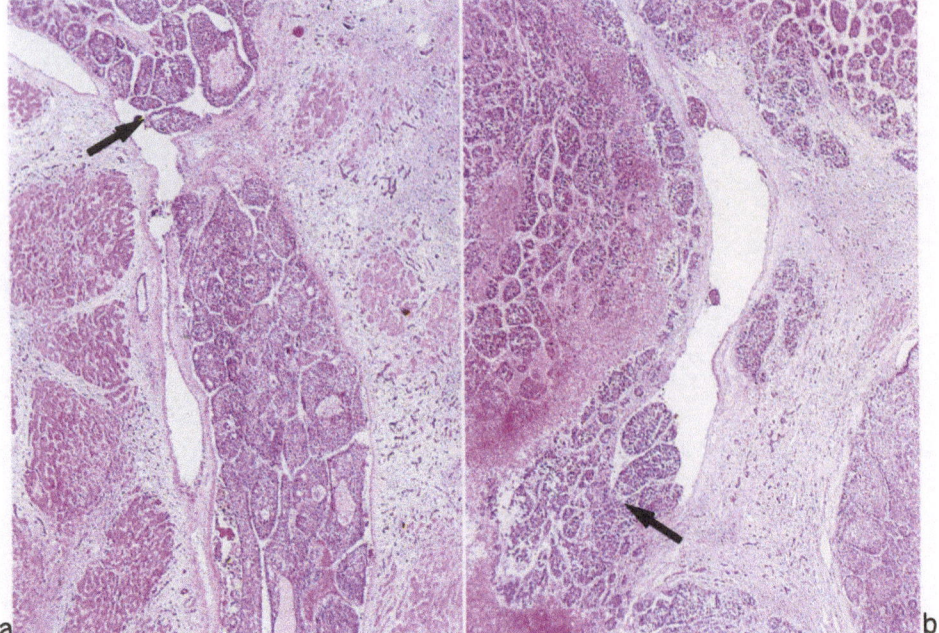

Fig. 6.6a, b. Artery-portal vein shunt, type II. Rapidly expanding tumor thrombi directly destroy the dilated arterial branches (*arrows*) around the portal vein. HE, × 20

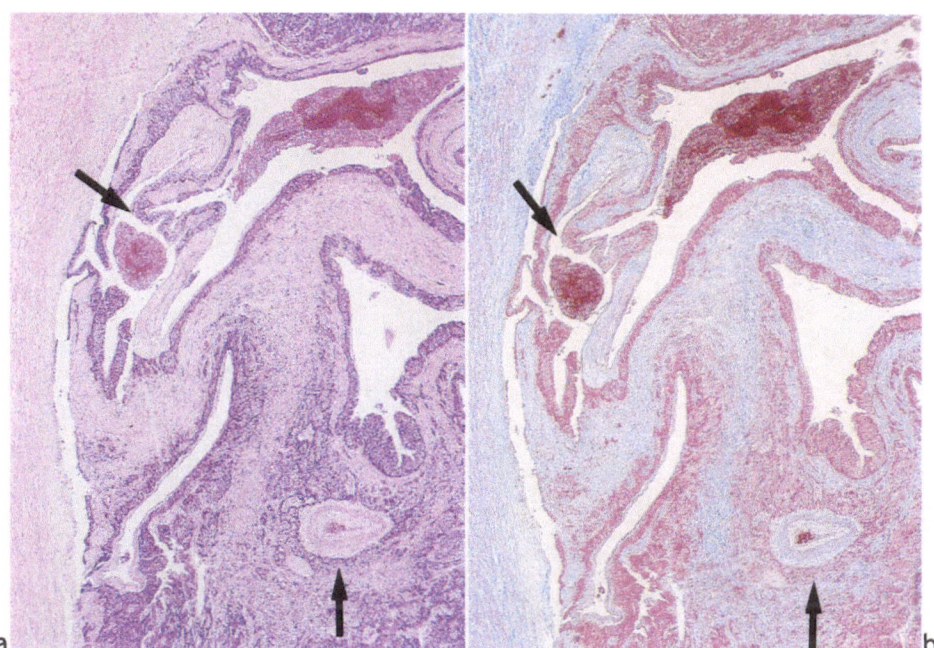

Fig. 6.7a, b. Artery-portal vein shunt, type III. Destruction of the entangled interlobular arteries (*arrows*) in the tumor thrombus results in shunt formation. **a** HE, **b** Azan-Mallory; × 20

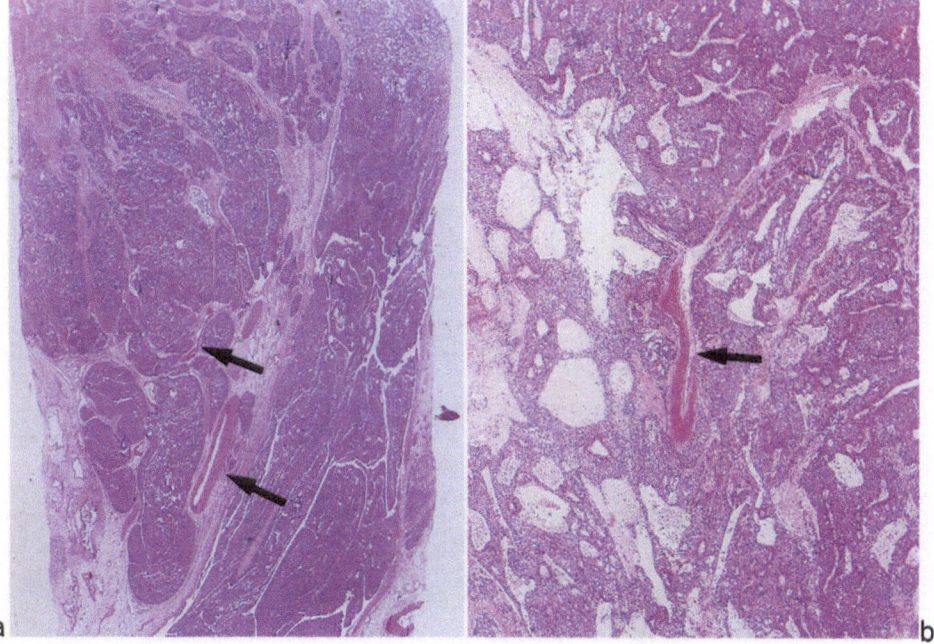

Fig. 6.8a, b. Artery-portal vein shunt, type III. **a** Relatively large interlobular arteries (*arrows*) are entangled in the tumor thrombus. **b** An entangled interlobular artery (*arrow*) shows necrotic change. HE, × 20

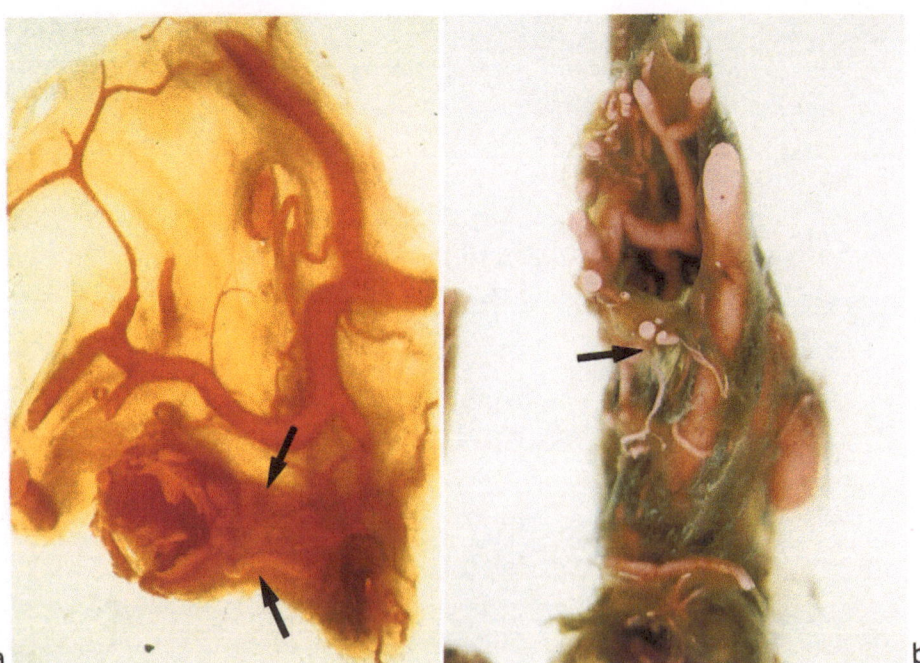

Fig. 6.9a, b. Angioarchitecture of the tumor thrombus of the portal vein. Marked dilatation and proliferation of the periportal arterial branches (*arrows*) due to occurrence of tumor thrombus. Transparent preparations

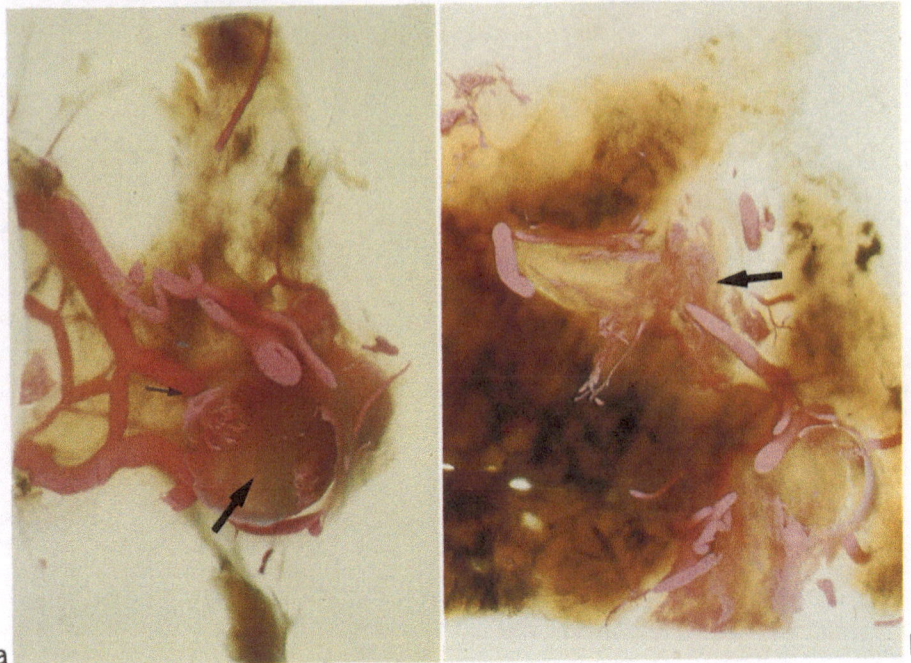

Fig. 6.10a, b. Angioarchitecture of tumor thrombi of the portal vein. The tumor thrombi receive the arterial tumor vessels from the dilated and proliferated periportal arterial branches. **a** Hypovascular tumor thrombus (*arrow*). **b** Hypervascular tumor thrombus (*arrow*). Transparent preparations

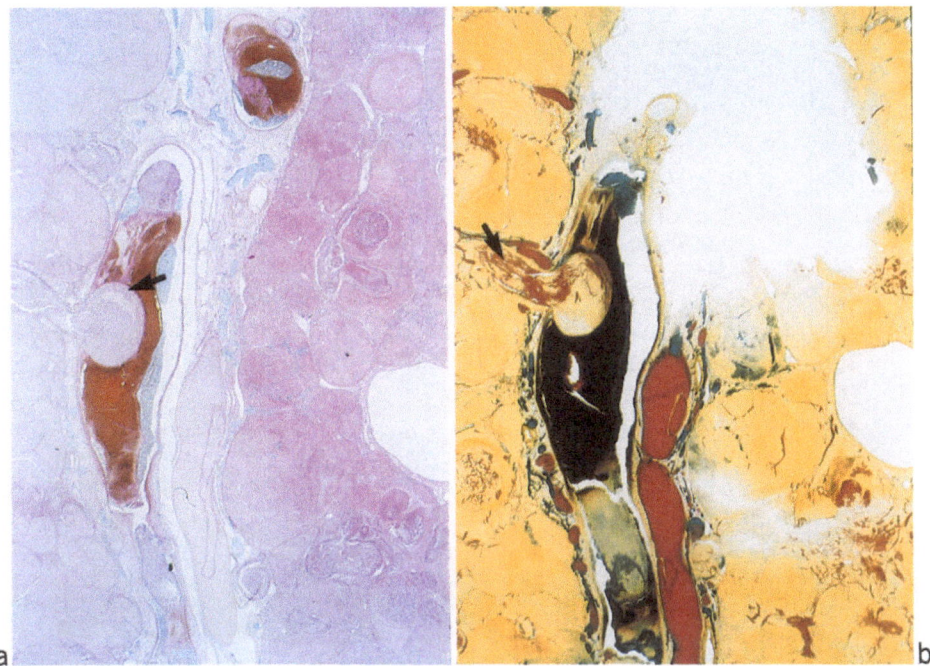

Fig. 6.11a, b. Tumor with retrograde proliferation in portal vein. Tumor thrombus in small branch proliferates to larger branch. **a** Protruded tumor surface in portal vein covered by endothelial cells. HE. **b** Tumor thrombus receives arterial tumor vessels (*arrow*). Transparent preparations

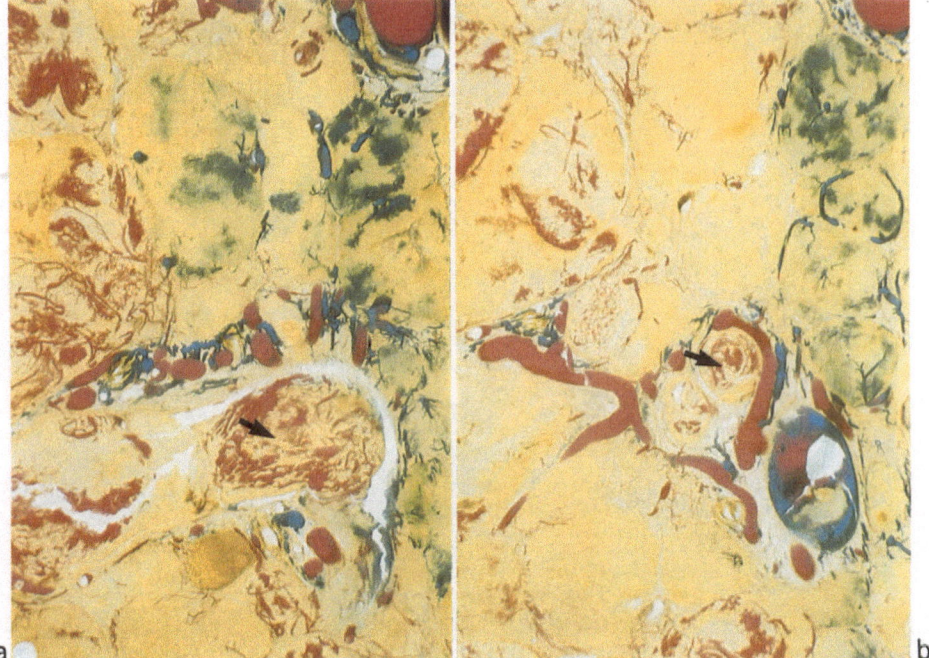

Fig. 6.12a, b. Angioarchitecture of tumor thrombi of the portal vein. The tumor thrombi receive the arterial tumor vessels (*arrow*) from the interlobular artery. Intrahepatic metastatic foci also receive the arterial tumor vessels. Transparent preparations

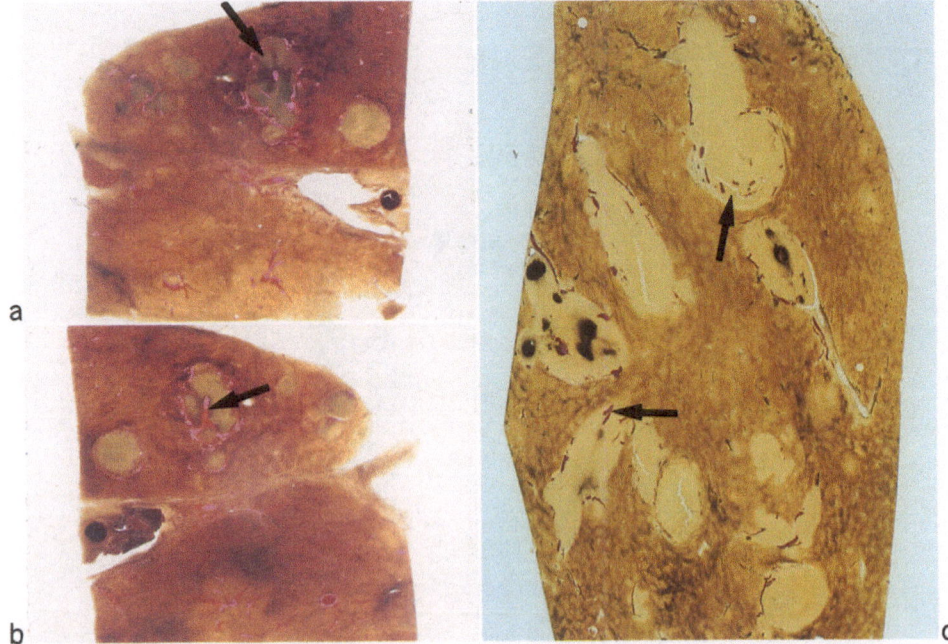

Fig. 6.13a–c. Angioarchitecture of a tumor thrombus of the portal vein. **a–c** Entangled interlobular arteries (*arrows*) in the tumor thrombus. Transparent preparations

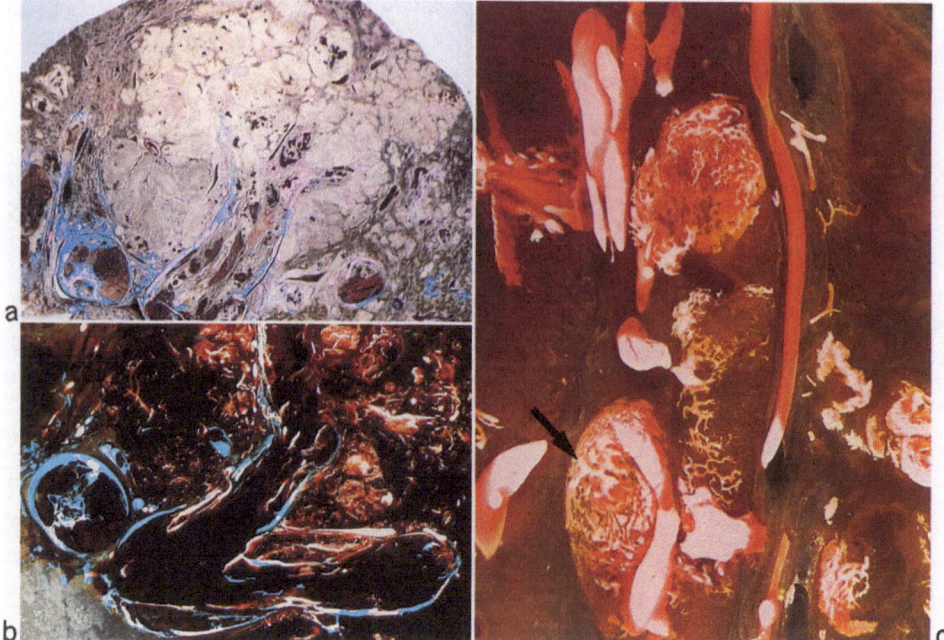

Fig. 6.14a–c. Angioarchitecture of tumor thrombus of the portal vein. **a** A massive tumor thrombus of the dilated portal vein contains red gelatin injected from the artery. **b, c** The arterial tumor vessels (*arrow*) branch into periportal metastatic foci from the dilated arteries around the portal vein. **a–c** transparent preparations

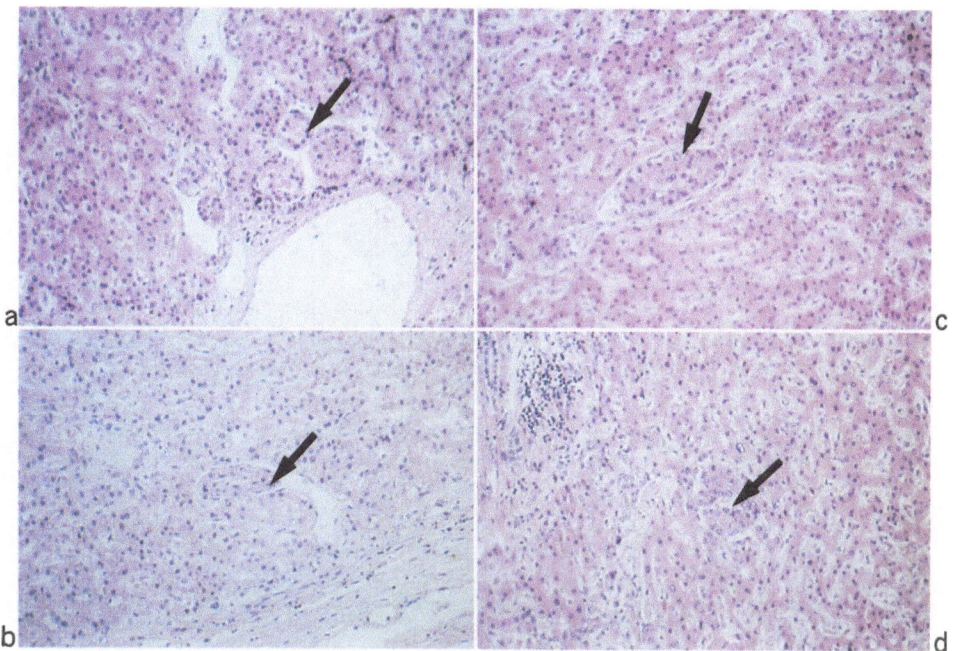

Fig. 6.15a–d. Tiny tumor nests (*arrows*) in dilated sinusoids. HE, × 50

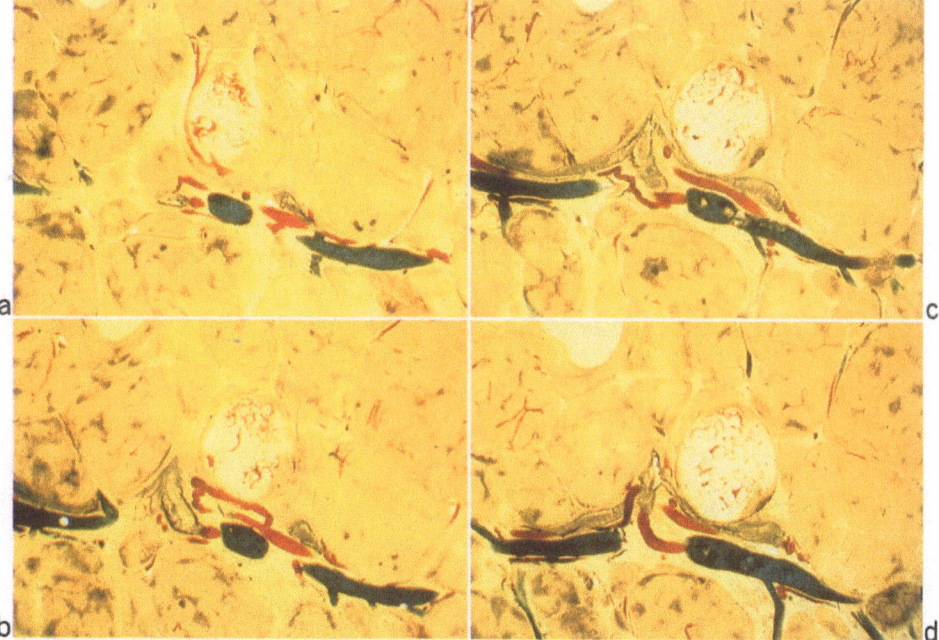

Fig. 6.16a–d. Intrahepatic metastasis through tumor thrombus of the portal vein. Serial section. The metastatic nodule receives the arterial tumor vessels from the interlobular artery. Transparent preparations: *red*, artery; *blue*, portal vein

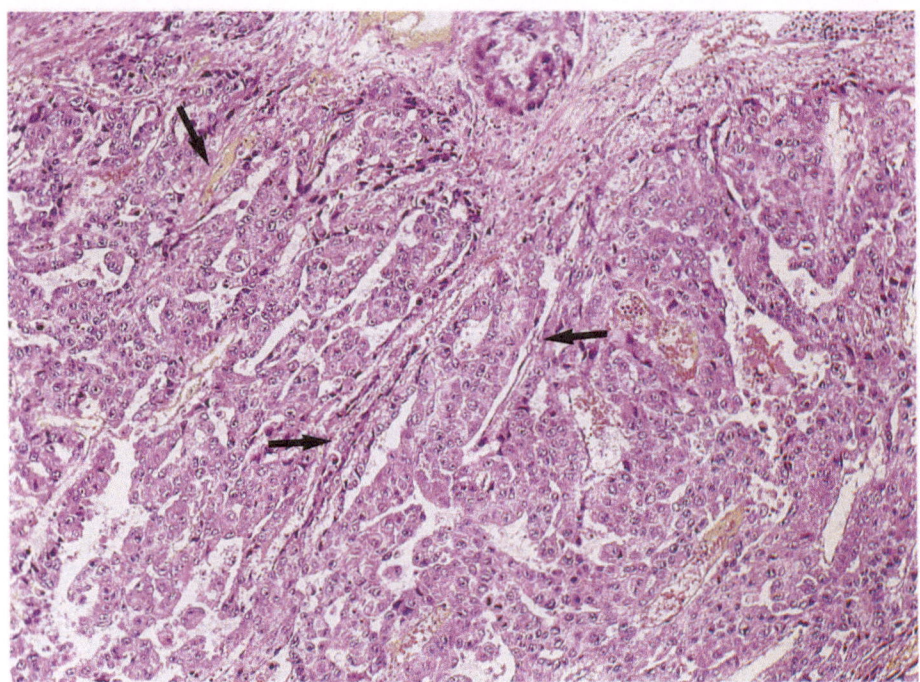

Fig. 6.17. Organization of tumor thrombus of the portal vein, type I. Organization has begun around the arterial tumor vessels (*arrows*). HE, × 100

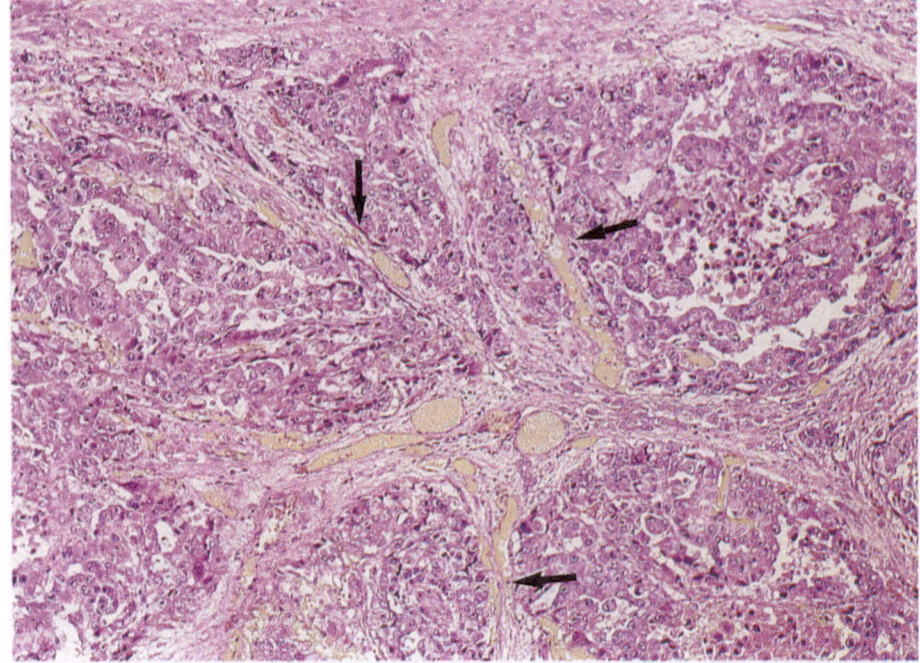

Fig. 6.18. Organization of tumor vessels of the portal vein, type I. Division of tumor thrombus by organization. Arterial tumor vessels (*arrows*) are dominant in the organized area. HE, × 100

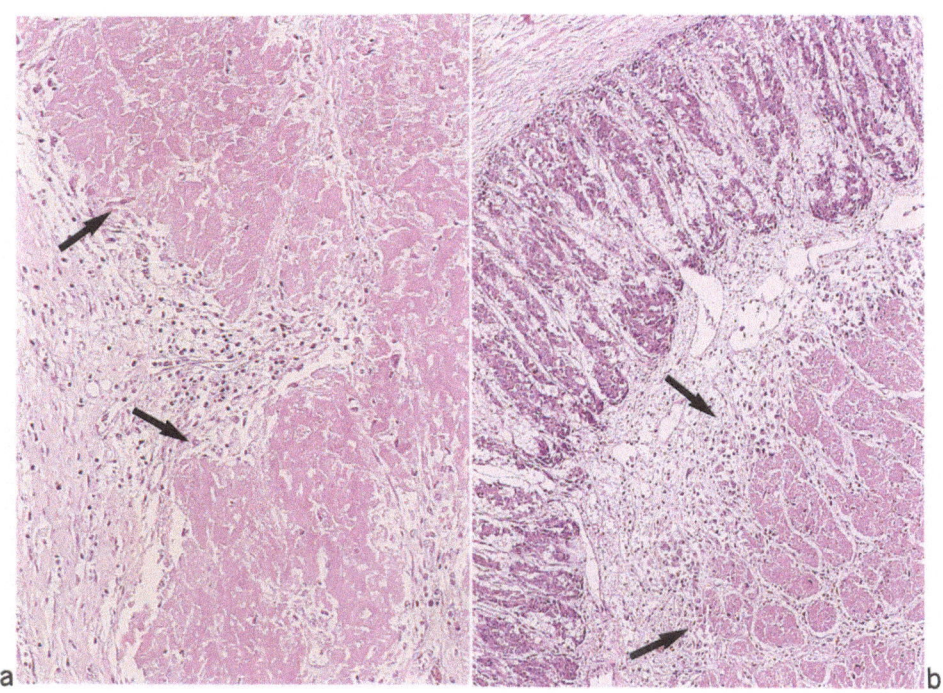

Fig. 6.19a, b. Organization of portal vein tumor thrombus, type II. **a** Necrosis of tumor thrombus (*arrows*). **b** Organization around necrosis of tumor thrombus (*arrows*). HE, × 50

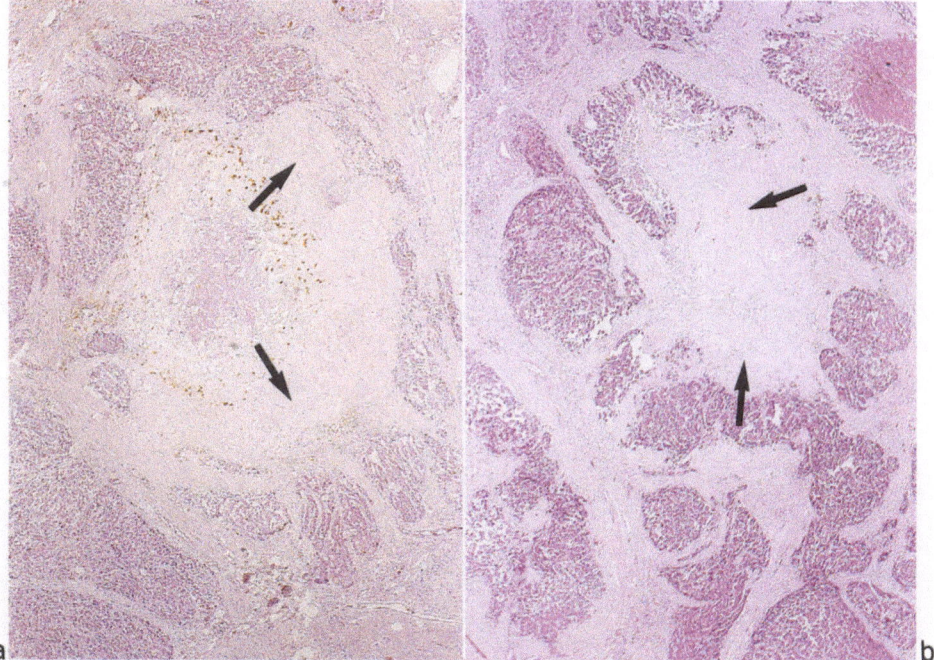

Fig. 6.20a, b. Organization of tumor thrombus of the portal vein, type II. Organization is seen around the necrotic area of the tumor thrombus. Hyalinization is seen in the organized area (*arrows*). HE, × 20

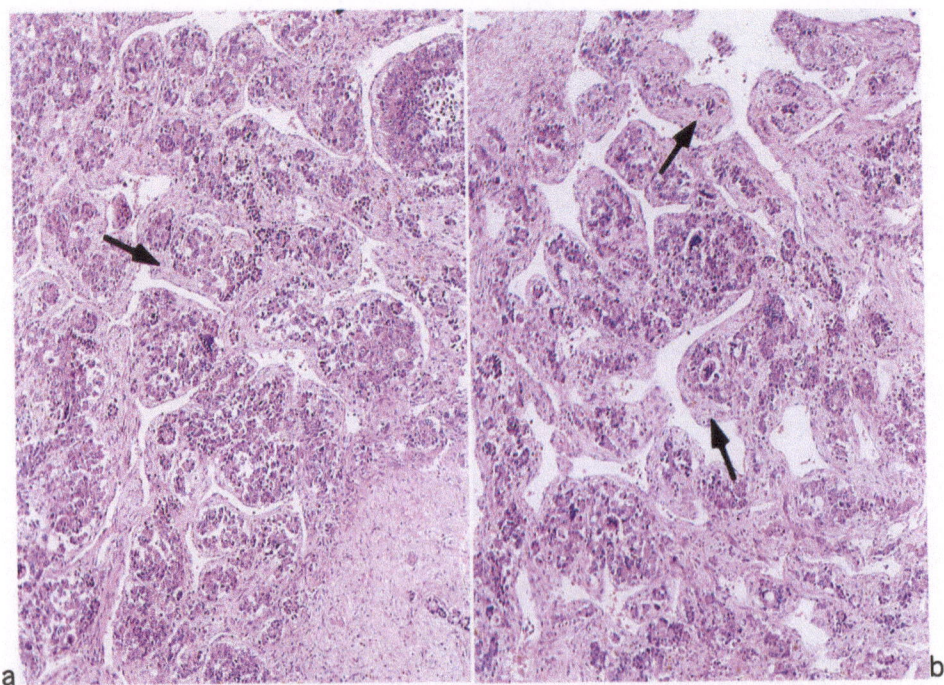

Fig. 6.21a, b. Organization of tumor thrombus of the portal vein, type III. Organization has begun in the subendothelial spaces (*arrows*) of the tumor nests. HE, × 20

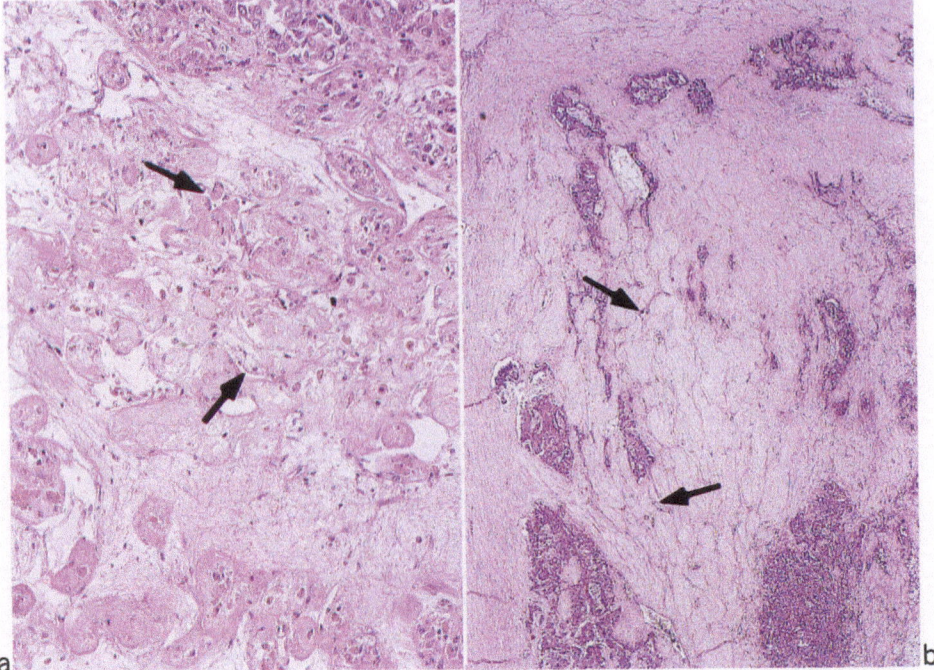

Fig. 6.22a, b. Organization of tumor thrombus of the portal vein, type III. **a** The tumor nests are completely organized and blood spaces remain in the organized area. **b** The blood spaces remaining in the organized area are markedly narrowed (*arrows*). HE, **a** × 50, **b** × 20

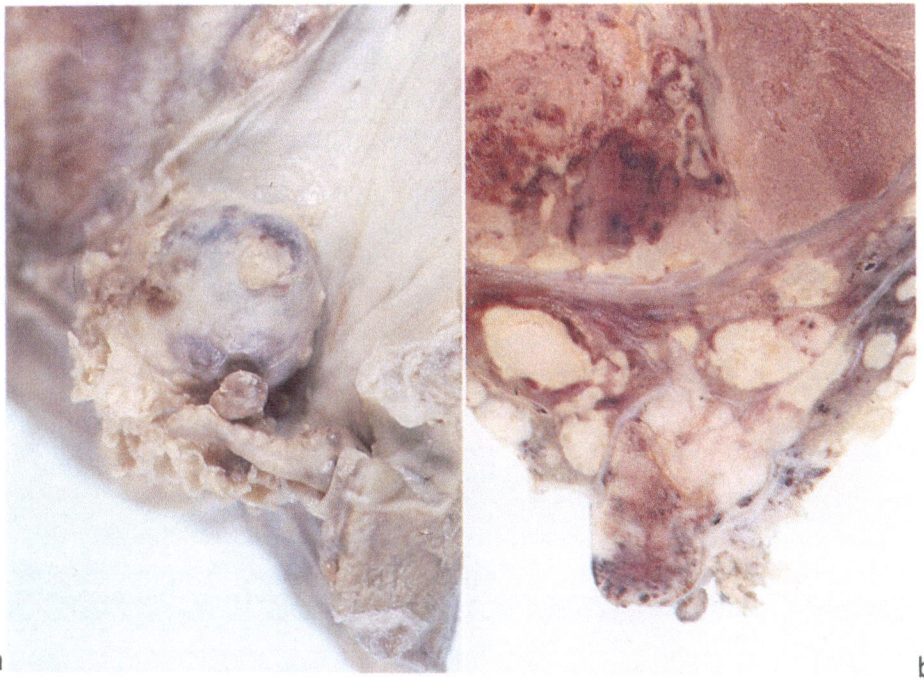

Fig. 6.23a, b. Tumor thrombus of the hepatic vein. **a** The surface of the tumor thrombus is covered with endothelial cells and looks smooth. **b** Cut surface of the tumor thrombus of the hepatic vein. The tumor thrombus is highly necrotic

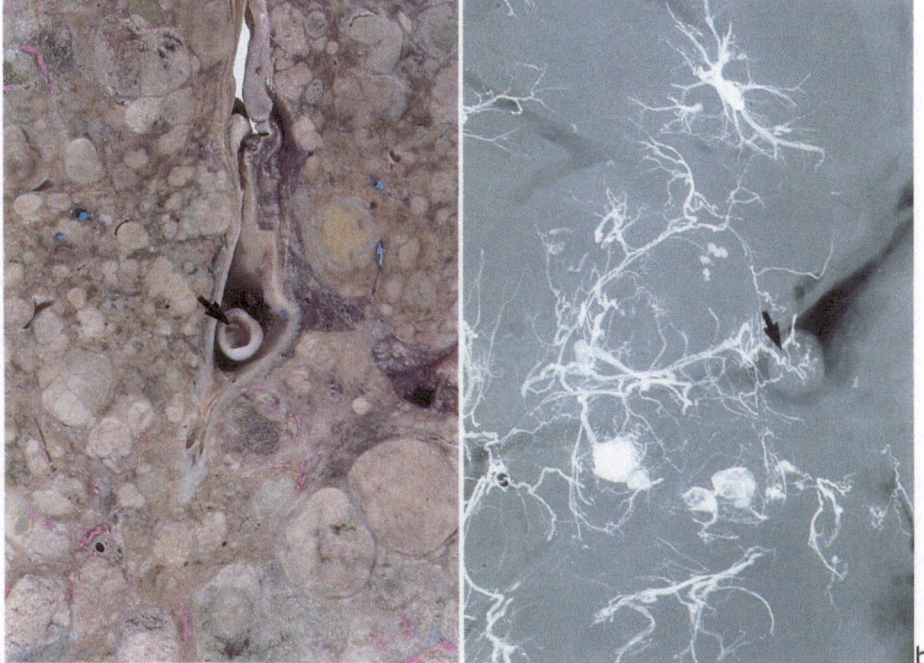

Fig. 6.24a, b. Tumor thrombus of the hepatic vein. **a** The surface of the thrombus looks smooth (*arrow*). **b** Soft X-ray finding in the same specimen. The tumor thrombus receives the arterial tumor vessels

Chapter 7
Intra-Atrial Tumor Invasion in Hepatocellular Carcinoma

Frequency of Intra-Atrial Tumor Growth

When HCC affects the venous system, it is not uncommon for a tumor thrombus to extend to the hepatic vein or inferior vena cava. Occasionally, such extension results in Budd-Chiari syndrome secondary to HCC [124, 125]. Ball-valve thrombus syndrome following an intra-atrial tumor growth has been described in some cases where sudden death ensued from extension of the tumor invasion into the right atrium [126]. Although extension of the tumor thrombus to the inferior vena cava and/or right atrium is first disclosed at autopsy in most cases, there are some cases in which the intra-atrial tumor growth could have been diagnosed by echocardiography or angiography 3–4 months prior to death. According to a survey of 78 cases of tumor thrombus in the inferior vena cava by Simpson [127], the tumor thrombus most commonly originated in malignancies of the kidney or adrenal gland; a tumor thrombus secondary to HCC was noted in only seven cases. According to Gustafson [128], of 62 cases of HCC, two had a tumor thrombus in the inferior vena cava extending into the right atrium. According to Gregory [129], of 234 cases of HCC described in the literature, only six had a tumor thrombus in the inferior vena cava or right atrium. Edmondson and Steiner [9] encountered a tumor thrombus of the hepatic vein in 11 of 100 cases of HCC. The tumor thrombus had extended up to the inferior vena cava in seven and the right atrium in one of the eleven cases. According to MacDonald [130], the thrombus extended into the inferior vena cava or right atrium in 3 of 108 cases of HCC. As the incidence of HCC in Japan is about ten times higher than that in Western countries, such extension is encountered more frequently. According to Kika [131], who studied 79 cases of HCC, tumor thrombus extending up to the right atrium was found in one of ten cases in which tumor invasion involved the inferior vena cava. The frequency of a tumor thrombus in the hepatic vein was reported to be significantly high by Kikuchi et al. [132], who noted it in 6 (40%) of 15 cases of HCC, and by Shikata [133], who noted it in 19 (39.5%) of 48 cases of HCC. In our series of 439 cases of HCC, a tumor thrombus in the hepatic vein was seen in 72 (16.4%) cases, in the inferior vena cava in 48 (10.9%) cases, and in the right atrium in 18 (4.8%) cases [134]. The tumor bolus crossed the tricuspid valve and entered the ventricle in 5 of these 18 cases. In 88 cases of HCC without associated liver cirrhosis, tumor thrombus of the hepatic vein, inferior vena cava, and right atrium was seen in fifteen (13.0%), ten (11.3%), and four (4.5%) cases, respectively. In 351 cases of HCC with associated liver cirrhosis, 55 (15.6%), 37 (10.5%), and 14 (3.9%) had a tumor thrombus in the hepatic vein, inferior vena cava, and right atrium, respectively. The frequencies do not vary significantly according to the presence or absence of liver cirrhosis (Figs. 7.1–8).

Tumor Growth in the Hepatic Vein, Inferior Vena Cava, and Right Atrium in Gross HCC

The hepatic vein was affected in 43 (14.9%) of 288 cases of the infiltrative type and in 5 (6.4%) of 78 cases of the noninfiltrative type of HCC. The frequency for the infiltrative type is significantly higher than that for the noninfiltrative type ($P < 0.05$). Of 18 cases of HCC with intra-atrial tumor growth, 17 were of the infiltrative type and one of the noninfiltrative type, the frequencies being 94.4% and 5.8%, respectively. Thus, intra-atrial tumor growth is closely related to the gross type of HCC. Tumor thrombus in the portal vein was also seen in 17 (94.4%) of the 18 cases with intra-atrial tumor growth.

Tumor Growth in the Hepatic Vein, Inferior Vena Cava, and Right Atrium: the Frequency of Extrahepatic Metastasis

In HCC of the infiltrative type, extrahepatic metastasis was encountered in 52 (85.2%) of 61 cases involving tumor growth in the hepatic vein, 38 (88.3%) of 43 cases involving the inferior vena cava, and 15 (83.3%) of 18 cases involving the right atrium. In HCC of the noninfiltrative type, seven (63.6%) of eleven cases involving the hepatic artery and three (60%) of five cases involving the inferior vena cava underwent extrahepatic metastasis; the one case involving the right atrium did not undergo extrahepatic metastasis. The frequencies do not vary significantly according to the extent of intravenous invasion of thrombus in either of the two groups.

Tumor Thrombus and Budd-Chiari Syndrome

With regard to Budd-Chiari syndrome, consisting of ascites, edema, hepatomegaly, splenomegaly, and collateral circulation resulting from blocked blood flow in the hepatic vein, Nakamura et al. [135] reported 23 cases in which membranous obstruction of the inferior vena cava was intrahepatically noted; these accounted for 32% of 71 cases of Budd-Chiari syndrome of unknown cause. In Japan, however, the majority of cases of Budd-Chiari syndrome seem to result from tumors, mostly HCC.

In many instances, Budd-Chiari syndrome secondary to HCC results from continuous extension of the tumor invasion from the hepatic vein to the inferior vena cava [136, 137]. Despite the presence of a tumor thrombus in the hepatic vein and inferior vena cava, a considerable proportion of cases are asymptomatic. In addition, Budd-Chiari syndrome is diagnosed relatively seldom because of the masking effects of symptoms of liver cirrhosis, which are commonly associated with HCC. Among our autopsy cases, Budd-Chiari syndrome was recorded in only 6 of 48 cases with a thrombus in the inferior vena cava.

Tumor Thrombus in the Right Atrium and Ball-Valve Thrombus Syndrome

In 18 cases of HCC with an intra-atrial tumor thrombus [138], there were no serious clinical cardiovascular symptoms in most cases, and ball-valve thrombus syndrome was suspected in only two cases. In the remaining 16 cases, the tumor thrombi, which were connected with tumor thrombi in the hepatic vein and inferior vena cava, were loosely adherent to the endocardium.

Tumor Thrombus and the Direct Cause of Death in HCC

In our 48 cases with a tumor thrombus in the inferior vena cava, death ensued most commonly from gastrointestinal hemorrhage and hepatic failure, in 12 and 11 cases respectively; however, hepatic failure and gastrointestinal hemorrhage are inseparable. In 47 of the cases, tumor thrombus of the portal vein and secondary hepatic congestion associated with necrosis and hemorrhage in the central zone of the cirrhotic lobules were noted together with advanced hepatic insufficiency. In addition, a tumor thrombus of the portal vein may cause portal hypertension and subsequently result in gastrointestinal hemorrhage and rupture of esophageal varices. Extensive bleeding from the digestive tract constitutes one of the major causes of death in HCC. In addition, intraperitioneal hemorrhage following rupture of the hepatic tumor and rupture of esophageal varices caused six and five deaths, respectively.

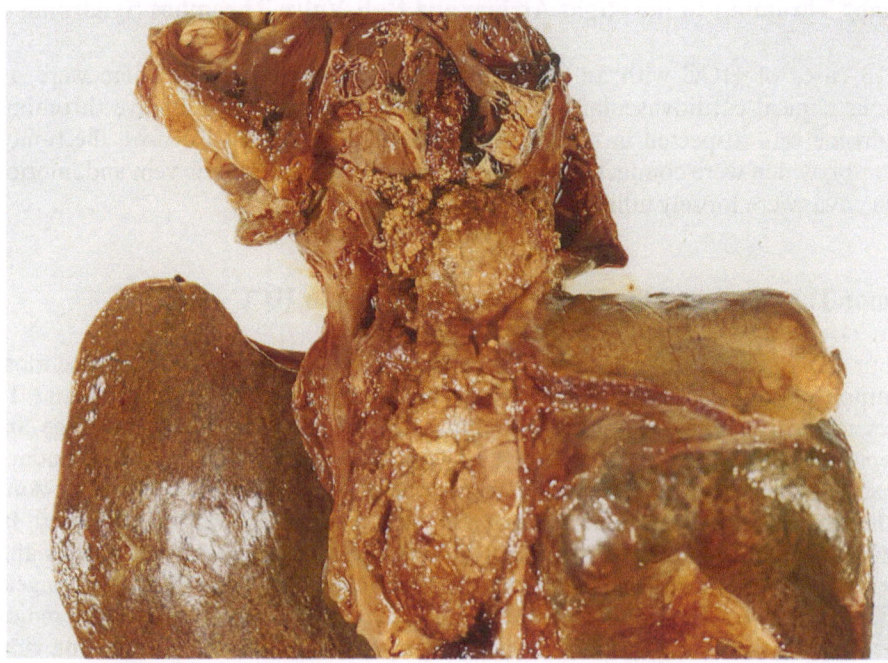

Fig. 7.1. Massive tumor casts in the inferior vena cava and the right atrium

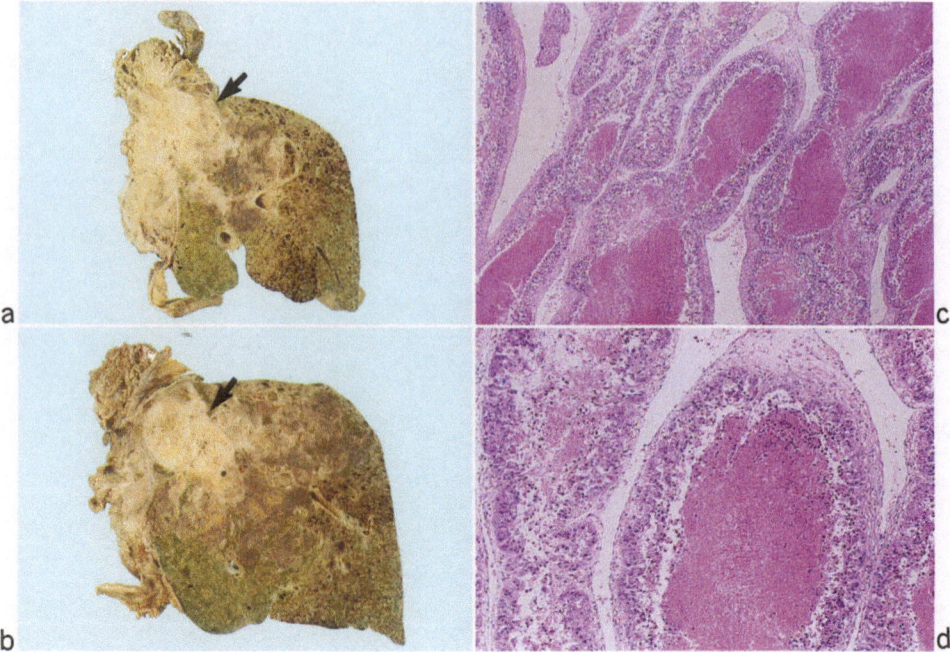

Fig. 7.2a–d. Same case. **a, b** Infiltrative HCC is invading the hepatic vein (*arrow*). **c, d** Histological findings of the tumor cast in the right atrium. Marked central necrosis of the tumor nests. HE; **c** × 10, **d** × 20

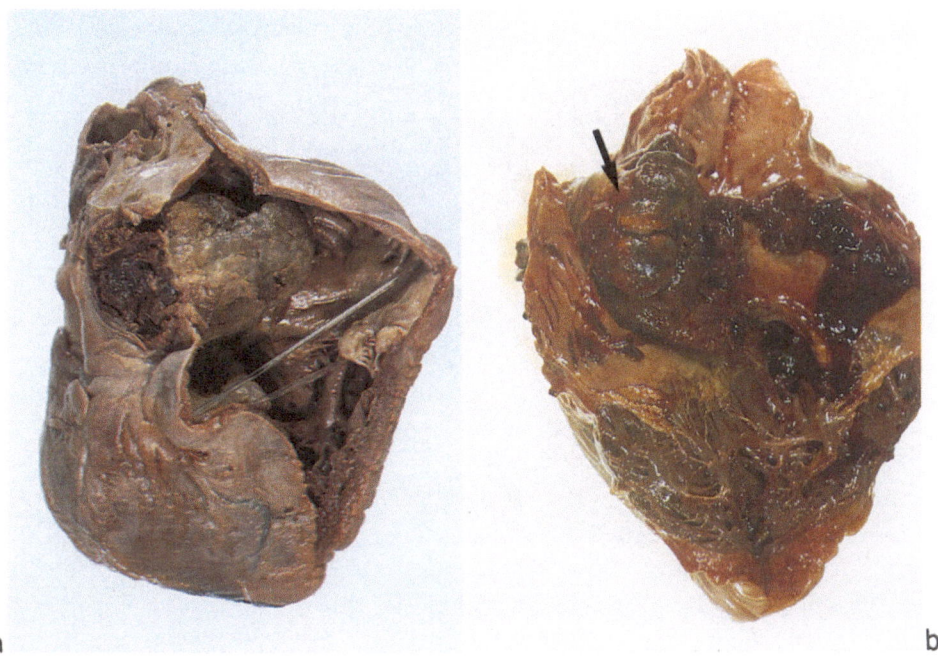

Fig. 7.3. **a** A tumor cast in the right atrium is covered by endothelial cells; its surface is smooth. **b** Ball-shaped tumor thrombus (*arrow*) in the right atrium

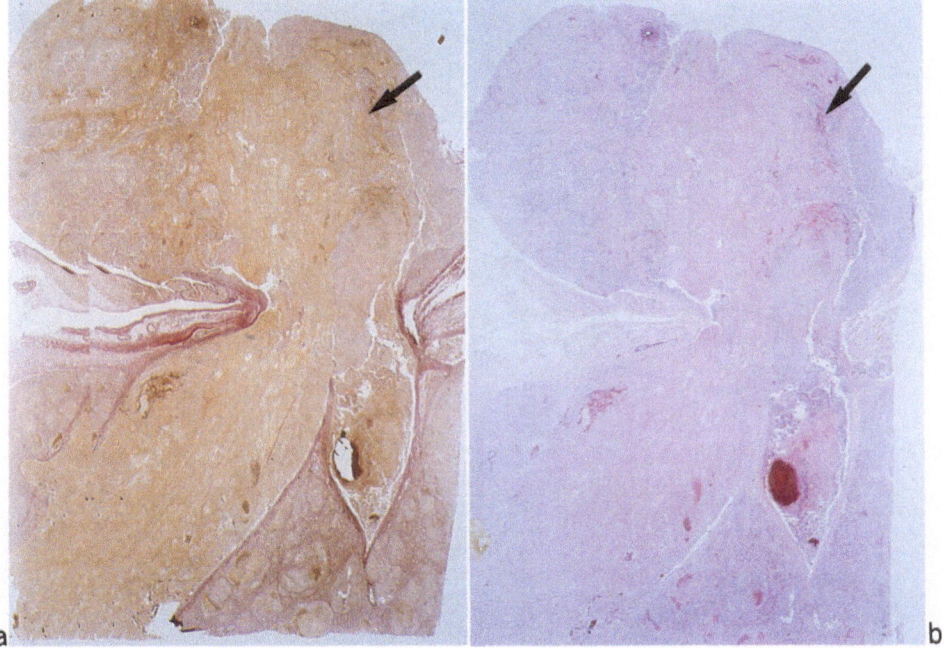

Fig. 7.4a, b. Tumor thrombus in the inferior vena cava protruding into the right atrium (*arrow*). **a** Van Gieson, **b** HE; × 1

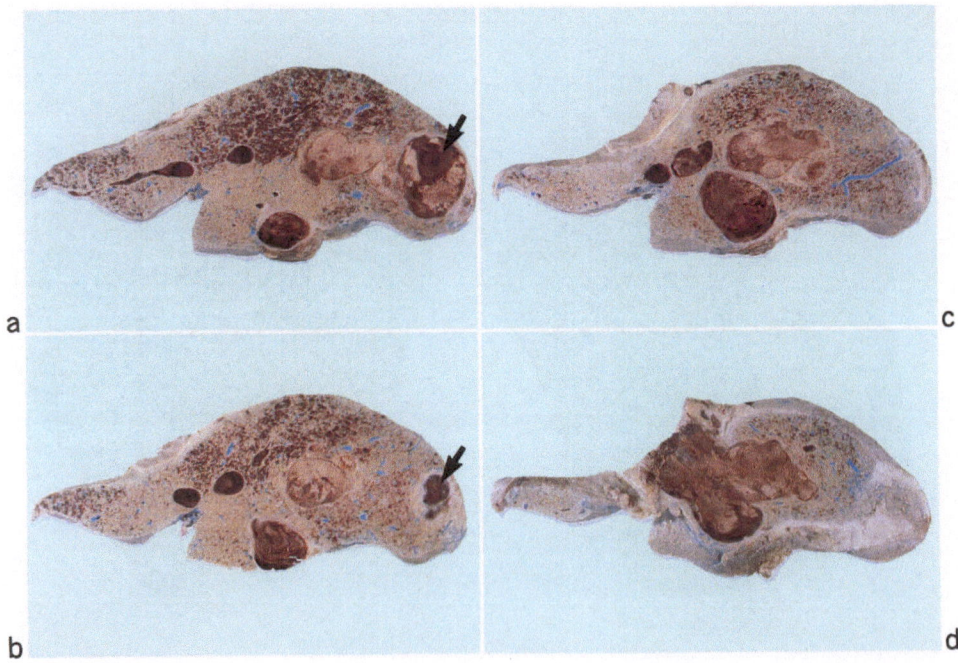

Fig. 7.5a–d. Expansive HCC with intra-atrial tumor growth. **a, b** The tumor is encapsulated (*arrows*) and is invading the hepatic vein. **c, d** The hepatic vein is filled with tumor cast and is markedly dilated

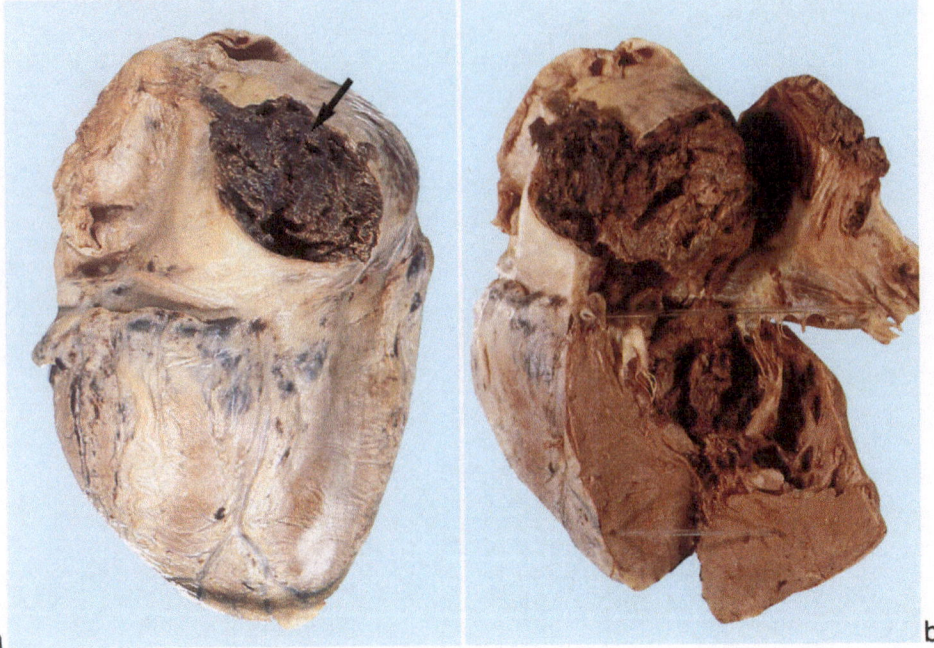

Fig. 7.6a, b. Same case. **a** Massive tumor cast in the right atrium (*arrow*). **b** The right atrium is filled by massive tumor cast

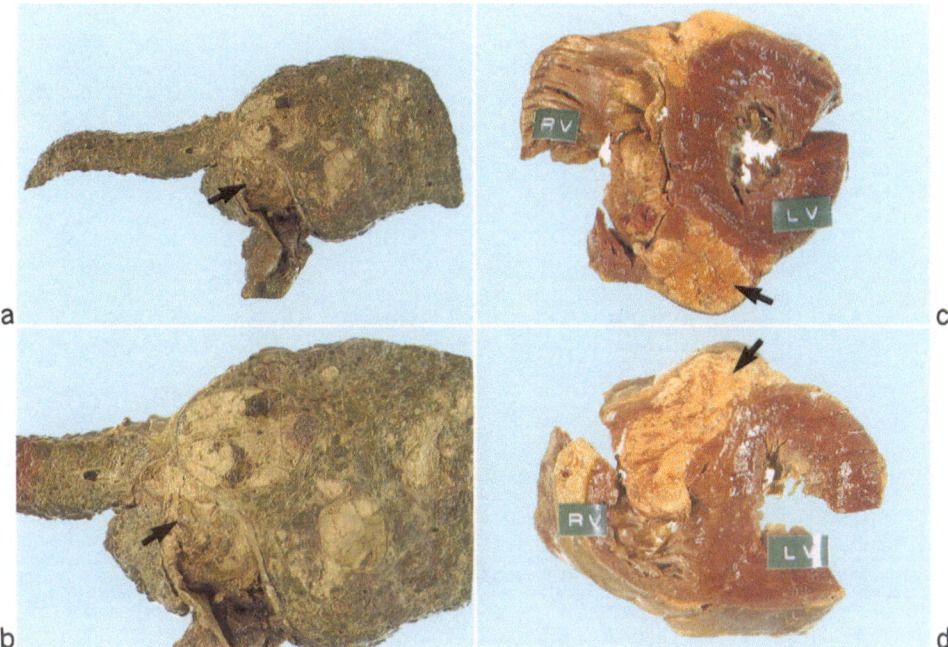

Fig. 7.7a–d. Infiltrative HCC with intra-atrial tumor growth and direct invasion into the myocardium. **a, b** Massive tumor casts in the hepatic vein and the inferior vena cava. **c, d** Intra-atrial tumor cast showing direct invasion into the myocardium (*arrows*)

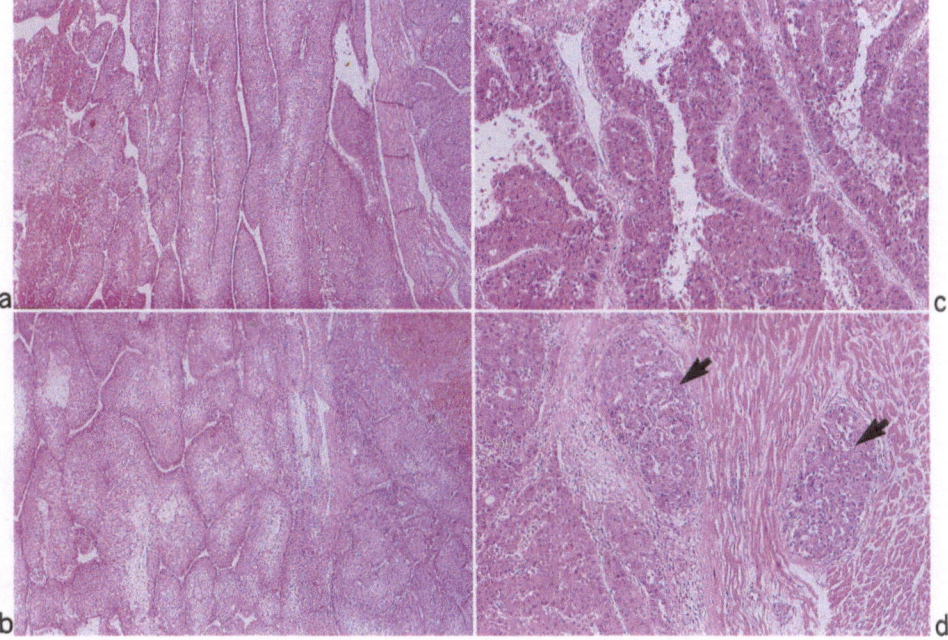

Fig. 7.8a–d. Histological findings of tumor casts. **a, b** Tumor cast in the inferior vena cava showing a finger-like column appearance, **c, d** Tumor cast invading the myocardium (*arrows*). HE; **a, b** × 10, **c, d** × 20

Chapter 8
Tumor Growth in the Bile Ducts in Hepatocellular Carcinoma

Tumor invasion in the bile ducts has been considered rare in HCC and has thus received little attention. Tumor growth in the bile ducts presents a variety of clinical and pathological features [139–141]. In cases in which obstructive jaundice develops, tumor invasion in the hepatic duct and/or common bile duct is frequently found at autopsy. In some cases, invasion by a tumor occurring in the porta hepatis into the adjacent bile duct results in obstructive jaundice as the initial sign, although the HCC itself is still in the early stage. Occasionally, necrotic cancerous tissue in the bile duct lodges at the papilla of Vater, resulting in severe obstructive jaundice. The bile duct is obstructed by hemorrhage and blood clotting in addition to the tumor.

Neither the series of 83 Japanese cases of HCC described by Kika [131] nor the 75 cases of HCC among the Bantu described by Berman [1], who classified HCC into five clinical types, includes cases suggesting bile duct involvement. Edmondson [10], who encountered a case of HCC invading the common bile duct, stated that apart from his cases there was only one other reported case in which extensive tumor invasion into the common bile duct was evident. Generally, the case of HCC associated with tumor growth in the gallbladder reported by Mallory [142] in 1947 is regarded as the first known case of HCC involving the bile duct system. Further cases have since been increasingly reported, but such tumor growth in the bile duct is relatively rare in Western countries.

Incidence of Intraductal Tumor Growth

Lin [143] classified HCC with severe icterus clinicopathologically as the "icteric" type, and Okuda and Nakashima [144] termed this the "cholestatic" type.

Cases of tumor invasion of the bile duct system can be divided into two groups on the basis of the clinical signs.

Group 1. HCC is manifested by progressive obstructive jaundice as an initial sign or during the course of the disease. In our series of 439 autopsy cases of HCC, 27 (6.1%) were considered to be of this type. Obstructive jaundice was the initial clinical sign in 13 of these 27 cases (2.7% of the total cases). Among the cases presenting with obstructive jaundice, instances of undetectable or low alpha-fetoprotein levels were thought to be due to biliary carcinoma or cholelithiasis. Tumor growth in the bile ducts often represents direct invasion from the primary tumor, occasionally invasion from an adjacent tumor thrombus in the portal vein (Figs. 8.1, 2, 5). Only when the tumor growth occurs in the hepatic duct and/or common bile duct does obstructive jaundice arise as a clinical problem.

Group 2. In our series, the gross and histological results at autopsy indicate tumor invasion of the small bile ducts at their periphery in 38 (8.1%) of the 439 cases.

Structure of Blood Vessels in Tumor Casts of the Bile Ducts

Morphological and angioarchitectural studies are the most suitable for specimens taken from tumor casts of group 2 invasion. In the case of advanced portal vein tumor thrombosis, in the peripheral region, the tumor thrombus extends upstream from the thrombus into the capillaries which constitute a plexus around the bile duct; tumor thrombi of the capillaries are seen immediately below the epithelium in the wall of the bile duct. These intracapillary tumor thrombi progressively protrude into the lumen of the bile duct in a hemispheric or papillary form, and most of them become covered with flattened bile duct epithelium (Fig. 8.6). Postmortem angiography with injection of colored gelatin into the hepatic artery reveals a direct connection between the tumor cast in the bile duct and the tumor thrombus in the portal vein, which is nourished by arterial tumor vessels. This indicates that tumor casts in the bile duct are also nourished by the arterial tumor vessels (Fig. 8.4). As there is no evidence that the tumor vessels empty directly into the bile duct or that the tumor undergoes necrosis, tumors localized within the bile duct seem to be furnished from the beginning with both afferent and efferent tumor vessels (Fig. 8.7). These increase in number and form a network of the arterial tumor vessels which play a part in tumor growth. Most tumor vessels are found to arise from the arterial branches constituting the capillary plexus around the bile duct.

HCC and Hemobilia

The term "hemobilia" is derived from "traumatic hemobilia," which Sandblom [145] used to describe hemorrhage in the bile duct due to subcapsular injury of the liver. The diagnosis of hemobilia depends on: (1) hematemesis or melena, (2) colic pain of the bile duct, (3) obstruction of the bile duct, and (4) tumor in the gallbladder. Growth of the tumor into the lumen may cause hemobilia by the mixing of blood with bile when the tumor necroses. We have encountered one case in which sudden death resulted from severe hemobilia (Figs. 8.3, 8b)

Gross HCC and Tumor Growth in the Bile Ducts

Of 27 cases of the first group, 25 were of the infiltrative type and two of the expansive type. The frequency of tumor growth in the bile ducts varies significantly depending on whether the HCC is of the gross type, suggesting that tumor growth in the bile ducts is not only a terminal feature of HCC. In one case in our series, a minute HCC of the infiltrative type arose in the porta hepatis close to the common bile duct and invaded the duct; this patient was first thought to have a stone in the common bile duct and underwent surgery.

Tumor Growth in the Biliary Tract and Extrahepatic Metastasis in HCC

Extrahepatic metastases are observed in 78.4% of cases of HCC involving the bile ducts. This incidence is significantly higher than that of extrahepatic metastases among all cases of HCC (63.3%; $P < 0.025$). Similar comparisons between the routes of extrahepatic metastasis reveal that only the difference between the incidence of the two hematogenous routes is significant ($P < 0.05$); that between the incidence of lymphatic metastasis and direct infiltration or dissemination is insignificant. This significant correlation of the incidence of hematogenous extrahepatic metastasis with the presence of a tumor in the bile duct may indicate that a tumor thrombus in the portal vein participates significantly in tumor spread to the bile duct.

Prognosis

Victims of HCC with intraductal tumor growth have shorter survival after diagnosis than other HCC patients. Survival after the total bilirubin level exceeds 20 mg/dl is extremely short, averaging 15.5 days.

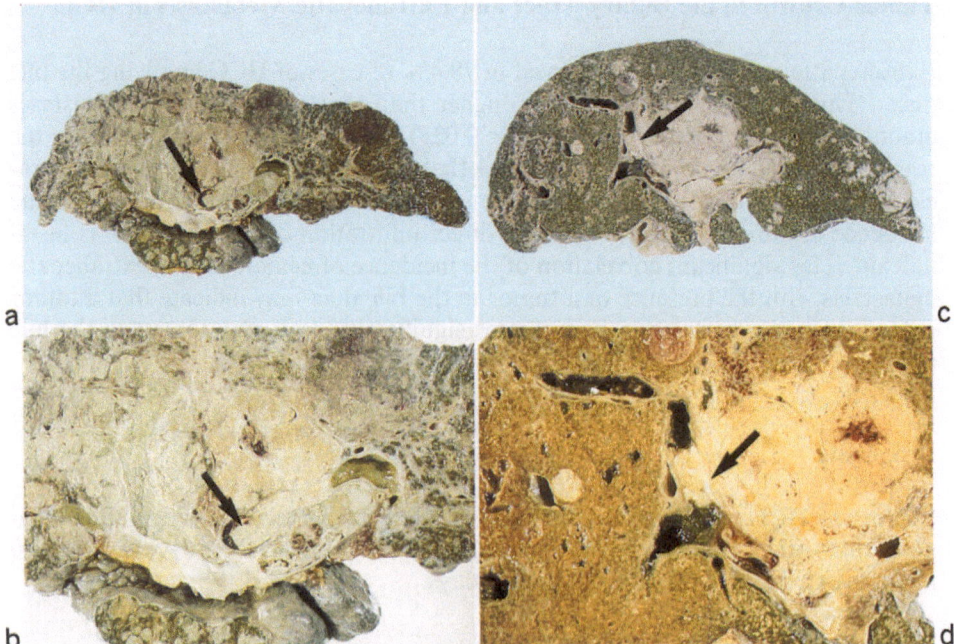

Fig. 8.1.a, b. Tumor invasion into the left hepatic duct (*arrows*). **c, d** Tumor invasion into the bile duct (*arrows*) in the right lobe with marked dilatation of the peripheral bile ducts

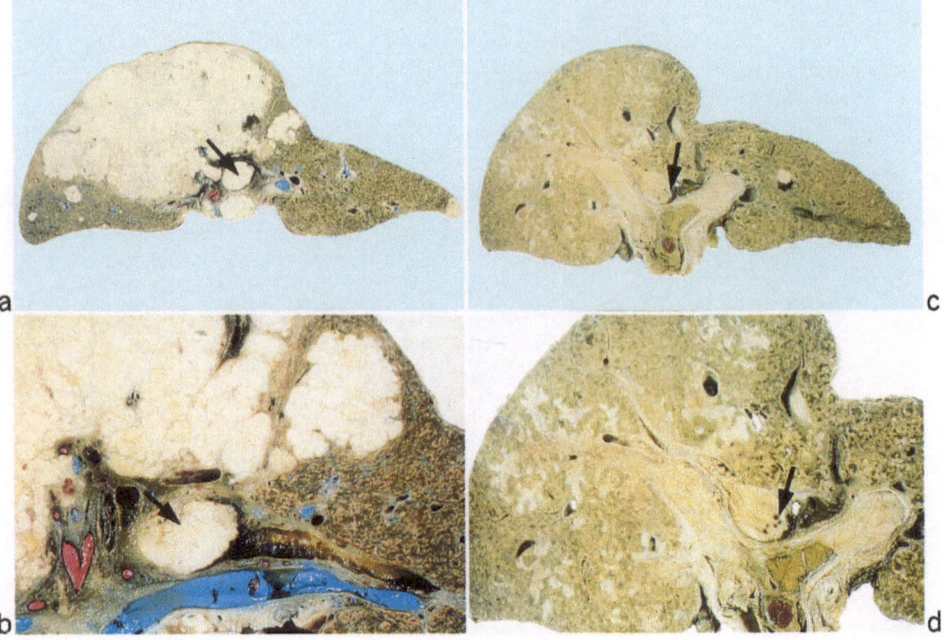

Fig. 8.2.a, b. Infiltrative HCC invading the bifurcation of the hepatic duct (*arrows*). **c, d** Tumor invasion at the bifurcation of the hepatic ducts from a massive tumor thrombus in the adjacent portal vein (*arrow*)

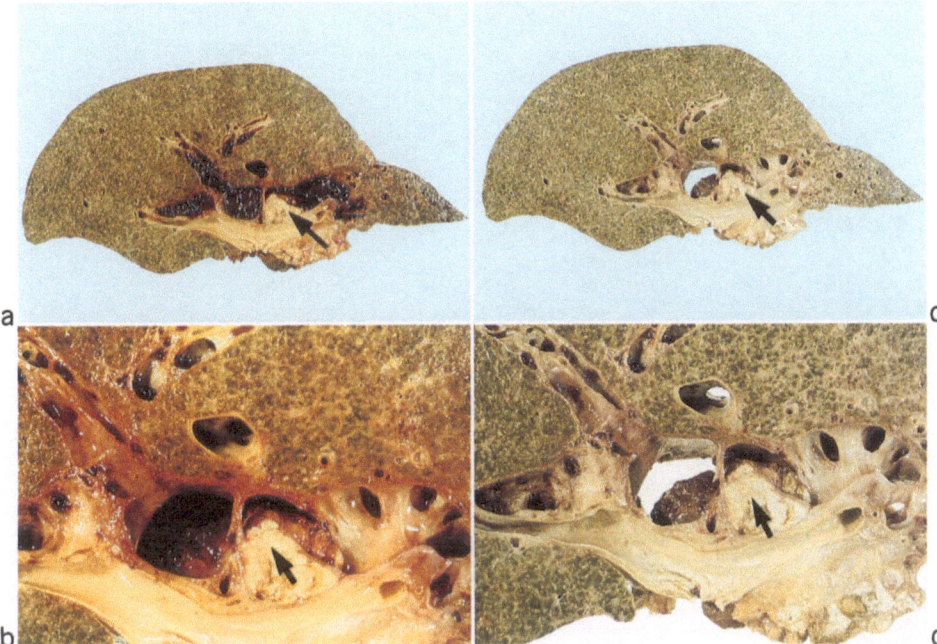

Fig. 8.3a–d. Hemobilia due to tumor growth in the bile ducts. A walnut-sized tumor growing at the bifurcation of the hepatic duct with massive hemorrhage into the dilated bile ducts (*arrows*). The main tumor is located behind this slice

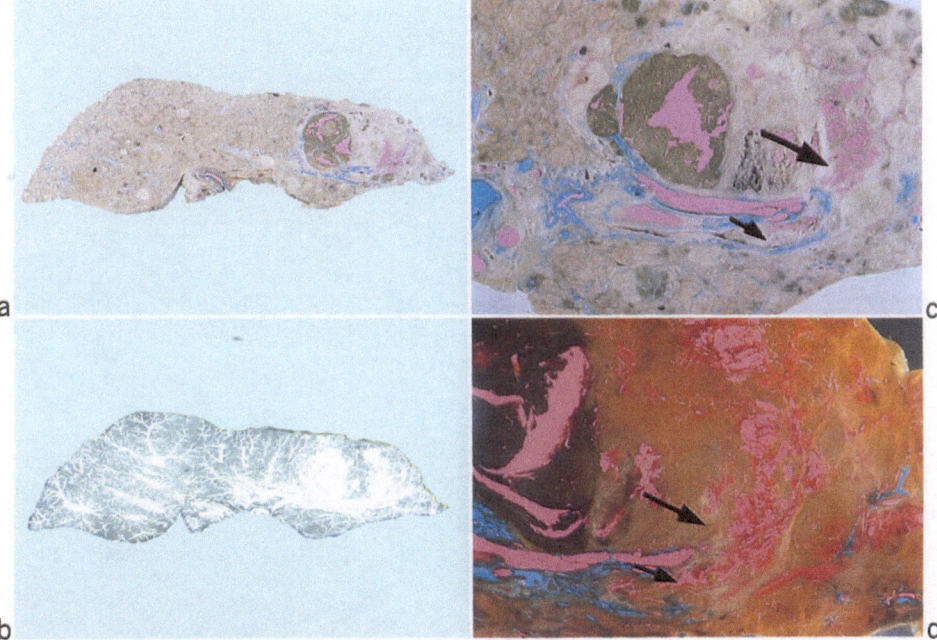

Fig. 8.4a–d. Angioarchitecture of a tumor cast in the bile duct. **a, b** The tumor casts in the portal vein and bile duct are hypervascular. **c, d** The arterial tumor vessels of the tumor cast in the bile duct (*short arrows*) are continuous with those of the tumor cast in the portal vein (*long arrows*)

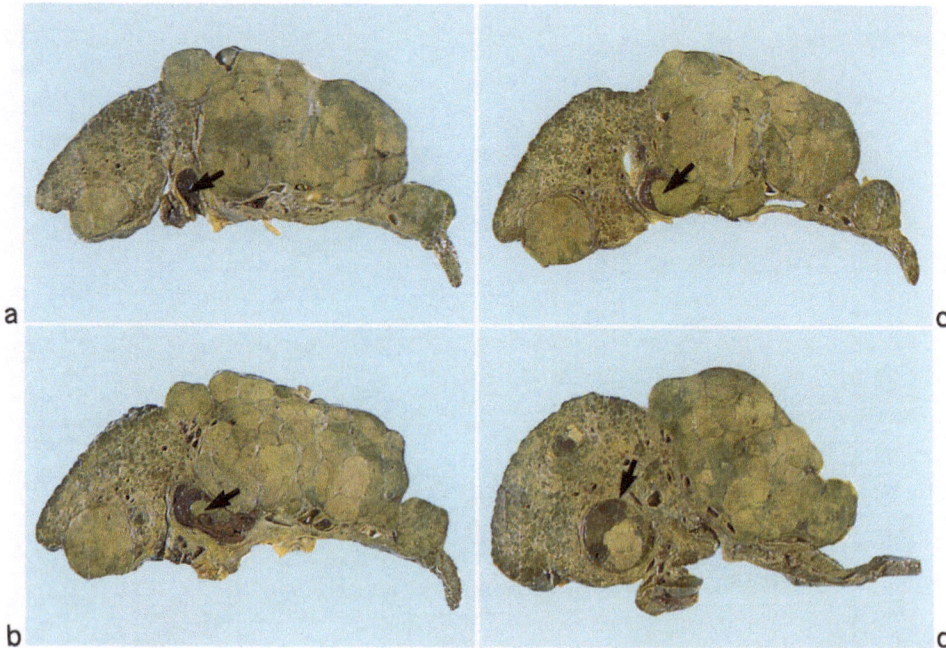

Fig. 8.5a–d. Massive tumor casts in the hepatic duct and the common bile duct (*arrows*). The diagnosis of HCC was made 2 years prior to death and the patient died of severe obstructive jaundice, due to the tumor growth in the bile ducts, which occurred shortly before death

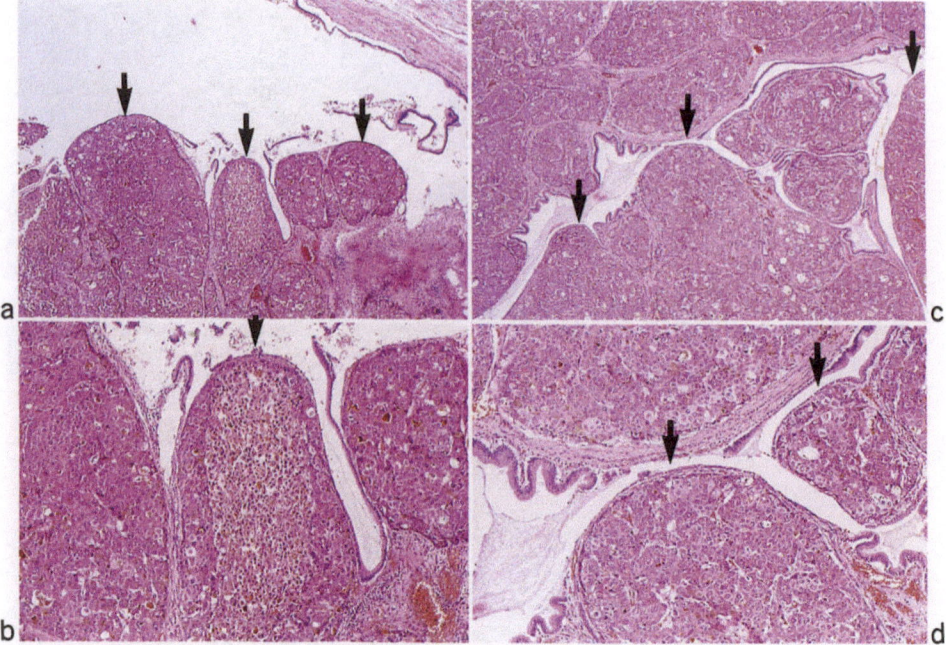

Fig. 8.6a–d. Tumor thrombi in the periductal portal veins protrude into the lumen of the bile duct, but bile duct epithelium covers the protruding tumor casts (*arrows*). HE; **a, c** × 20, **b, d** × 50

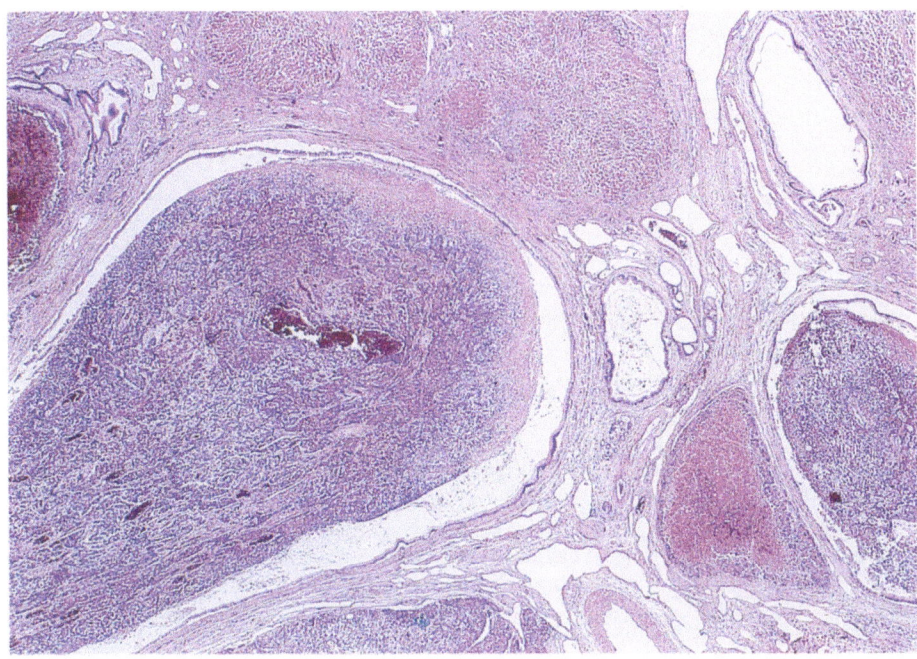

Fig. 8.7. Tumor cast in the bile duct with little necrosis. This finding suggests sufficient blood supply in the tumor cast. HE, × 20

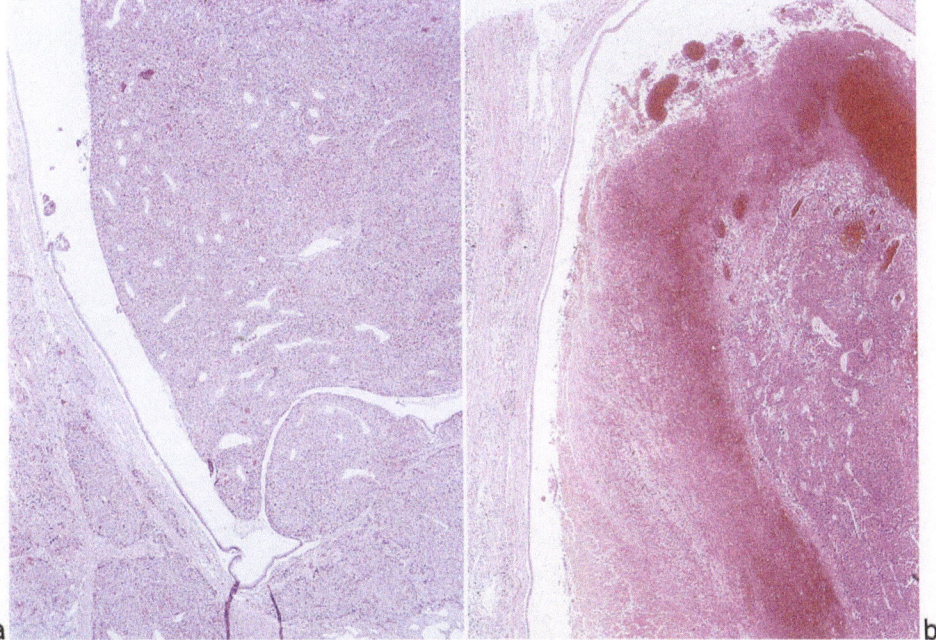

Fig. 8.8. a Tumor cast in the bile duct and protruded tumor thrombus in the periductal portal vein. **b** Tumor cast in the bile duct with hemorrhage. HE, × 20

Chapter 9
Extrahepatic Metastasis of Hepatocellular Carcinoma

Not a few reports have dealt with metastasis of HCC, drawing somewhat varying conclusions. In general, HCC has been known as a tumor which metastasizes outside the liver only at a rather late stage, despite the occurrence of widespread intrahepatic metastasis at a relatively early stage.

Kika [131], who undertook a statistical study of 110 cases of HCC, found extrahepatic metastasis in 62.0% of cases and stated that the HCC might have been spread hematogenously. Rates of 70.0% and 74.4% were reported by Mori [40] and Miyaji et al. [41], respectively. Extrahepatic metastases were evident in 63.3% of our present 439 cases of HCC. The reported rates range from 48% to 75% in Western countries [1, 9, 146–148] and a figure of 59% has been reported in South Africa [97].

According to Mori [40], who evaluated the correlation between associated liver cirrhosis and extrahepatic metastasis in HCC in 104 autopsy cases, hematogenous metastases were found in 46.1% of HCC cases without cirrhosis and in 56.2% of cases with liver cirrhosis. Thus, the rate of metastasis for HCC in cirrhotic liver is higher than that for HCC without cirrhosis. In contrast, Peters [66] reported that the rate of metastasis was higher in HCC without cirrhosis than in HCC with cirrhosis—67.0% and 46.2%, respectively. In our series of extrahepatic metastases in the cases with and without associated liver cirrhosis being 60.1% and 76.1%, respectively. The latter is significantly higher than the former ($P < 0.01$).

According to Mori [40], in Japanese patients with HCC, 52.8% of all metastases were hematogenous, commonly involving the lungs, adrenals, and bone, and 29.8% were lymphatic, commonly involving the hepatic hilar lymph nodes, periportal vein lymph nodes, retroperitoneal lymph nodes, and mediastinal lymph nodes. HCC has been known frequently to invade the portal and hepatic veins to metastasize to a variety of extrahepatic organs and tissues, as well as metastasizing within the liver. Hematogenous metastasis thus occurs more frequently than lymphatic metastasis. According to Miyaji et al. [41], hematogenous metastases were noted in 52.9% and lymphatic ones in 42.0% of cases involving metastasis, the former proportion being apparently higher than the latter. In our series, the corresponding figure for hematogenous metastasis was 48.7%, significantly higher than the figure for lymphatic metastasis (29.4%; $P < 0.01$). The proportion of infiltrative or disseminated metastasis was 23.3%. As described in Chap. 4, the incidence of extrahepatic metastasis is related to the histological growth pattern of HCC. Extrahepatic metastasis occurs earlier and more frequently in HCC of the sinusoidal type than in other kinds of HCC.

Hematogenous Metastasis

The lung is the most common site of hematogenous metastasis. In addition, the adrenals, bone, gastrointestinal tract, spleen, heart, and kidney may be involved.

It has been widely accepted that HCC may metastasize to tissues outside the liver in a selective manner. The mechanical factor has been mentioned as one of the reasons for this selectivity. It is beyond doubt that the mechanical factor is operative in the selective metastasis of HCC to the lung, but this factor alone is not sufficient to explain the selectivity. The "seed and soil" factor also operates to some degree [149, 150]: The microenvironment of the particular organ may be more or less suitable for the implantation and multiplication of tumor cells.

About 80% of HCC arise in a cirrhotic liver, suggesting that hematogenous metastasis may depend on intrahepatic and extrahepatic collateral circulation, resulting from advanced circulation disturbance in the portal and hepatic veins. In a cirrhotic liver, the portal bed is diminished markedly, occasionally to such a degree that the ratio of the arterial bed to the portal bed in the liver may be inverted. Shunt formation between the hepatic artery branches and the portal vein branches has also been demonstrated in cirrhotic livers. The resulting retrograde portal circulation through the shunt constitutes the major cause of portal hypertension. As HCC frequently occurs in a cirrhotic liver in which the blood circulation is markedly distorted in the way detailed above, hematogenous metastases of HCC may spread not only via the ordinary portal vein system, but also via other more complicated circulatory systems. According to Kika [131], two major routes, intrathoracic collateral circulation and visceroparietal collateral circulation, can be considered. Not all cancer cells which enter the circulation are necessarily implanted, and the majority of cancer cells (entering the circulation perish due to various factors such as mechanical barriers, immunological mechanisms, and biochemical mechanisms.

Lungs

Incidence. In our series, metastasis to the lung (Figs. 9.1–12) occurred in 46.0% of patients with HCC and accounted for 94.3% of all hematogenous metastases. The rates of pulmonary metastasis range from 43% to 46% among reports [9, 40, 41, 130, 147, 151–154]. Berman [151] reported that lung metastasis was found in 89% of cases with extrahepatic metastasis. Peters [66] stated that pulmonary metastasis was observed in 38.8% of cases with liver cirrhosis and 41.0% of cases without cirrhosis. In our series, the rates of pulmonary metastases were 45.2% and 48.8% with and without liver cirrhosis, respectively. The rates for HCC without associated liver cirrhosis were somewhat higher than those for HCC with liver cirrhosis, but the difference was not significant.

Among the 202 HCC cases with pulmonary metastasis in our series, 52.0% were grossly of the infiltrative type and 38.6% of the expansive type ($P < 0.05$).

Size and distribution of metastatic foci. No reports have given complete information on size and distribution of pulmonary metastases of HCC. MacDonald [130] stated that metastatic foci in the lung were generally small and located in the peripheral region. Tull [155] stated that the few foci which attained broad-bean size were largely found in the region close to the pleura. In our series, most metastatic foci were between 5 and 10 mm in diameter. In 28.9% of cases the foci were distributed densely in the lungs, in 38.0% moderately, and in 32.9% sparsely (Figs. 9.1, 2).

Macroscopic and histological features of metastatic foci. Most metastatic foci are gray-white, regardless of their size. Foci with marked necrosis have a yellowish gray-white hue. Depending on the degree of intrafocal bile production, the color changes from greenish gray-white to greenish (Figs. 9.1, 2, 11). Therefore, metastasis of HCC is grossly evident in some cases. In cases where the tumor tissue is rich in blood vessels (angiomatous type), the necrotic focus is red-brown.

HCC often consists of various histological types, and it is rather rare to encounter tumors which are histologically uniform. This also applies in pulmonary metastases. In our series, 53.3% of pulmonary metastases were exclusively trabecular in pattern. The solid and sclerotic patterns seldom occur alone. In 96.4% of pulmonary metastases which are histologically of mixed type, the trabecular pattern is dominant. The histological features of pulmonary metastases may be modified by the structure peculiar to the lung. A few examples of such lung-specific modifications are as follows.

Angiomatous appearance. The stroma of the primary foci consists mainly of blood spaces, but numerous dilated blood spaces stemming from alveolar capillaries, simulating hemangioma, are occasionally seen in pulmonary metastases. The angiomatous appearance is evidence that the metastatic foci are nourished by oxygen-rich blood from alveolar capillaries (Figs. 9.7, 8).

Sclerotic changes. The lung is an organ in which the lymphatics are highly developed. In cases in which tumor invasion extends to the lymphatic vessels, the histological features may vary markedly. Because the superficial lymphatics form a network in the subpleural tissue, sclerotic areas with abundant connective tissue, which result from carcinomatous lymphangitis, are often seen in pulmonary metastatic foci. As part of the pulmonary lymphatics run along the bronchus or pulmonary artery to the hilus, a tumor thrombus of the pulmonary artery may induce carcinomatous lymphangitis by damaging the vascular wall. In such a case, the cancer cells proliferate in infiltrating fashion into the tissues, occasionally producing cancer foci of sclerotic HCC characterized by the presence of abundant stromal connective tissue around the blood vessels (Fig. 9.10c, d).

Necrotic changes. In occasional cases, all the pulmonary metastatic foci are found to be completely necrotic. Additional hemorrhage is also noted. These metastatic foci are all thickly covered with connective tissue. Most of them are located on the surface of the lung.

Clinical signs. Only in two of our cases, involving metastatic tumors larger than 20 mm in diameter, were respiratory symptoms the first manifestation of HCC. In one of the two patients, with a single large metastatic focus, the first clinical sign was the development of a cough and production of sputum. In the other case, the metastatic tumor, which had an angiomatous appearance, penetrated into the bronchus to produce a mass in the bronchial lumen, and subsequent rupture of blood vessels led to the initial clinical sign of hemosputum (Fig. 9.5, 6). HCC first manifested by hemosputum is relatively seldom. In 1951, Berman [1] described a rare case with pulmonary metastasis manifested by hemosputum as an initial sign. Okuda [156] in 1976 reported one case of HCC in which hemoptysis was the major sign.

Adrenals

The incidence of adrenal metastasis (Figs. 9.13–16) is low, but they occupy second place after pulmonary metastasis. The incidence of adrenal metastasis varies markedly among reports, ranging from 1.2% to 21% [9, 40, 41, 128, 130, 131, 152, 157, 158] In our series, the rate although including cancer infiltration of the adrenal capsule, is 8.8%.

Smith [158] reported that 4 of 25 cases with adrenal metastasis in his series involved the right adrenal. Meyer [152] found adrenal metastasis in 3 of 75 cases of HCC; two involved the right adrenal and one the left adrenal. Our series includes a total of 34 cases of adrenal metastasis. Of these 34 cases, in 17 (50%) the metastatic foci were in the right adrenal, in seven (20.5%) they were in the left adrenal, and in ten (29.4%) they were bilateral. The rate of metastasis to the right adrenal is significantly higher than that to the left adrenal. Adrenal metastasis occurs in 7.6% and 13.6% of HCC cases with and without associated liver cirrhosis, respectively.

The adrenal metastatic foci in our series are predominantly gray-white in color. None of them have the greenish hue which suggests bile production. Histologically, 46.6% of adrenal metastatic foci display the trabecular pattern and 33.3% are of the free-cell type. the free-cell type is thus more frequent in adrenal metastasis than in pulmonary metastasis ($P < 0.01$).

Bone

Bone metastases of HCC (Figs. 9.17–20) are believed mostly to result from hematogenous spread. Edmondson [10] mentioned vertebral involvement as the most common form, possibly due to retrograde circulation from the portal vein to the vertebral vein. Metastases to the bone other than the vertebrae may include those by way of the pulmonary or systemic circulation or due to direct expansion from metastatic foci in adjacent organs or tissues.

The incidence of bone metastasis also varies markedly among reports, ranging from 3.0% to 16.4% [9, 40, 128, 130, 131]. In our series, it is 5.2%. Goveia and Bahn [159] stated that in general, malignant tumors tend to metastasize more often to the bones with active marrow, such as the ribs, sternum, vertebrae, pelvis, skull, and the proximal end of the femur. In cases of HCC, metastases to the vertebra and sternum are particularly prominent. Of 71 cases with metastases to the bone in our present series, 46.3% involve metastasis to the vertebrae, 29.5% to the ribs, and 14.0% to the sternum. All of these bones contain active marrow and are vulnerable due to their position. The bone metastasis of highest incidence is that to the vertebrae, which are subjected to the burden of body weight.

Macroscopic and histological features. Berman [1] reported that bile production was found in some metastatic foci in the bone. Of his 23 cases with bone metastases, 16 could be examined histologically, and bile production was demonstrated in four of them. In one of our cases, at autopsy, metastatic foci of the thoracic vertebra had a green hue, which was imparted by focal bile production (Fig. 9.17a). Histologically, as also seen in metastatic foci in organs other than bone, the trabecular pattern of HCC is dominant (77.7%). This is higher than the corresponding rates for other sites, e.g., pulmonary and adrenal metastases, (53.3% and 46.6%, respectively), but the difference is not significant. Metastatic lesions in the bone have been believed to be osteolytic, as evaluated by X-ray film and histologically. All the bone metastases in our series were found to be osteolytic on X-ray (Fig. 9.17). In one case of metastasis to the lumbar vertebra, both osteoblasts and osteoclasts were observed in the metastatic foci, indicating absorption of the bone. The appearance of osteoclasts in bone metastasis suggesting bone absorption could be related directly to the bone metastasis.

Clinical features. HCC was first manifested by the development of symptoms attributable to bone metastasis in 39.1% of the patients with bone metastasis in our HCC series, representing 2.0% of the whole series. The major symptoms include pain and the formation of bone tumor. Chest pain, hypochondriac pain, and back pain are common. Occasionally the metastasis causes neurological disorders. In one such case, HCC first metastasized to the cervical vertebra and the tumor then extended to the adjacent tissues, resulting in paralysis of cranial nerves VII and XII [160, 161]. Metastases to the vertebrae were found in as many as 14 (60.8%) of 23 cases with bone metastasis. Of these 14 patients, 6 had symptoms of section of the spinal cord.

Gastrointestinal tract

Metastasis to the gastrointestinal tract (Figs. 9.21–24) is relatively rare and has been reported only sporadically [162–165]. Gastrointestinal tract metastases were found in 30 cases (6.8%) in our series, consisting of 17 cases of hematogenous metastasis, three cases of possible lymphatic metastasis, nine cases of infiltration or dissemination, and one case in which the route was unknown. In the study by Mori [40], the incidence of hematogenous metastasis to the esophagus, stomach, and duodenum was 0.9%, 3.8%, and 0.9%, respectively. Miyaji et al. [41] reported that metastasis to the stomach was found in 5.5% of cases. In our series, metastasis to the stomach was found in 14 cases (3.1%), of which eight were hematogenous. Tumor thrombus of the portal vein is assumed in all eight cases.

The incidence of duodenal metastasis is lower. Only a small number of cases with duodenal metastasis were reported by Kimura et al. [166] and Wada et al. [167]. Our series includes three cases, in all of which direct infiltration from metastatic foci of the peripancreatic lymph nodes and/or disseminated metastasis from the primary tumor are assumed.

Pancreas

Metastasis to the pancreas (Figs. 9.25–28) is also rather infrequent, the incidence ranging from 3% to 4.8% among reports [1, 40, 41, 128, 148]. In our series, pancreatic metastasis was seen in 30 cases (6.8%). In 16 (3.6%) of these cases metastasis was due to retrograde circulation through the portal vein, in seven (1.5%) it was the result of extension from lymphatic metastases, and in seven (1.5%) it possibly resulted from direct infiltration and/or disseminated metastasis from the primary focus.

Peters [66] evaluated the relationship between associated liver cirrhosis and pancreatic metastasis and reported that pancreatic metastasis occurred in none of his HCC cases without cirrhosis and in 1.1% of those with liver cirrhosis. In our 16 cases of hematogenous pancreatic metastasis, associated liver cirrhosis was present in two instances (3.2%) and absent in 14 (3.9%) in our series. The rates do not differ significantly.

Hematogenous metastasis to the pancreas is mediated mainly by way of retrograde circulation through the portal vein with the tumor thrombus. Macroscopically, intrapancreatic metastases are widespread diffuse lesions. A pancreatic vein is filled with tumor thrombus and dilated. Tumor invasion extends outside the vein infiltratively to the pancreatic tissues. Histologically, the lesions are mainly of the trabecular or the pseudoglandular type. Of nine cases examined in our series, four are trabecular and three are pseudoglandular. On the other hand, in cases where the pancreatic foci are due to direct invasion by lymphatic metastatic foci, macroscopically enlarged lymph nodes replace the pancreatic tissue and histologically the capsule of the pancreas is destroyed by the cancer, which grows in an infiltrative fashion. Most such foci are of the free-cell type.

Gallbladder

The incidence of metastasis to the gallbladder (Figs. 9.29–32) in Japanese patients with HCC was reported as 5.7% and 7.2% by Mori [40] and Miyaji et al. [41], respectively. It is 4.3% in our series. In the cases where histological determination was possible, metastasis was principally by the hematogenous route via the portal vein. In such cases, the tumor thrombus shows a trabecular pattern, but the extravascular infiltrative foci tend to be of the sclerotic type, characterized by the presence of abundant fibrous stroma, and the cancer cells are histologically similar to those of the free-cell type.

Occasionally, HCC invasion extends directly into the wall of the gallbladder from the fossa vesicae felleae, forming a tumor in the lumen. Histological examination, however, reveals that a tumor thrombus of the intrahepatic portal vein has extended in a retrograde fashion into a vein in the wall of the gallbladder and further extension, destroying the mucous membrane of the gallbladder, has resulted in a mass in the cavity. Hematogenous metastasis through the portal vein may thus be the principal cause of extrahepatic foci in the gallbladder, even if the foci seem grossly to result from direct invasion of HCC into the wall of the gallbladder.

Heart

Malignant tumors may metastasize to the myocardium via the coronary arteries in a hematogenous fashion. In addition, metastasis to the heart may involve several other processes, such as metastasis through the inferior vena cava to the myocardium, direct invasion of the pericardium, as seen in the case of carcinoma of intrathoracic organs (direct infiltration), and retrograde superficial lymphangitis through the mediastinal lymphatics or the paratracheal and peribronchial lymphatics.

The incidence of cardiac metastasis from HCC (Figs. 9.33, 34) ranges from 0% to 2.8% among reports [40, 130, 168]. Although MacDonald [130] found cardiac metastasis in 2 of 84 cases of HCC, these were intra-atrial extensions of the tumor thrombus into the inferior vena cava. We eliminated intra-atrial tumor extension through the inferior vena cava from cardiac metastases. Cardiac metastasis is seen in 11 (2.5%) of 439 cases in our series. The sites of metastasis are the endocardium in two cases, myocardium in two cases, pericardium in six cases, and both myocardium and pericardium in one case. Peters [66] evaluated the correlation between associated liver cirrhosis and cardiac metastasis and reported that cardiac metastasis occurred in 1.6% and 3.6% of HCC cases with and without liver cirrhosis, respectively. The rates are, respectively, 2.5% and 2.2% in our series; the difference is not significant. Intramyocardial metastases appear as firm nodules, but may also be of sarcomatous appearance or of the free-cell type, as well as trabecular.

Kidney

The incidence of renal metastasis (Figs. 9.35, 36) varies markedly among reports [40, 41, 130, 152, 155, 157], ranging from 0% to 7.4%. Edmondson and Steiner [9] and Peters found no renal metastasis in their series (90 and 223 cases, respectively). It is 1.1% in our series, with all cases considered as hematogenous.

Spleen

In Japan, the rate of metastasis of HCC to the spleen (Figs. 9.37–39) has been reported as 4.8% by Mori [40] and 4.7% by Miyaji et al. [41]. It is 2.2% in our series. According to Peters [66], the metastatic rate varied depending on the presence or absence of liver cirrhosis—7.7% without and 2.1% with liver cirrhosis. In our series, however, the two rates are the same at 2.2%. Besides retrograde hematogenous metastasis through the portal vein, metastasis may occur via the systemic circulation through the splenic artery or by dissemination [169]. In contrast to metastasis to the splenic parenchyma, metastatic foci in the splenic capsule are characterized by the free-cell type, lacking formation of tumor nests, and by abundant stromal connective tissue, possibly due to the infiltrative proliferation in the tissues and the remarkable proliferation of stromal connective tissues.

Thyroid

Metastasis to the thyroid gland was not found in most of the published studies of HCC. Kika [131], Mori [40], and MacDonald [130] found no cases of metastasis to the thyroid among their 79, 104, and 84, respectively, HCC cases. According to Edmondson and Steiner [9], the first case was reported by Rosenblatt and the second case was his own. It is seen only in one case in our series (Fig. 9.40).

Ovary

Metastasis of HCC to the ovary also occurs very seldom. Two instances were found among our 439 cases.

Lymphatic Metastasis

There is little noteworthy description of lymphatic metastasis in the literature, possibly because the overwhelming majority of extrahepatic metastases are hematogenous.

Frequency
In our series, the lymph nodes around the pancreas are the most common site of lymphatic metastasis (15.2%) followed by the nodes of the hepatic hilum (14.3%). The reported incidence of metastasis to the hepatic hilar lymph nodes ranges from 11.1% to 38.8% [10, 40, 41, 128, 131, 152, 170].

In our series (Figs. 9.41–48), lymphatic metastases are seen in 35.1% of cases of infiltrative HCC and in 20.4% of cases of expansive HCC (29.3% overall). Massive tumors resembling malignant lymphoma have been encountered in as many as 32 of the total of 129 cases.

Lymph nodes are involved in 39.7% of HCC cases without liver cirrhosis, while the rate is 26.7% in cases with associated liver cirrhosis. Lymphatic metastasis thus tends to favor HCC without liver cirrhosis ($P < 0.025$).

Histological features
Lymphatic metastatic foci are histologically of the trabecular type in 29.1%, the pseudoglandular type in 4.1%, the solid type in 0%, the sclerosing type in 1.3%, the free-cell type in 16.3%, the sacromatous type in 2.7%, and a mixture of these histological types in 53.5%.

Massive lymph-node metastasis resembling malignant lymphoma
Of the 439 cases of HCC in our series, 32 involved lymph node metastasis so massive as to lead to erroneous diagnosis of malignant lymphoma (Figs. 9.41, 42).

Kawabata [171] studied the clinical features, autopsy findings, and focal distribution of alpha-fetoprotein and albumin-positive cells in such massive lymph node metastases. According to his study, histologically the tumor tissue can be classified into the islet-cell type and the free-cell type. The former is characterized by the presence of cancer cells which proliferate to form a tumor nest and the latter by cells which are poorly adhesive and proliferate in a diffuse fashion without forming any distinct tumor nest. Such massive metastases are found in 19 of our 32 cases. Eleven cases (57.8%) were of the islet-cell type and eight (42.1%) of the free-cell type. In the remaining 13 cases, the lymph nodes were moderately enlarged. In 170 cases of HCC in which primary foci could be histologically examined, primary foci of the islet-cell type were found in 154 cases, foci of the free-cell type in 11 cases, and in five cases the two patterns were mixed. The free-cell type is more frequent in massive lymph node metastases than in primary foci, indicating that tumor tissues are considerably modified in the lymph node. Such massive tumors replace the entire lymph node in many cases. Massive lymph node metastases of the islet-cell type have primary foci of similar type in many instances. Free-cell type HCC may correspond to the "HCC in which tumor proliferates infiltratively in a diffuse fashion within a lymph node" described by Edmondson and Steiner [10]. The occurrence of the free-cell type may be attributed to the poor adhesiveness and the mobility of the cancer cells, although environmental factors cannot be excluded.

Metastatic routes
Before studying lymphatic metastasis of HCC, it is necessary to understand the circulation of lymph in the liver. The lymph vessels in the liver can be classified roughly into the superficial group in the hepatic capsule and the deep group inside the liver. Most vessels of both groups drain into the intra-abdominal lymphatics. The superficial lymphatics of the left hepatic lobe and part of the deep lymphatics of both lobes communicate with intrathoracic lymphatics across the diaphragm. This communication may be responsible for metastasis to the hilar, paratracheal, and mediastinal lymph nodes [172–174]. A network of intrahepatic lymphatics become entangled with the walls of the portal vein and the hepatic vein. As the formation of tumor thrombus of the portal vein or the hepatic vein is characteristically early in HCC, HCC may have a predilection for affecting the walls of blood vessels and then penetrating into the lymph circulation. As lymphatic metastasis occurs rather infrequently, however, portal vein tumor thrombus does not necessarily affect the lymphatics. Saitsu et al. [175] demonstrated the lymphatics connecting a tumor nodule in the liver and an abdominal lymph node by means of percutaneous injection of contrast medium (Lipiodol) into the hepatic tumor. They demonstrated lymph vessels extending from the tumor nodule to the abdominal lymph nodes immediately after the injection of Lipiodol in three cases of HCC and stagnant collections of Lipiodol in the abdominal lymph nodes by subsequent plain films of the abodmen and by abdominal computed tomography. Saitsu et al. also found many large and small fat droplets in the lymph nodes removed at partial hepatectomy or autopsy in the histological examination.

Retrograde hematogenous metastasis through a tumor thrombus of the portal vein and evidence supporting such metastasis have been found unexpectedly in many cases involving extrahepatic metastasis. This suggests that retrograde hematogenous metastasis of HCC to lymph nodes, in particular to nodes in the hepatic hilum, may be much more common than has been thought.

Disseminated Metastasis

Disseminated metastasis seems to occur at a rather late stage in HCC and may affect any part of the peritoneum, as may be expected from the position of the liver.

Diaphragm
Berman [1] and Orsos [176] described bile-stained metastatic foci in the diaphragm. Mori [40] and Miyaji et al. [41] reported the frequency of metastasis to the diaphragm in HCC to be 12.5% and 6.9%, respectively. In our series (Figs. 9.49, 50), it was seen in 14.7% of HCC with associated liver cirrhosis and 8.8% of HCC without cirrhosis.

Douglas' cavity
Metastasis to Douglas' cavity in HCC was reported to be 10.5% by Mori [40]. In our series (Figs. 9.51, 52), it was seen in 6.6% of cases.

Peritoneum, omentum
As metastases in the capsules of spleen and pancreas, serosa of gallbladder were
counted as metastases of the respective organ in our series, our figure for metastasis
to the peritoneum and omentum is lower (3.8%) than the 14.5% of Mori [40], the
5.6% of Meyer [152] the 6.1% of Miyaji et al. [41], and the 11.1% of Edmondson
and Steiner [9].

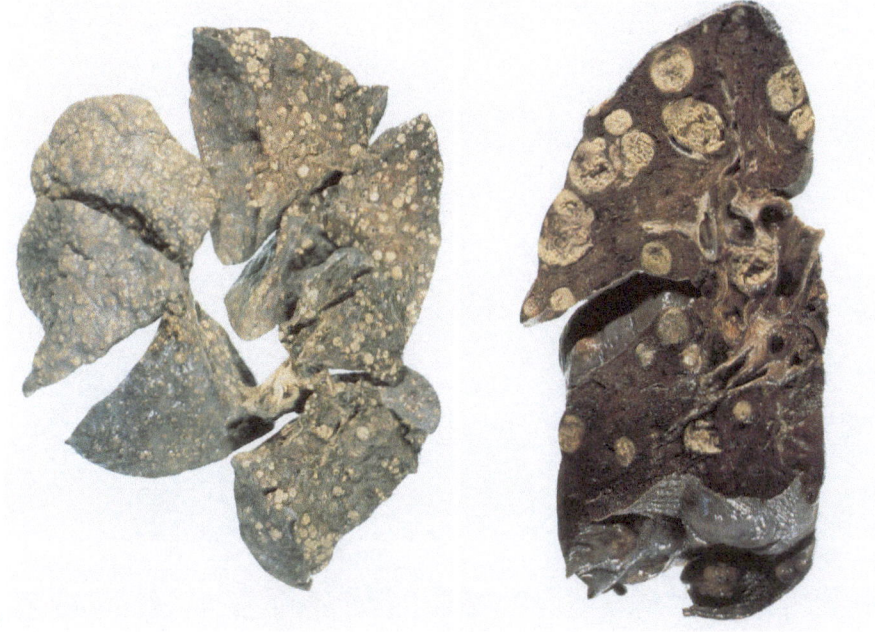

a   b

Fig. 9.1a, b. Metastasis to lung. **a** Numerous metastatic nodules ranging from 2 to 5 mm in diameter diffusely distributed throughout lung. **b** Well-demarcated metastatic nodules, 10–20 mm in diameter, are seen in the upper and lower lobes

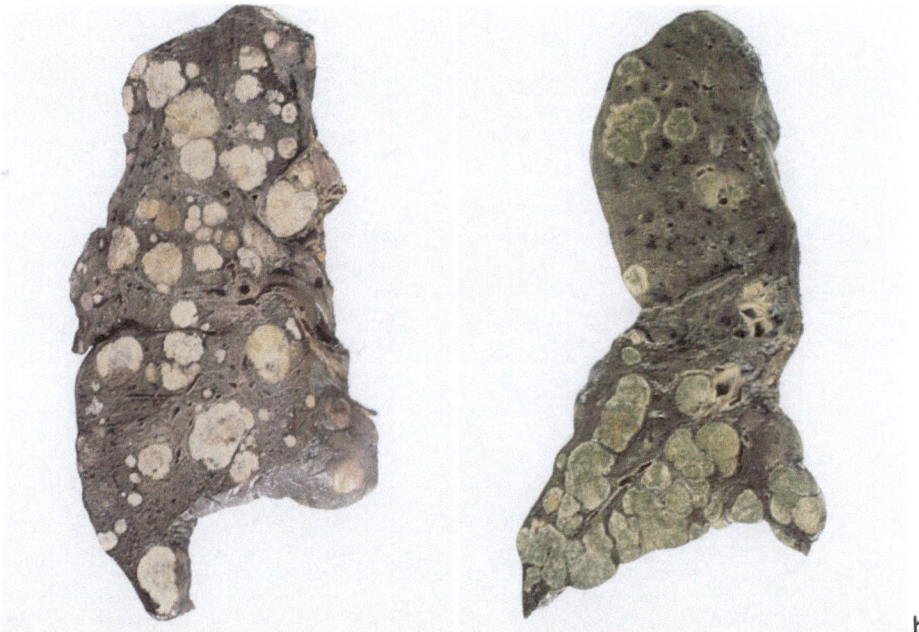

a   b

Fig. 9.2a, b. Metastasis to lung. **a** Varying sized metastatic nodules in lung. **b** Metastatic nodules with prominent bile production.

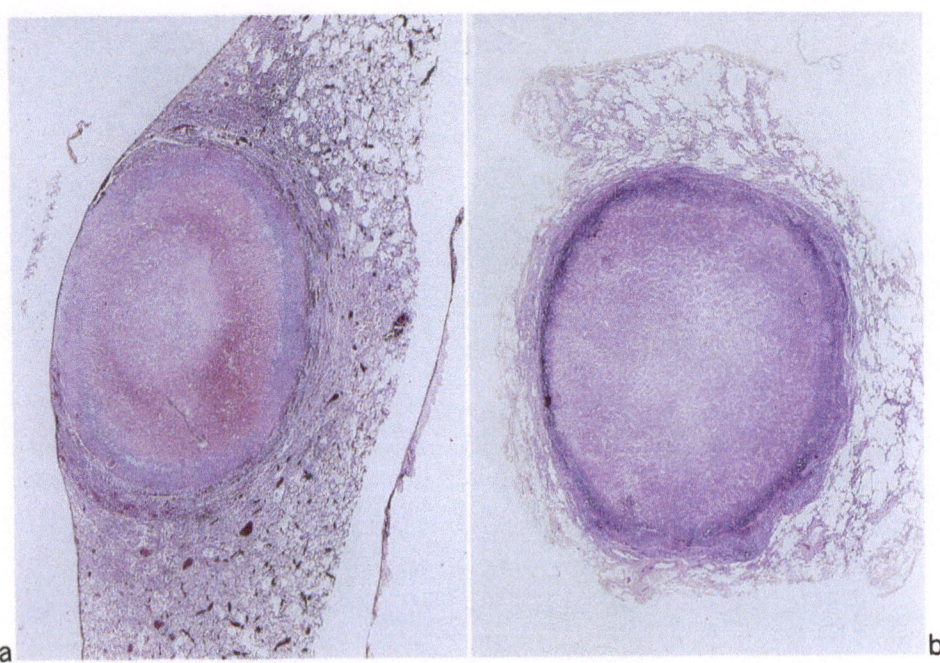

Fig. 9.3a, b. Metastasis to lung. Necrotized metastatic nodule. HE, × 1

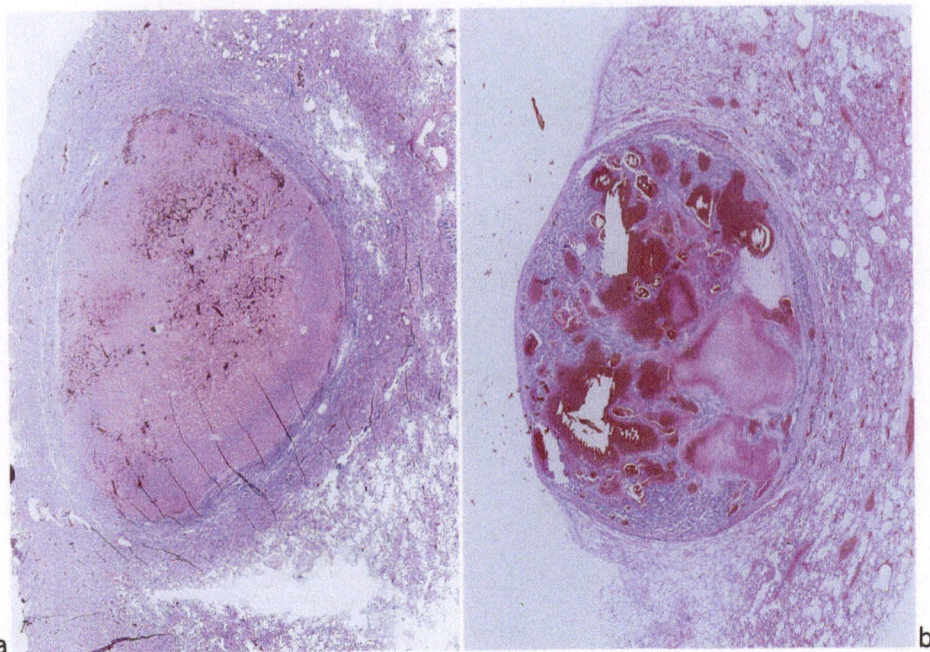

Fig. 9.4a, b. Metastasis to lung. Well-demarcated metastatic nodule with prominent hemorrhage and necrosis. HE, × 1

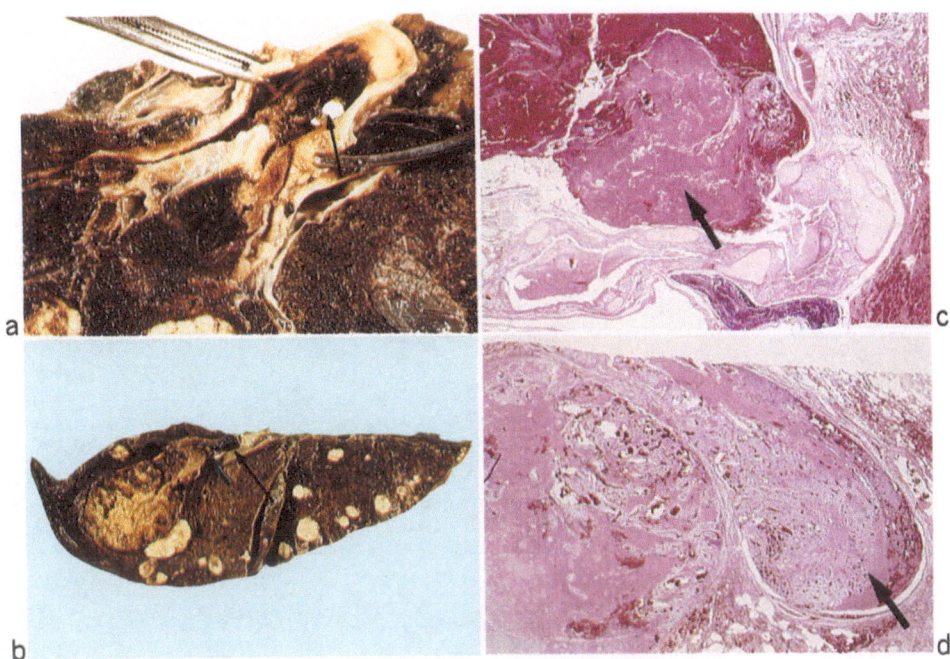

Fig. 9.5a–d. Metastasis to lung. Case with hemosputum as an initial sign. **a, b** The bronchus is filled with blood clot and tumor is seen in the bronchial wall (*arrows*). **c** Necrotized tumor in the bronchus (*arrow*). **d** Proliferating tumor in the bronchus (*arrow*). **c, d** HE stain, × 10

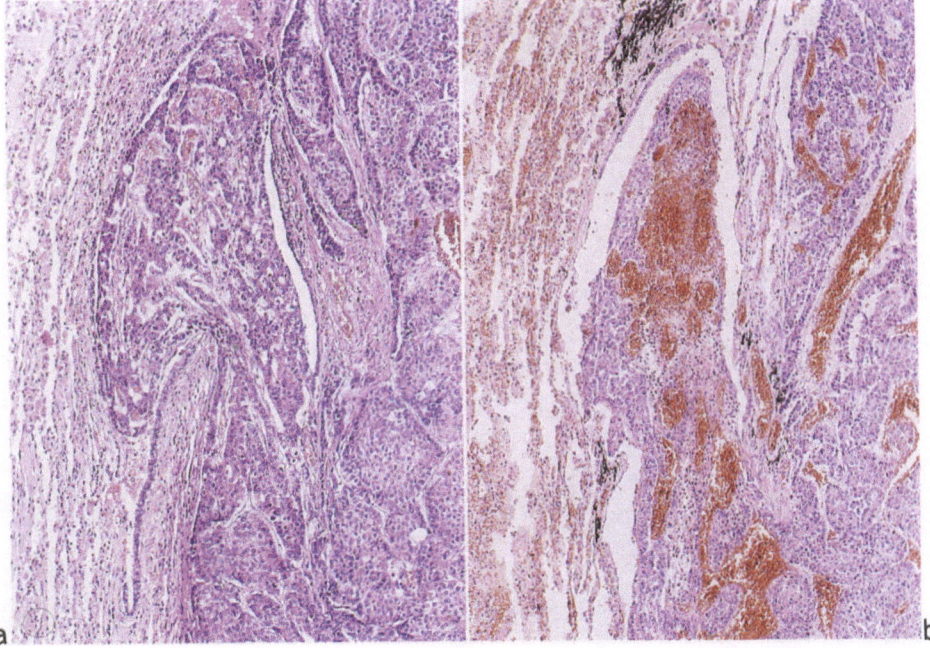

Fig. 9.6a, b. Metastasis to lung. Proliferating tumor in the bronchus. **a** Trabecular HCC with bile production in the bronchus. **b** Trabecular HCC with angiomatous appearance due to marked dilation of blood spaces. HE, × 50

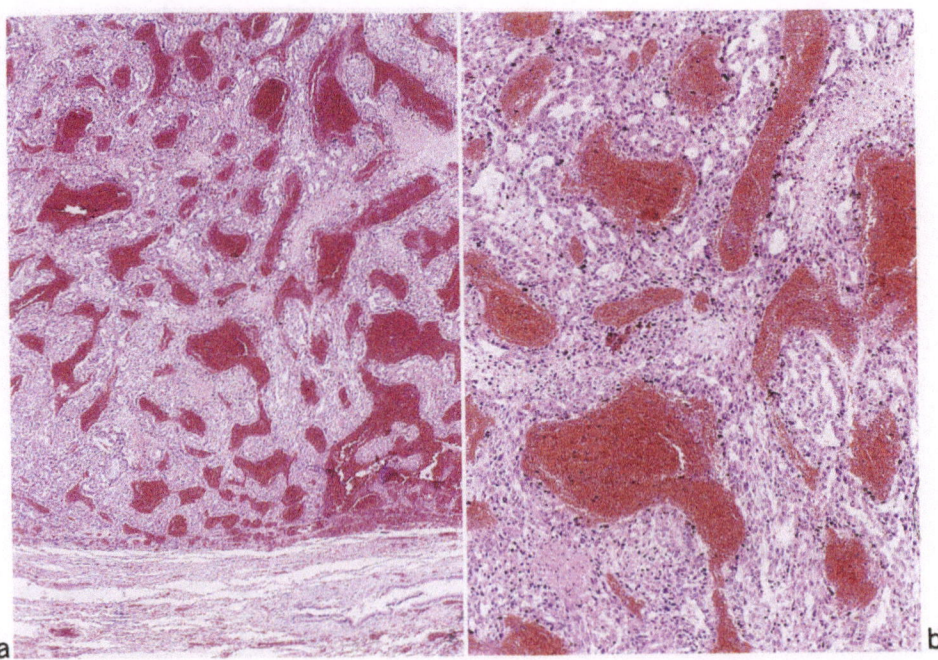

a   b

Fig. 9.7a, b. Metastasis to lung. Trabecular HCC showing angiomatous appearance due to marked dilation of blood spaces. HE; **a** × 20, **b** × 50

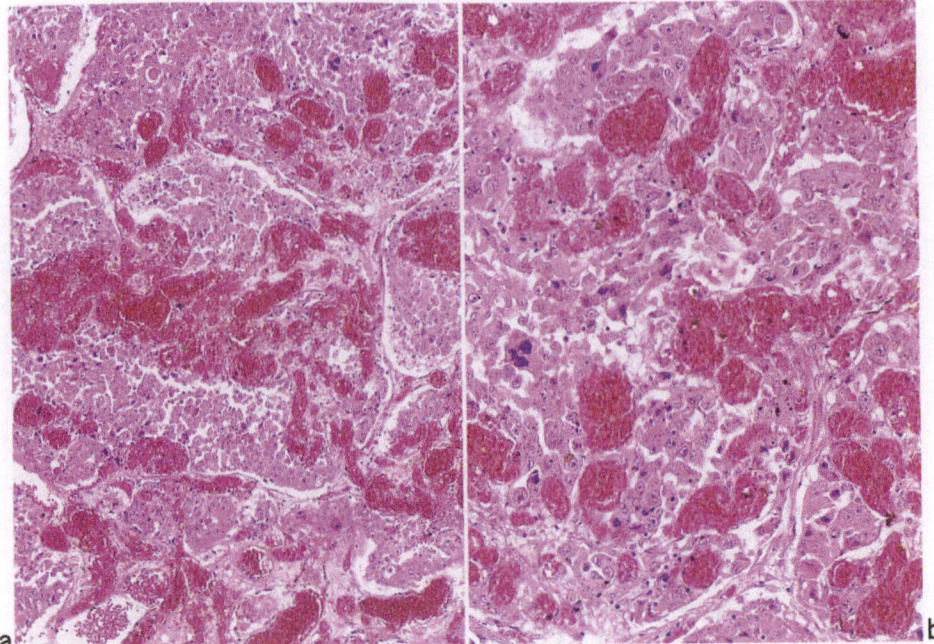

a   b

Fig. 9.8a, b. Metastasis to lung. Free-cell type HCC. The tumor receives the arterial tumor vessels from the dilated arteries in the alveoli. HE; **a** × 50, **b** × 100

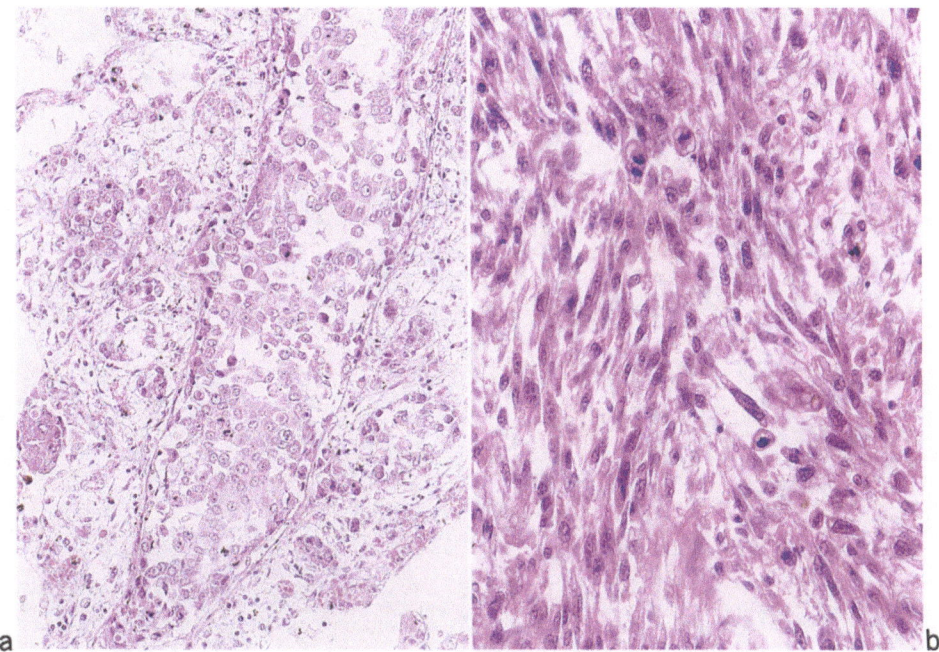

Fig. 9.9a, b. Metastasis to lung. **a** Free-cell type HCC. Tumor cells infiltrating into the lymphatic vessels. **b** A metastatic focus in the pleura showing sarcomatous features. HE; **a** × 100, **b** × 200

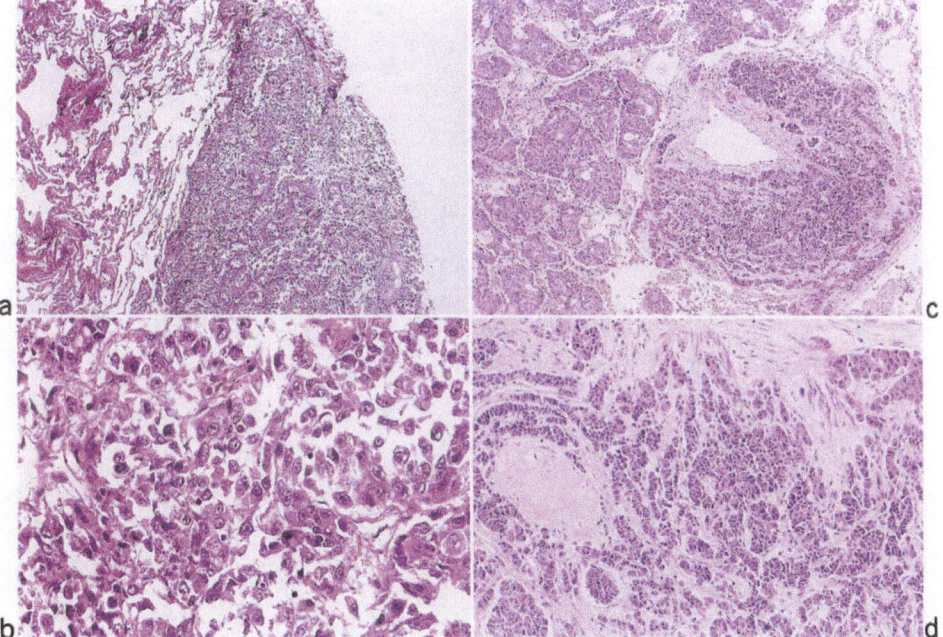

Fig. 9.10a–d. Metastasis to lung. Subpleural metastasis of free-cell type HCC. HE; **a** × 20, **b** × 100, **c** × 20, **d** × 50

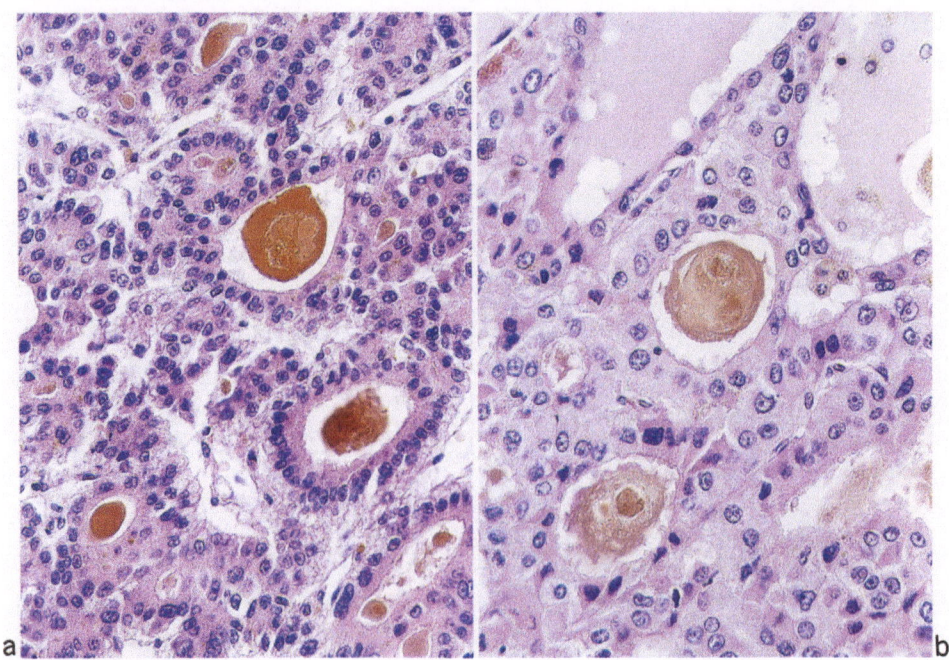

Fig. 9.11a, b. Metastasis to lung. Prominent bile production in metastatic HCC of the pseudo-glandular type. HE, × 200

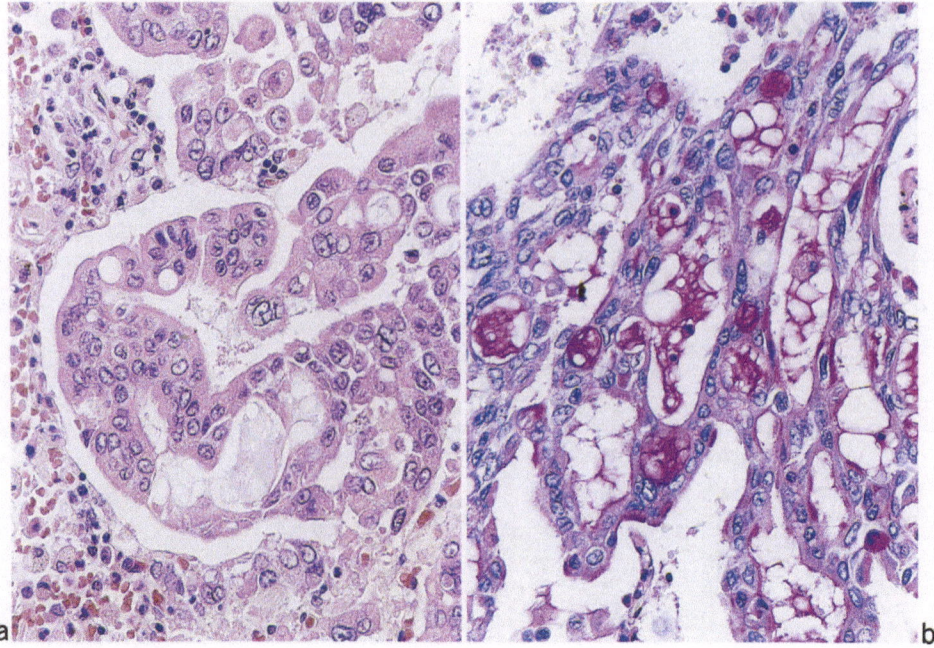

Fig. 9.12a, b. Metastasis to lung. **a** Mucin-like substances in metastatic HCC of the pseudoglandular type. HE, × 200. **b** The mucin-like substances are PAS-positive. PAS, × 200

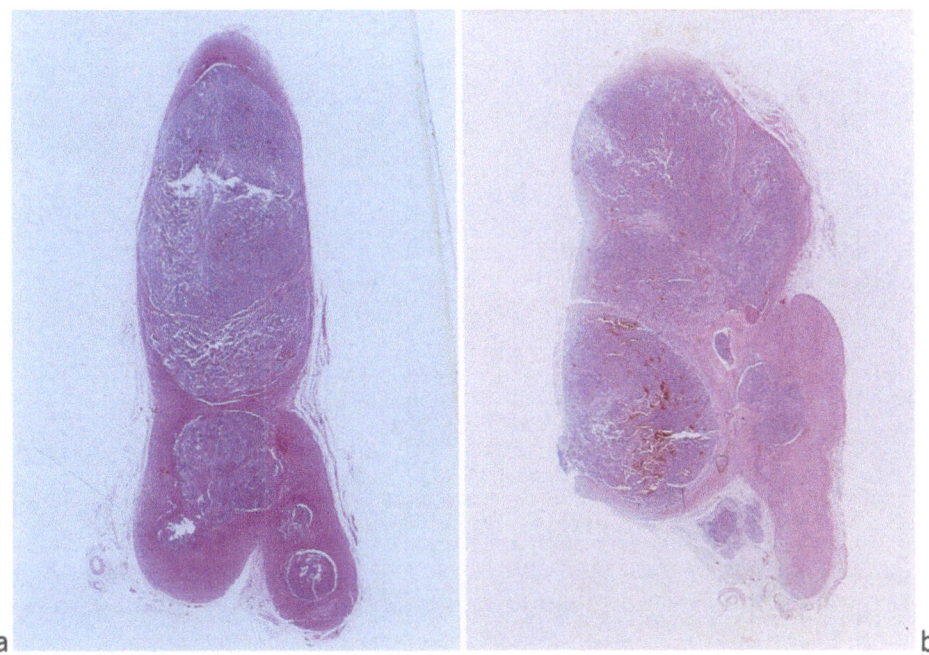

Fig. 9.13a, b. Bilateral metastasis to adrenal glands. **a** Left adrenal; **b** Right adrenal. HE, × 1

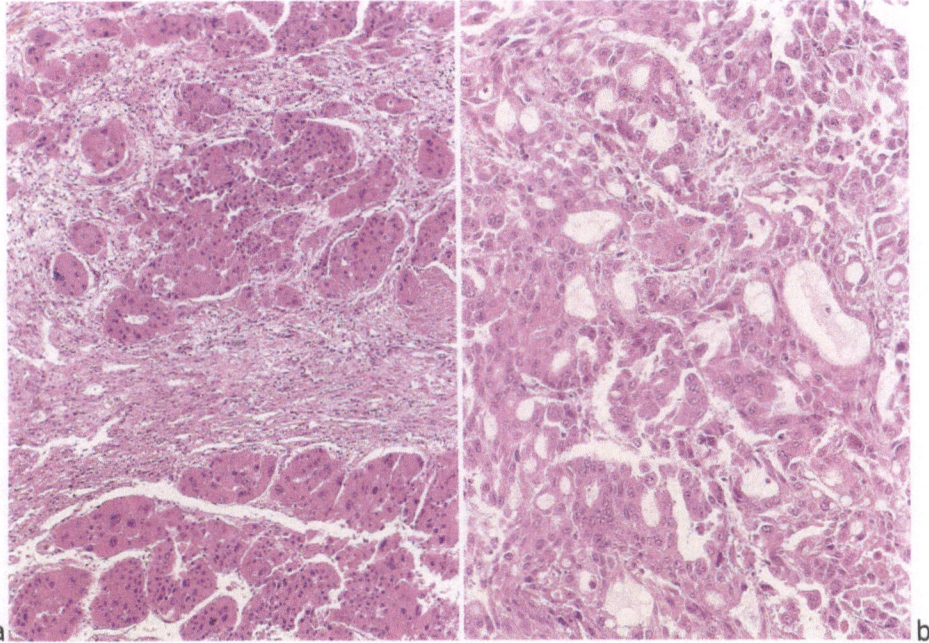

Fig. 9.14a, b. Metastasis to adrenal glands. **a** Trabecular HCC in the adrenal cortex. **b** Pseudo-glandular HCC. HE; **a** × 50, **b** × 100

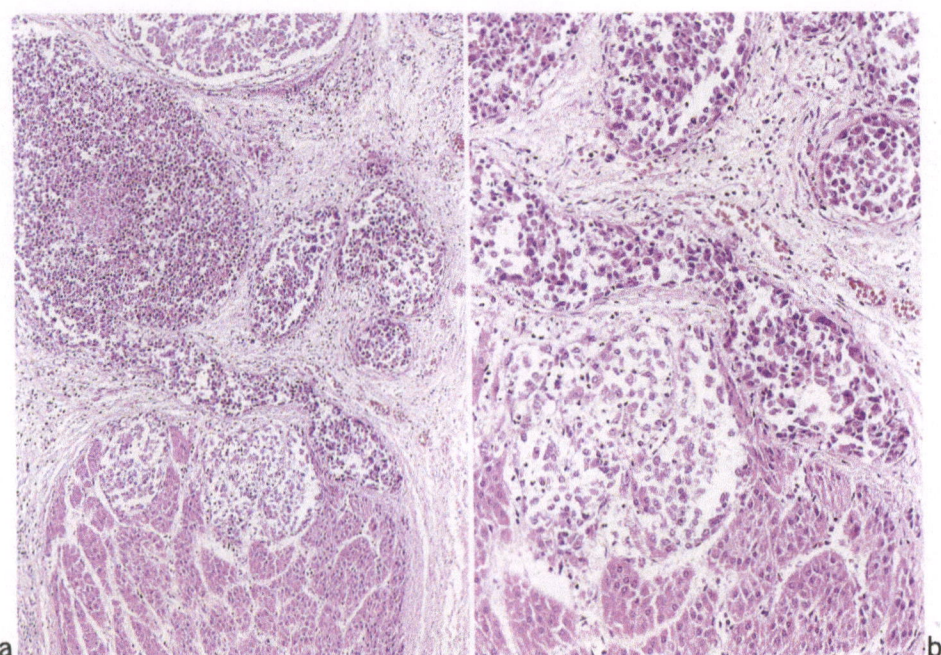

Fig. 9.15a, b. Metastasis to adrenal glands. Free-cell type HCC HE; **a** × 20, **b** × 100

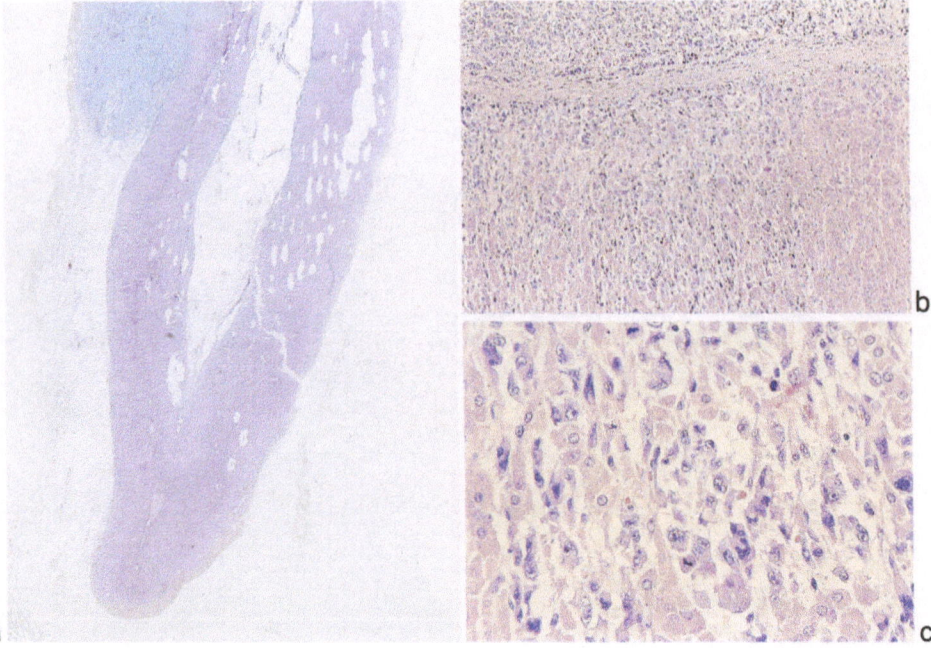

Fig. 9.16a–c. Metastasis to adrenal glands. Free-cell type HCC in the capsule is proliferating into the adrenal parenchyma

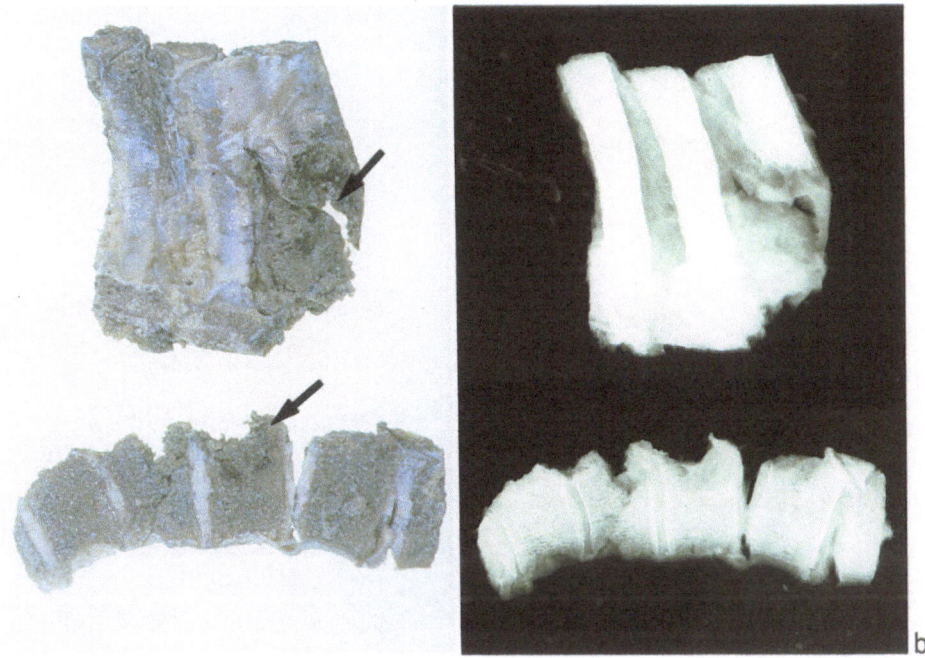

Fig. 9.17a, b. Bone metastasis. **a** Metastatic foci of thoracic vertebra (Th 7–9) (*arrows*). **b** Soft X-ray shows osteolytic features

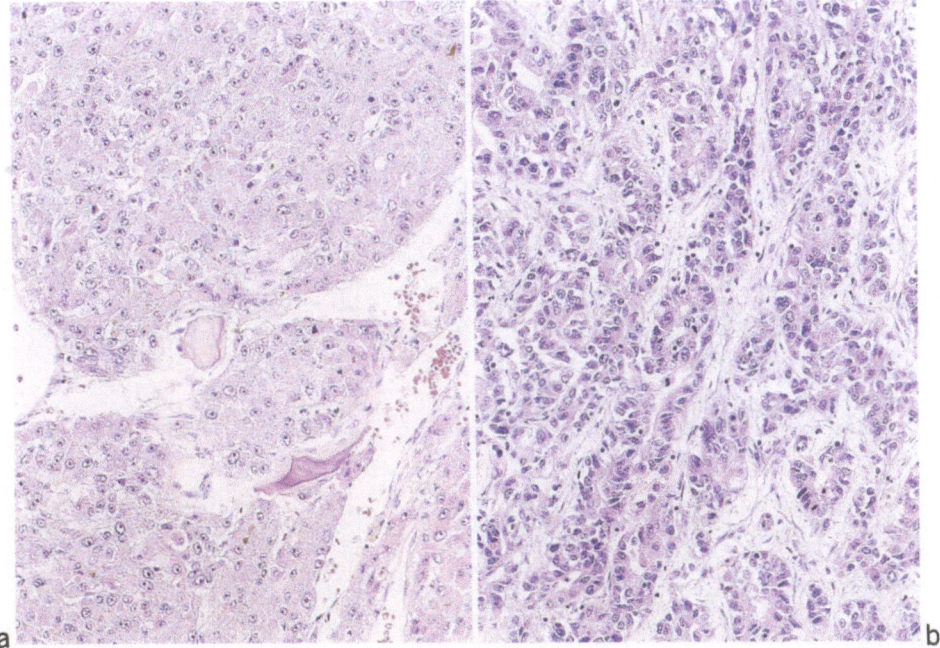

Fig. 9.18a, b. Bone metastasis. **a** Remnants of atrophied bone trabeculae in metastatic tumor. **b** Metastatic pseudoglandular HCC. HE, × 100

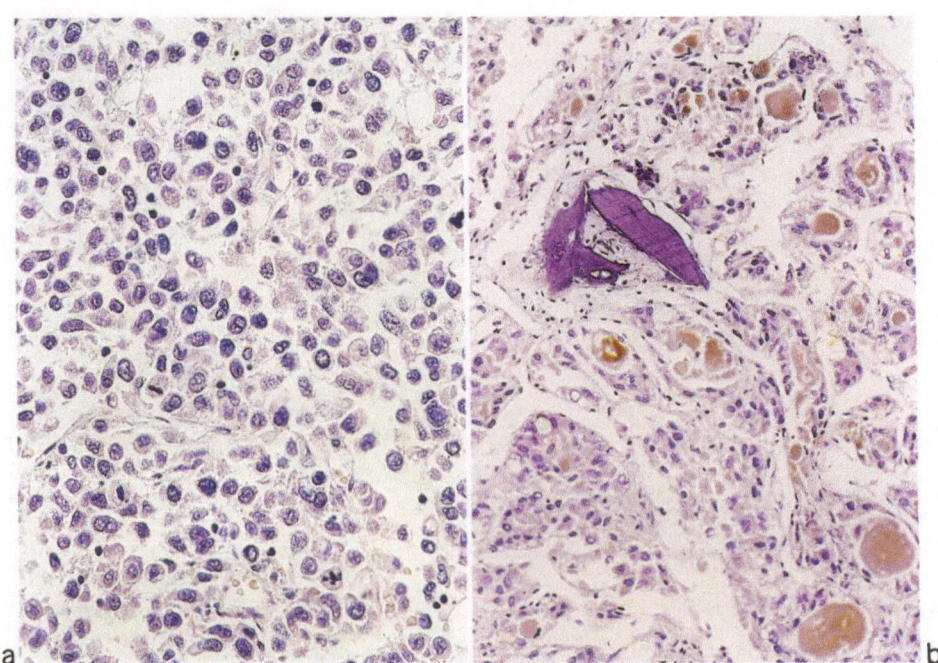

Fig. 9.19a, b. Bone metastasis. **a** Free-cell type HCC. **b** Remnant of atrophied bone trabecula in metastatized pseudoglandular HCC with bile production

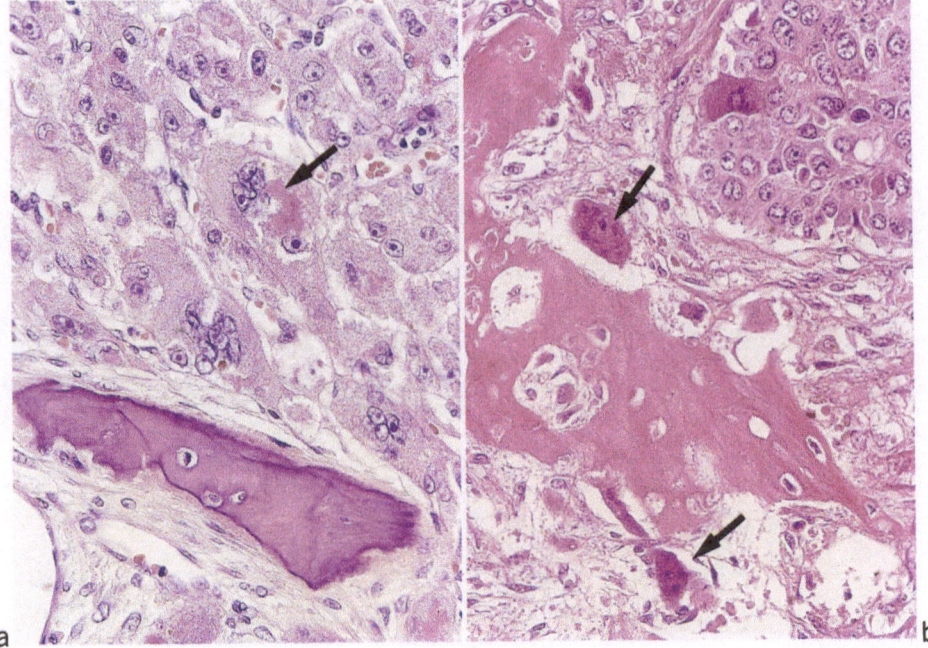

Fig. 9.20a, b. Bone metastasis. **a** Metastasized HCC with Mallory body (*arrow*). **b** Atrophied bone trabecula and osteoclasts (*arrows*) HE, × 200

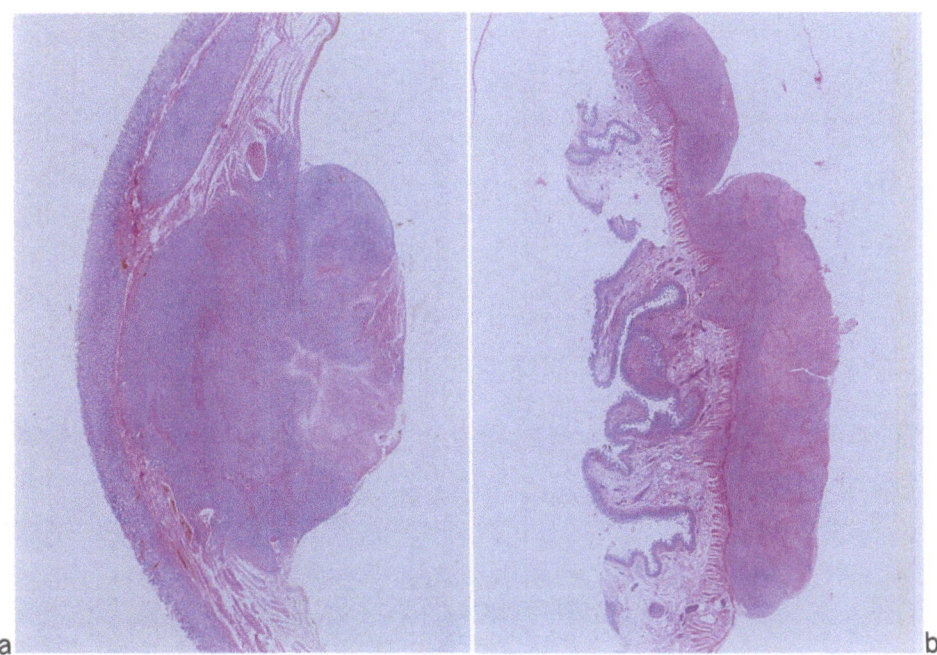

Fig. 9.21. **a** Metastasis to stomach. **b** Metastasis to ileum. HE, × 1

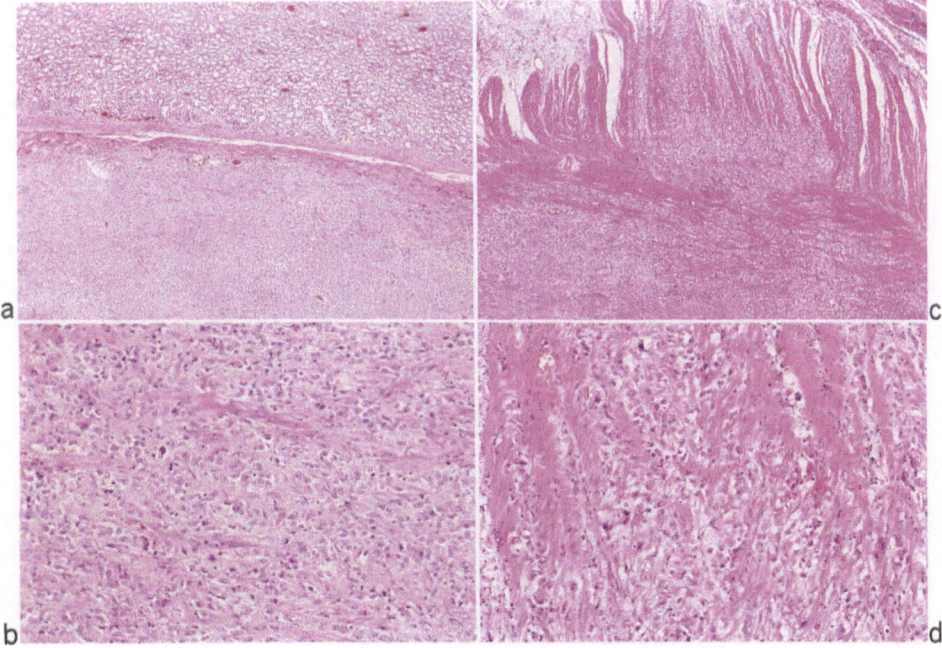

Fig. 9.22. a, b Metastasis to stomach. Free-cell type HCC is proliferating in the submucosal layer. **c, d** Metastasis to ileum. Free-cell type HCC is proliferating in the muscular layer. HE; **a, c** × 20, **b, d** × 50

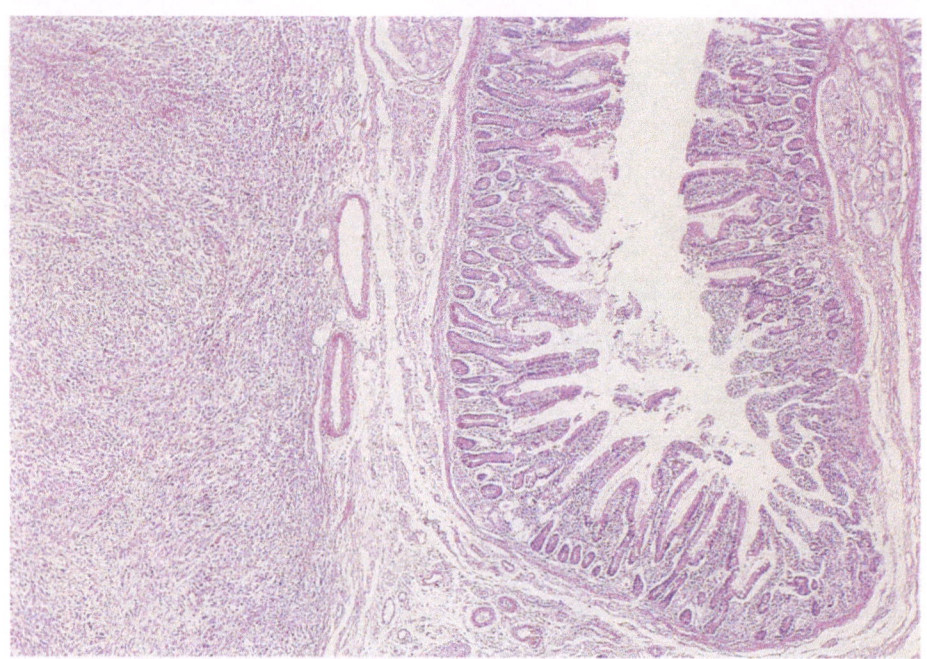

Fig. 9.23. Metastasis to ileum. Metastasized HCC with sarcomatous appearance in the submucosal layer. HE, × 20

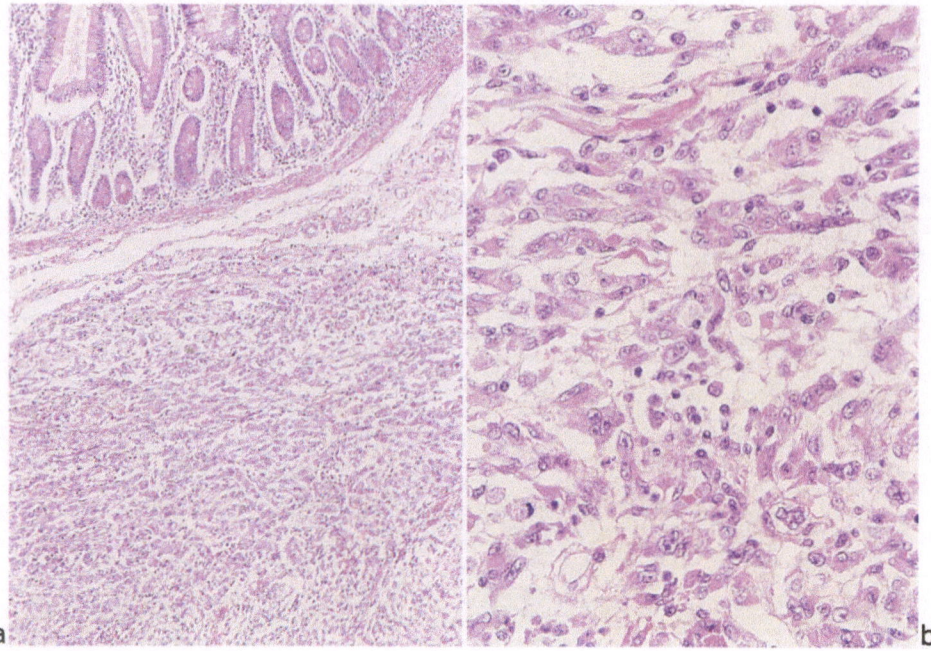

Fig. 9.24a, b. Metastasis to ileum (same case). Metastasized HCC showing sarcomatous appearance. HE; **a** × 50, **b** × 200

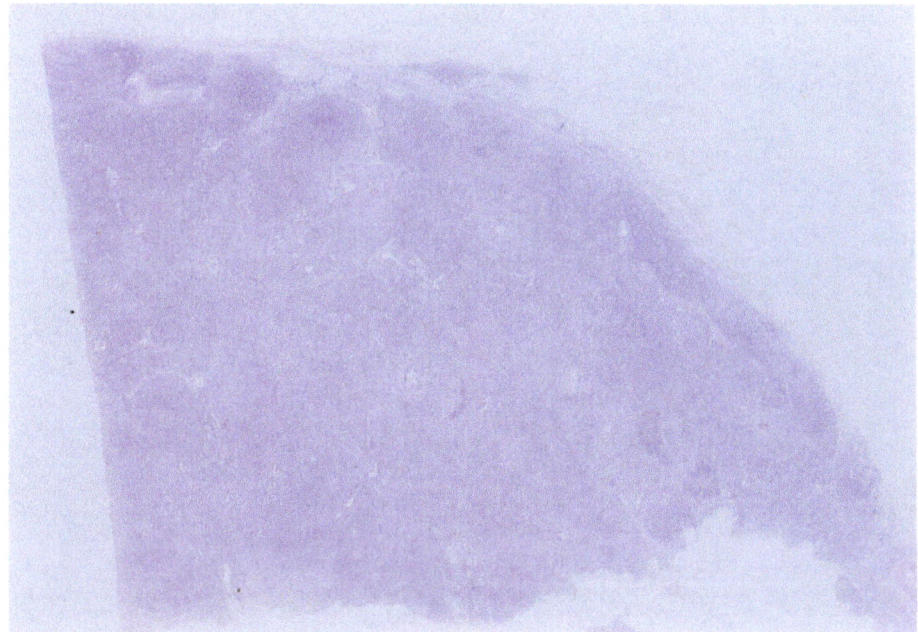

Fig. 9.25. Ill-defined metastasis to pancreas. HE, × 1

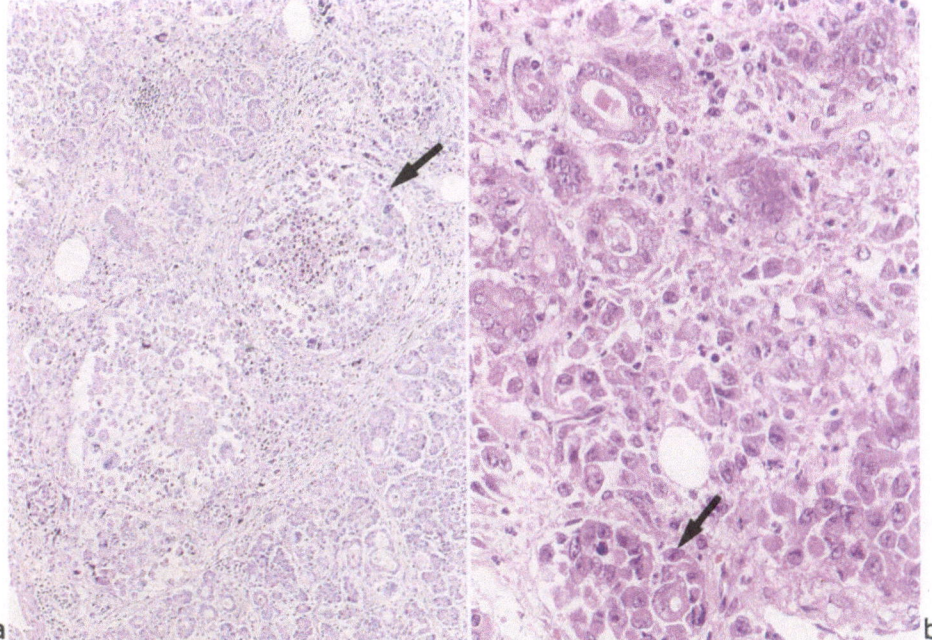

Fig. 9.26a, b. Metastasis to pancreas (same case). Free-cell type HCC is proliferating in the parenchyma. **a** Tumor thrombus in blood vessel (*arrow*) of pancreas. **b** Free-cell type HCC cells (*arrow*)

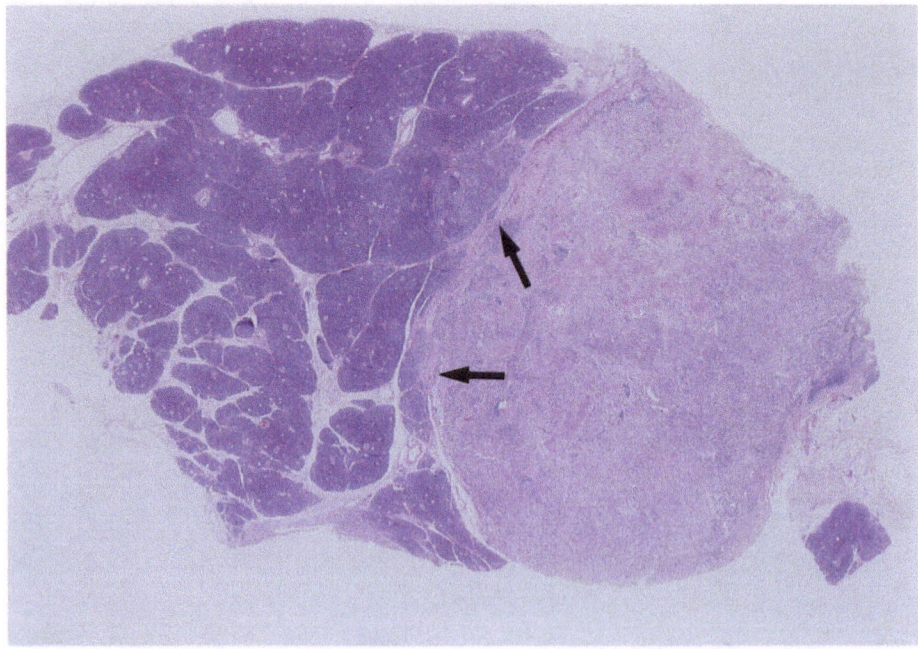

Fig. 9.27. Metastasis to pancreas. Tumor extension into the pancreas from metastasis of the peri-pancreatic lymph node (*arrows*). HE, × 1

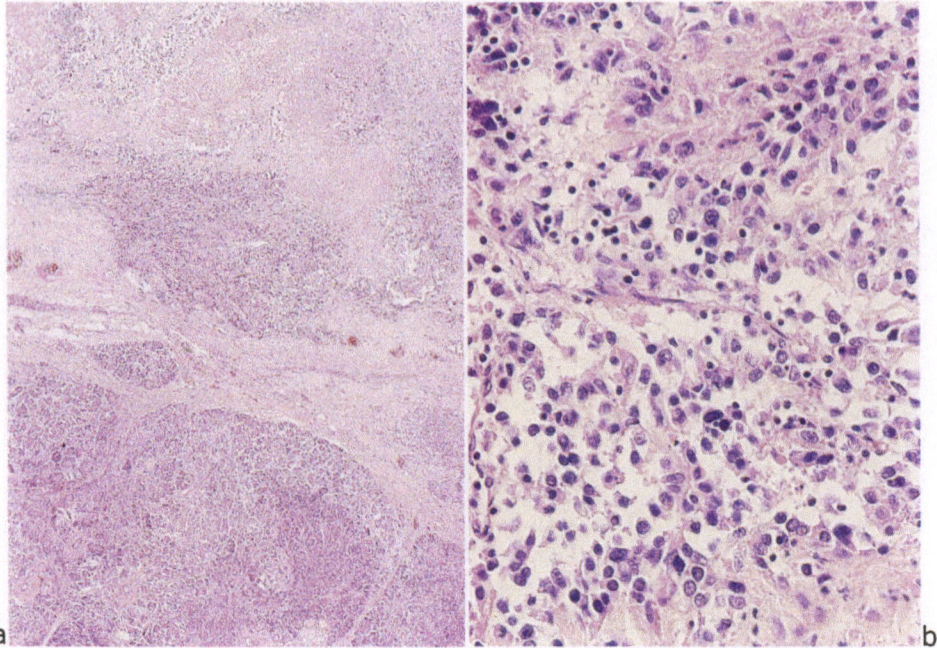

Fig. 9.28a, b. Metastasis to pancreas (same case). Infiltrating HCC cells of the free-cell type. HE; **a** × 20, **b** × 200

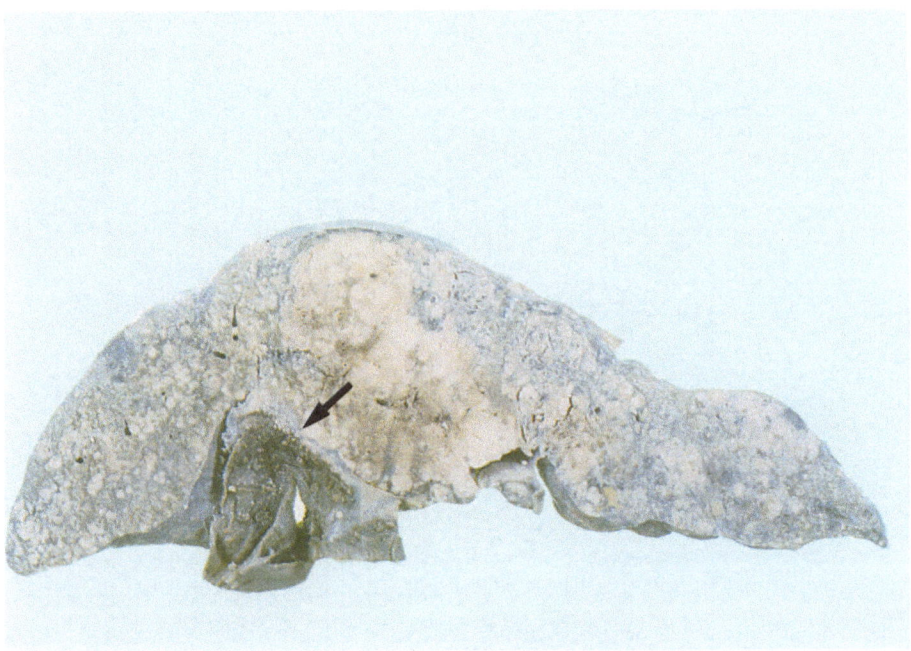

Fig. 9.29. Metastasis to gallbladder. The HCC tumor extends to the gallbladder (*arrow*)

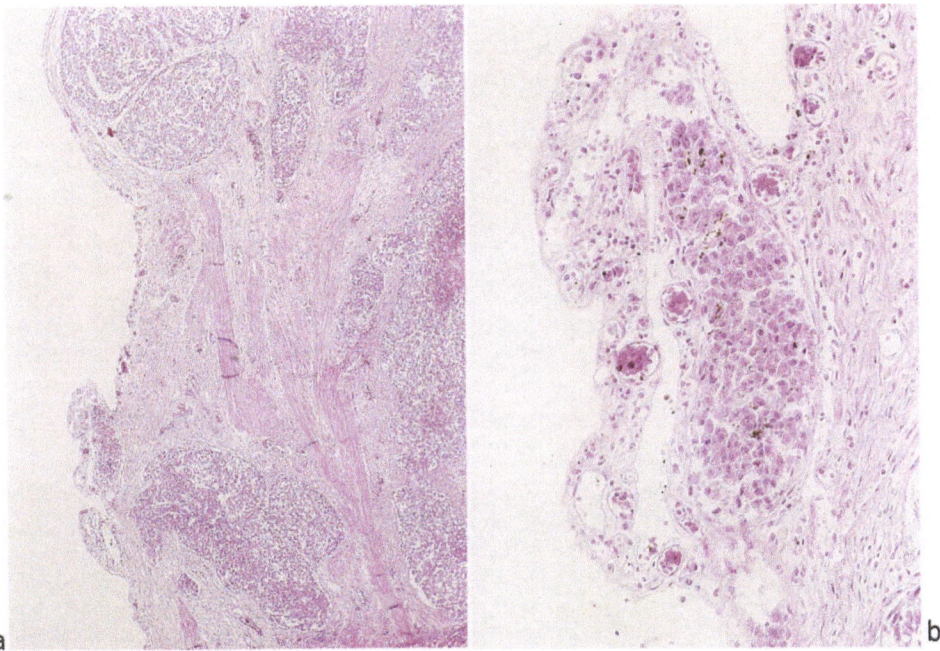

Fig. 9.30a, b. Metastasis to gallbladder. Prominent tumor thrombi in dilated vessels of mucosa

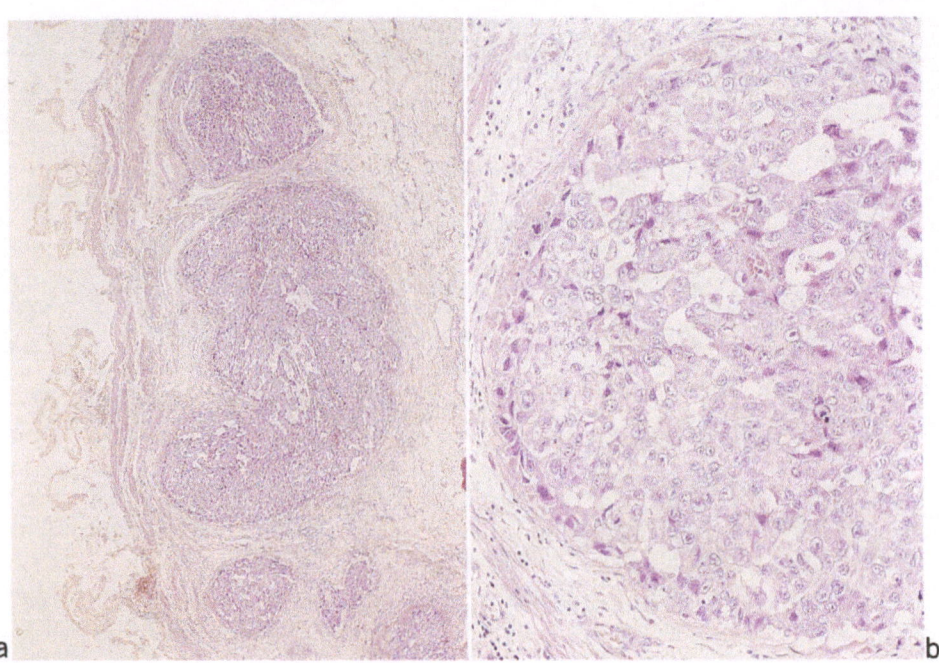

Fig. 9.31a, b. Metastasis to gallbladder. Prominent tumor thrombi of the veins in the subserosal tissue of the gallbladder. HE; **a** × 20, **b** × 200

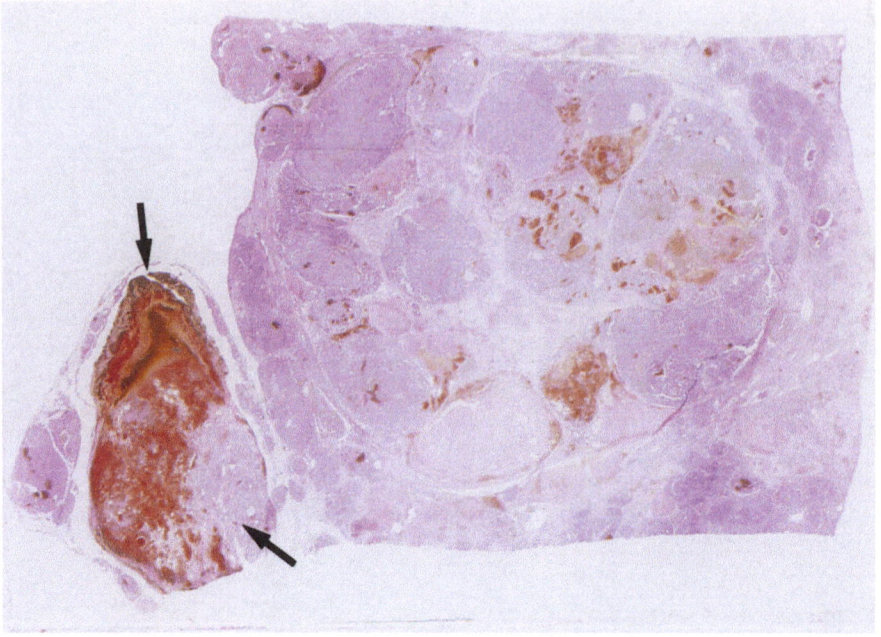

Fig. 9.32. Metastasis to gallbladder. Tumor and blood clots (*arrows*) fill the gallbladder. HE, × 1

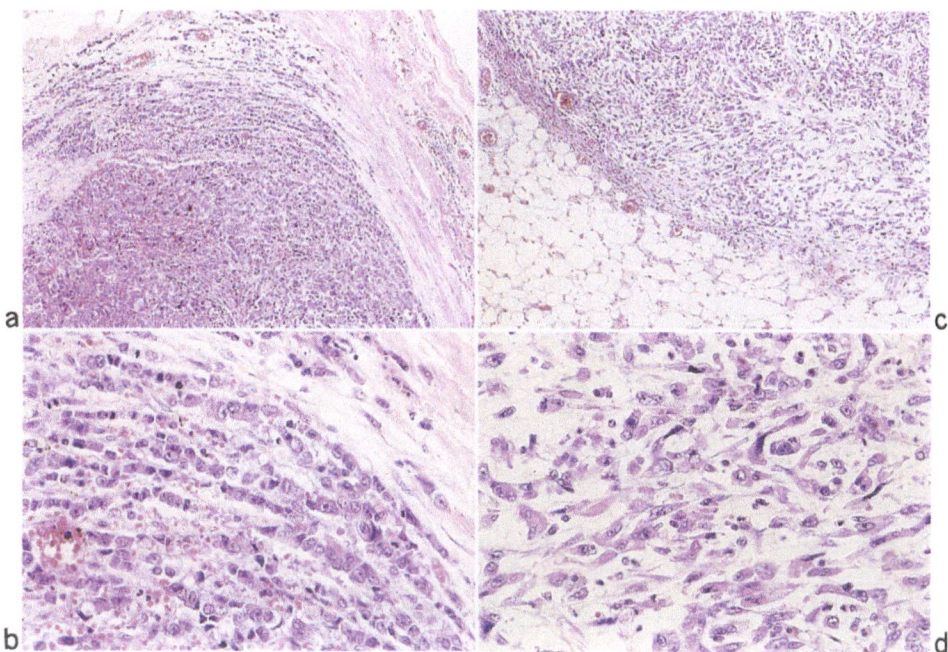

Fig. 9.33a–d. Metastasis to pericardium. Metastasized free-cell type HCC. HE; **a, c** × 20, **b, d** × 100

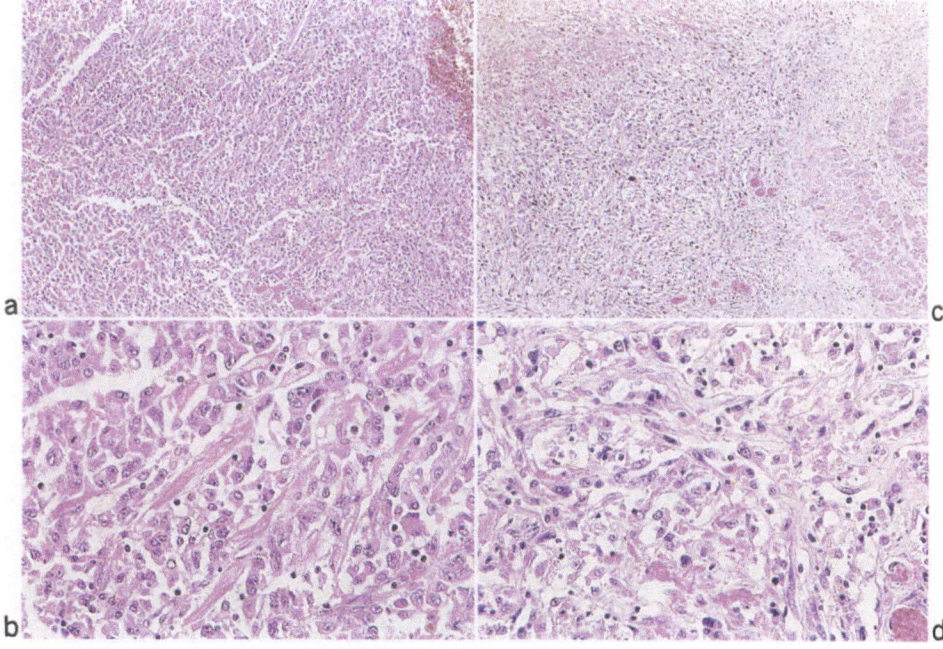

Fig. 9.34. a, b Metastasis to myocardium. Free-cell type HCC cells are proliferating between the myocardial fibers. **c, d** Metastasis to the endocardium. HE; **a, c** × 20, **b, d** × 100

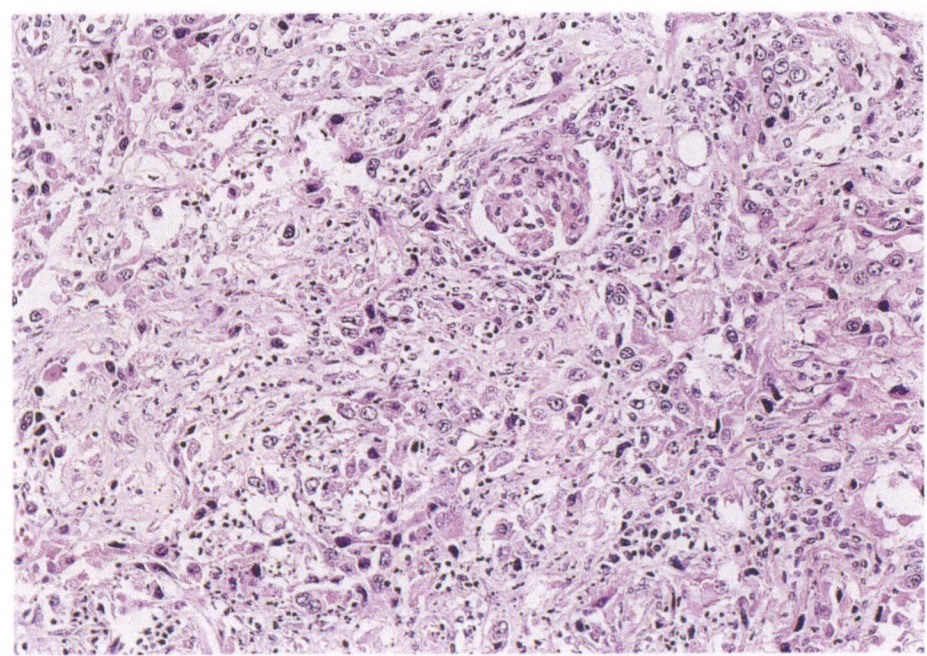

Fig. 9.35. Metastasis to kidney. Free-cell type HCC in the renal cortex. HE, × 100

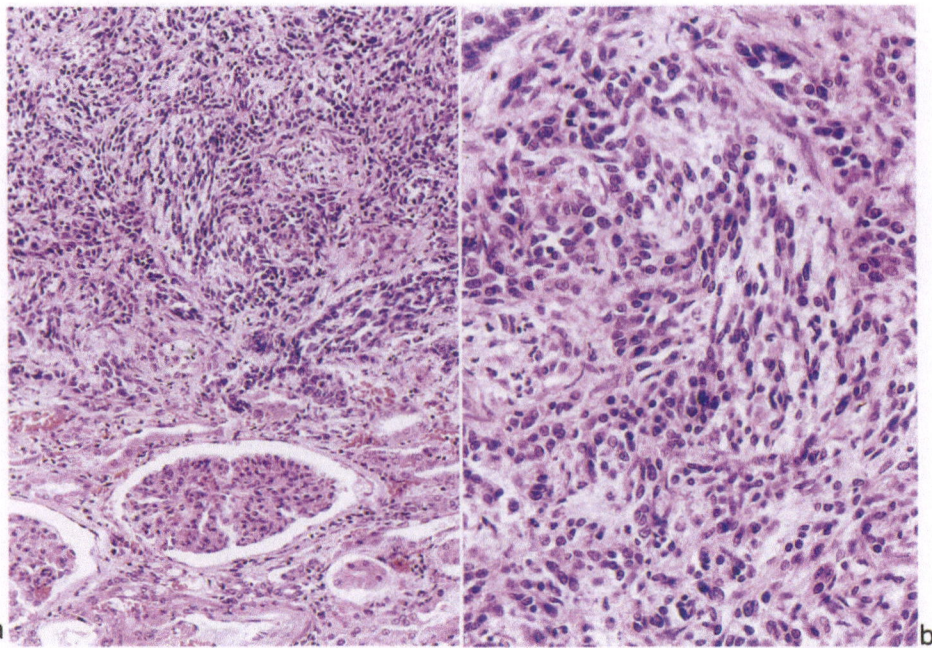

Fig. 9.36a, b. Metastasis to kidney. Sarcomatous HCC consisting of spindle-shaped tumor cells in the renal cortex. HE; **a** × 100, **b** × 200

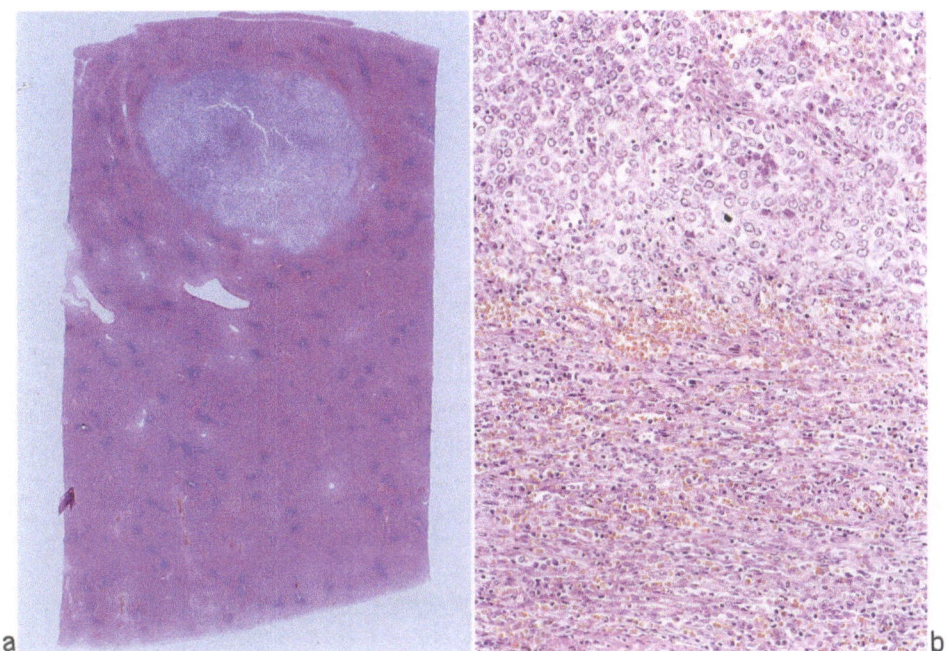

Fig. 9.37a, b. Metastasis to spleen. HE; **a** × 1, **b** × 100

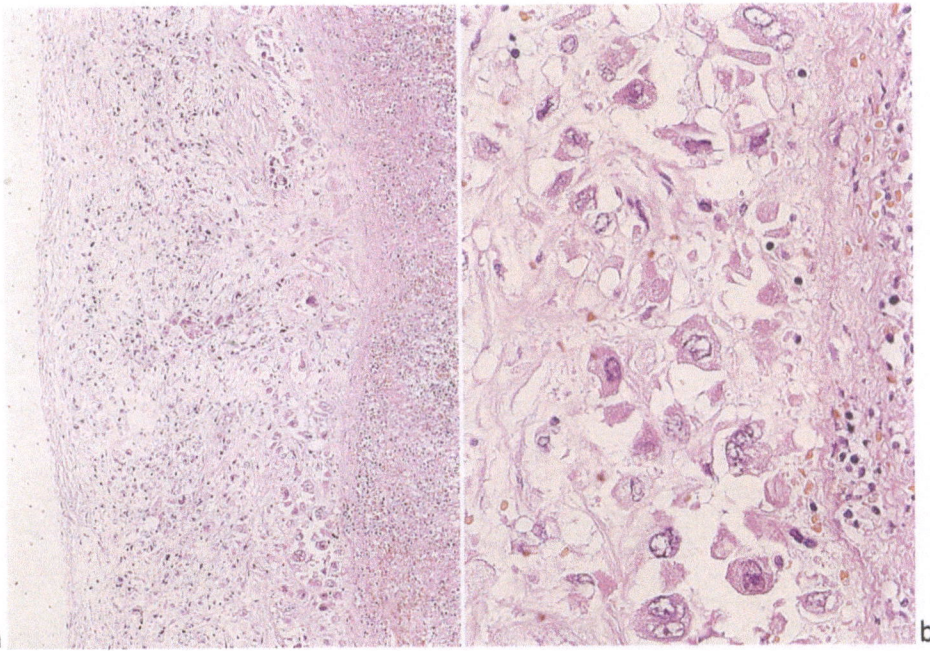

Fig. 9.38a, b. Metastasis to spleen. **a** Metastasized HCC in the splenic capsule. **b** The tumor cells show marked pleomorphism. HE; **a** × 50, **b** × 200

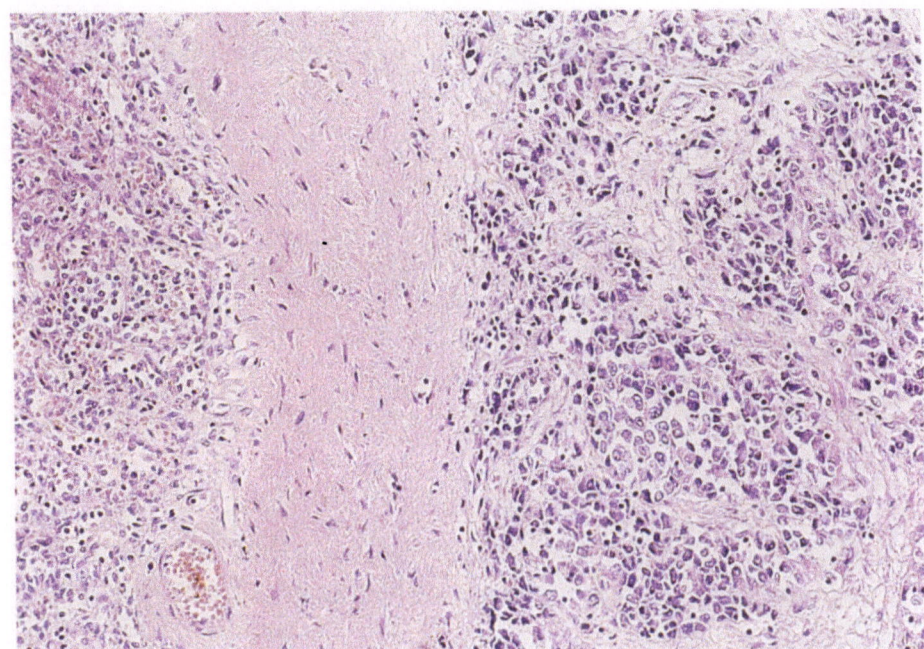

Fig. 9.39. Metastasis to spleen. Metastasis of free-cell type HCC in the splenic capsule. HE, × 100

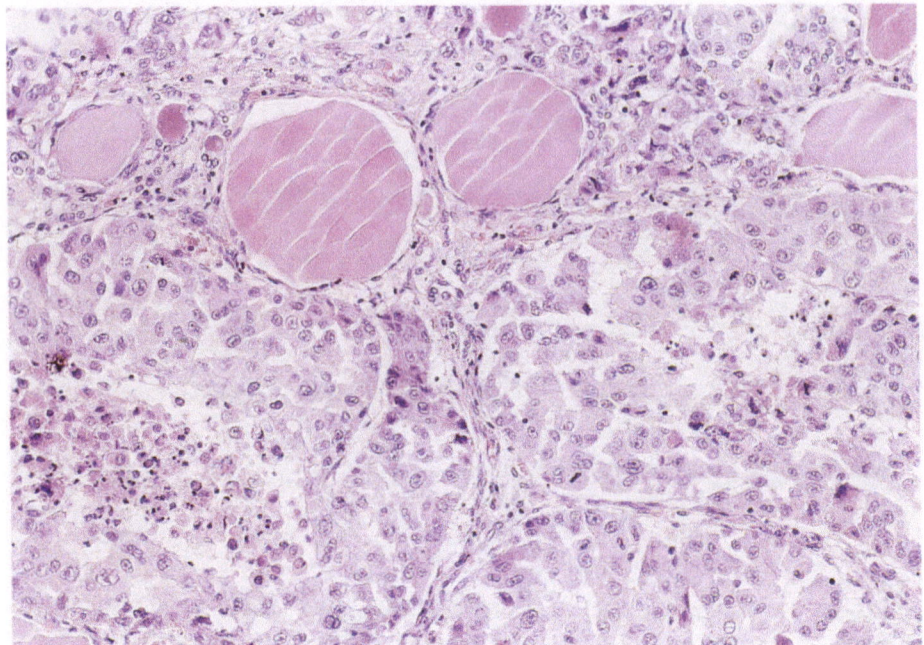

Fig. 9.40. Metastasis to thyroid. Trabecular type HCC is proliferating in the thyroid parenchyma. Residual thyroid follicles are seen among tumor nests. HE, × 200

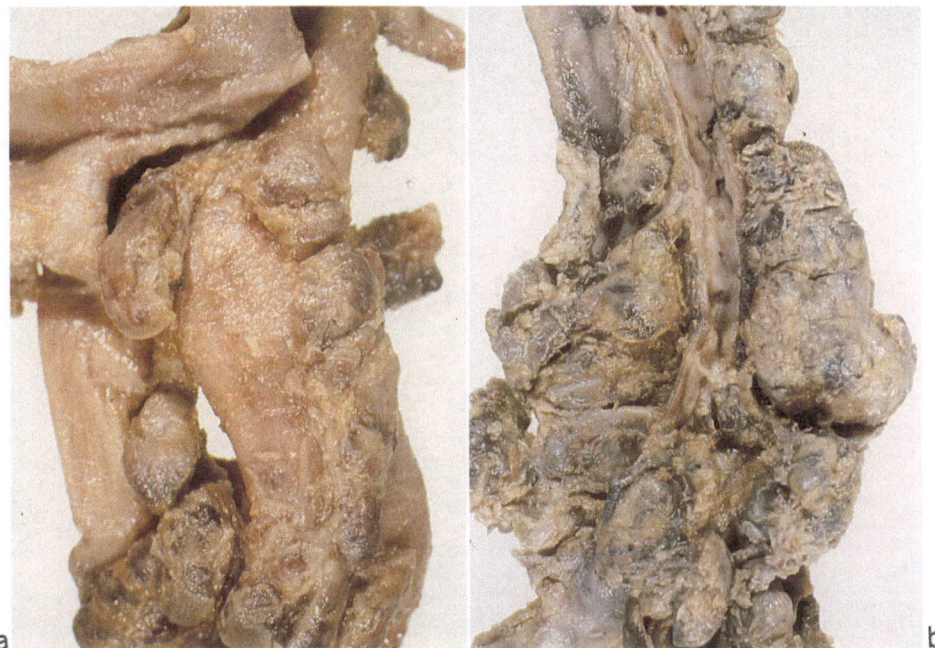

Fig. 9.41a, b. Lymph node metastasis. Massive metastasis in the periaortic lymph nodes

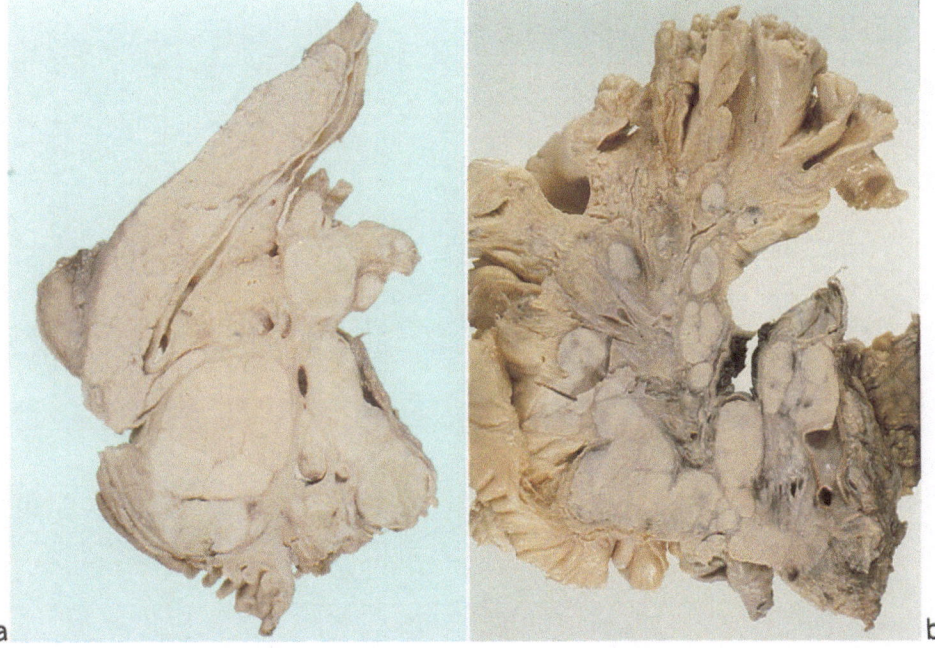

Fig. 9.42a, b. Lymph node metastasis. Massive metastasis in the peripancreatic lymph nodes (**a**) and the mesenteric nodes (**b**)

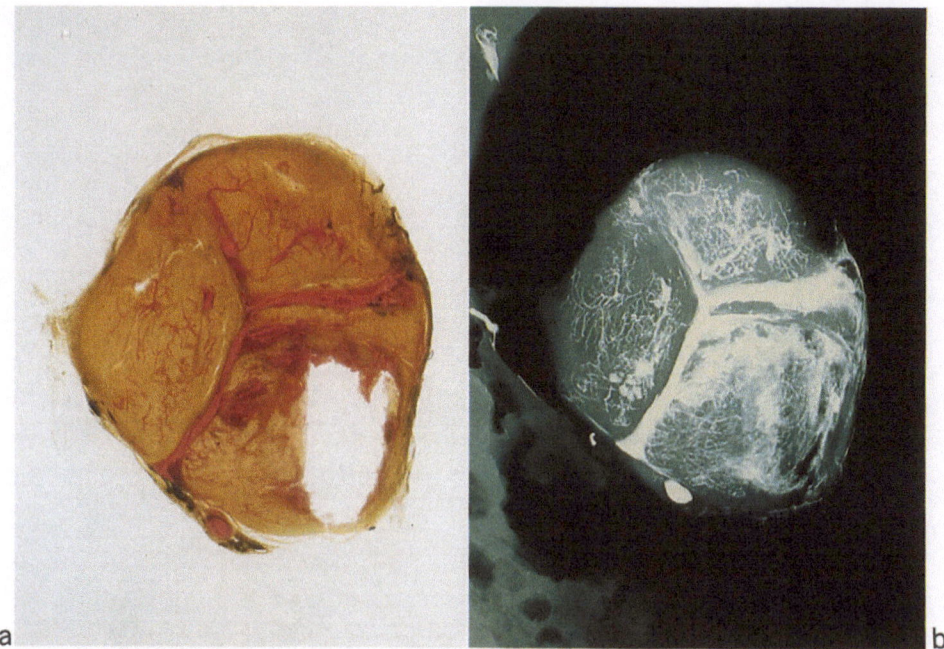

Fig. 9.43a, b. Hypervascular lymph node metastasis. **a** Metastasis in the lymph node of the porta hepatis. **b** Soft X-ray finding

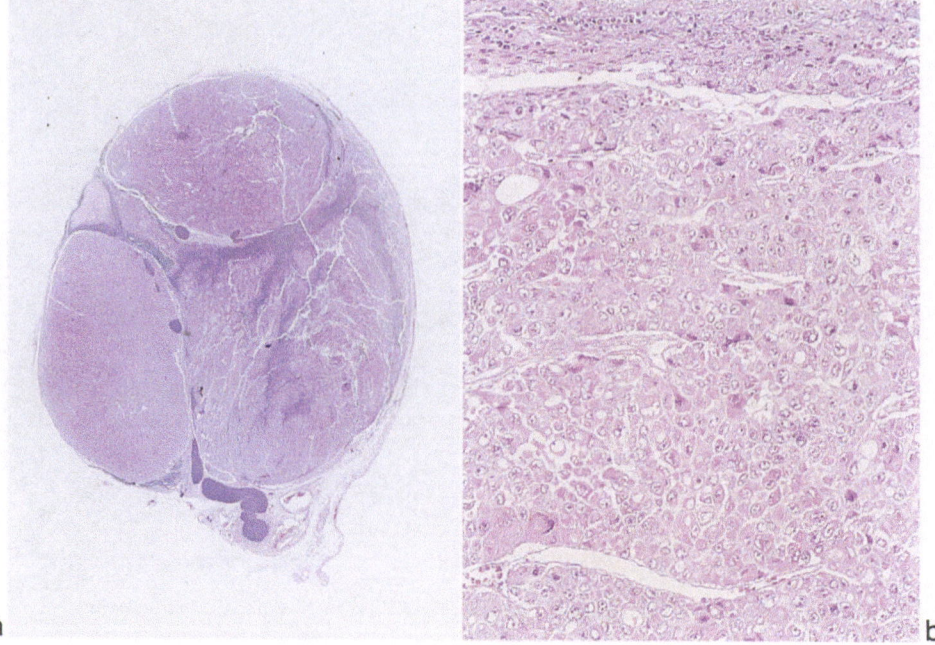

Fig. 9.44a, b. Same lymph node. Metastasis of trabecular HCC. HE; **a** ×1, **b** ×100

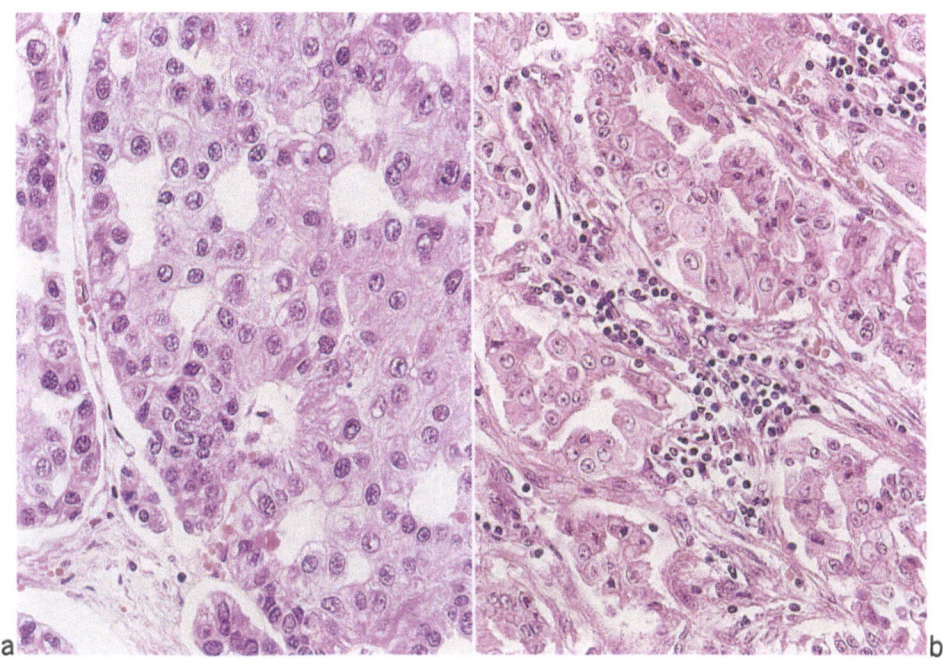

Fig. 9.45a, b. Lymph node metastasis. Metastasis of pseudoglandular HCC. HE, × 200

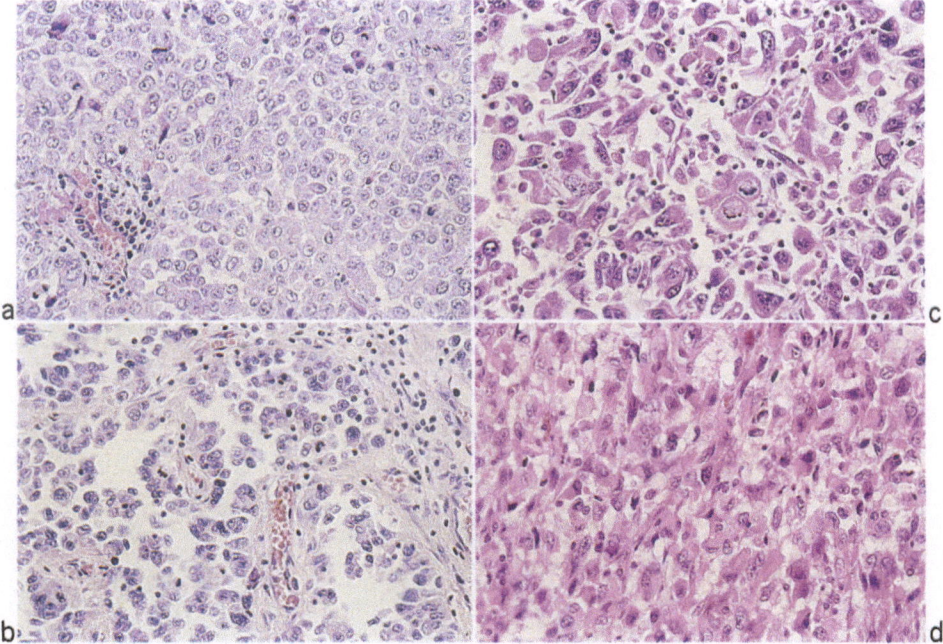

Fig. 9.46a–d. Lymph node metastasis. **a, b** Free-cell type HCC; **c, d** Sarcomatous HCC. HE, × 100

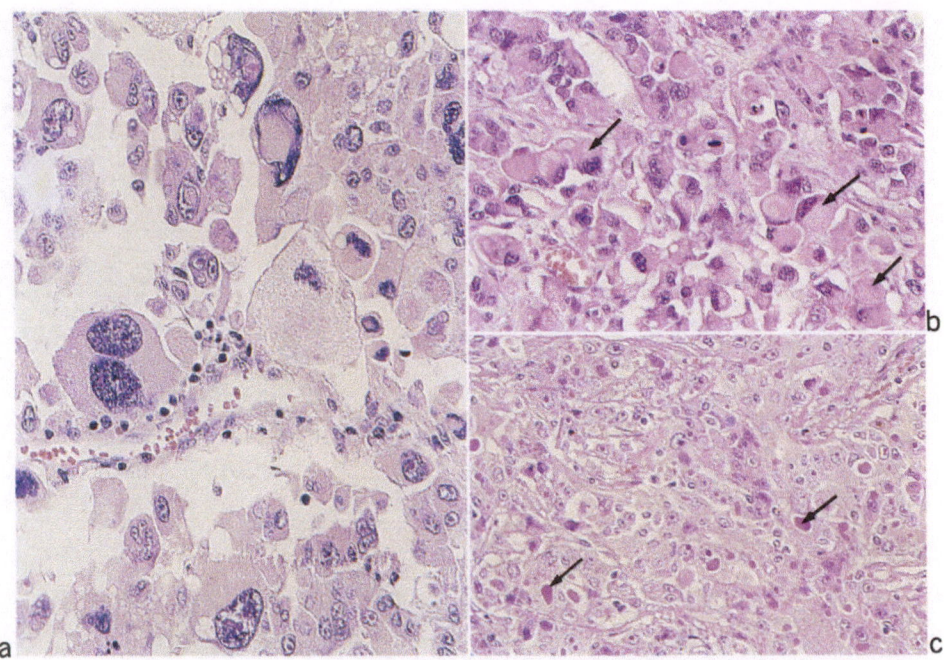

Fig. 9.47a–c. Lymph node metastasis. **a** Giant cell type HCC. **b** Metastatic HCC with ground-glass inclusions (*arrows*). **c** Metastatic HCC with hyaline inclusions (*arrows*). HE; **a** × 200, **b, c** × 100

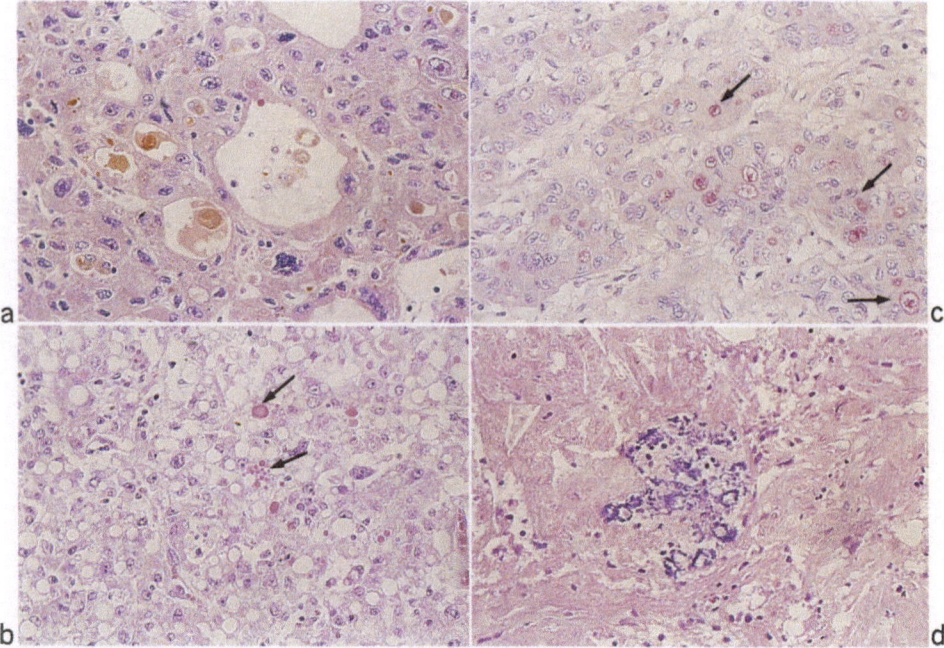

Fig. 9.48a–d. Lymph node metastasis. **a** Pseudoglandular HCC with bile production. **b** Marked fatty degeneration and hyaline inclusions (*arrows*) in metastatic HCC. **c** Metastatic HCC with mucin production (*arrows*). **d** Calcification in metastatic HCC. **a** HE, × 100; **b, d** HE, × 50; **c** Mayer's mucicarmin, × 100

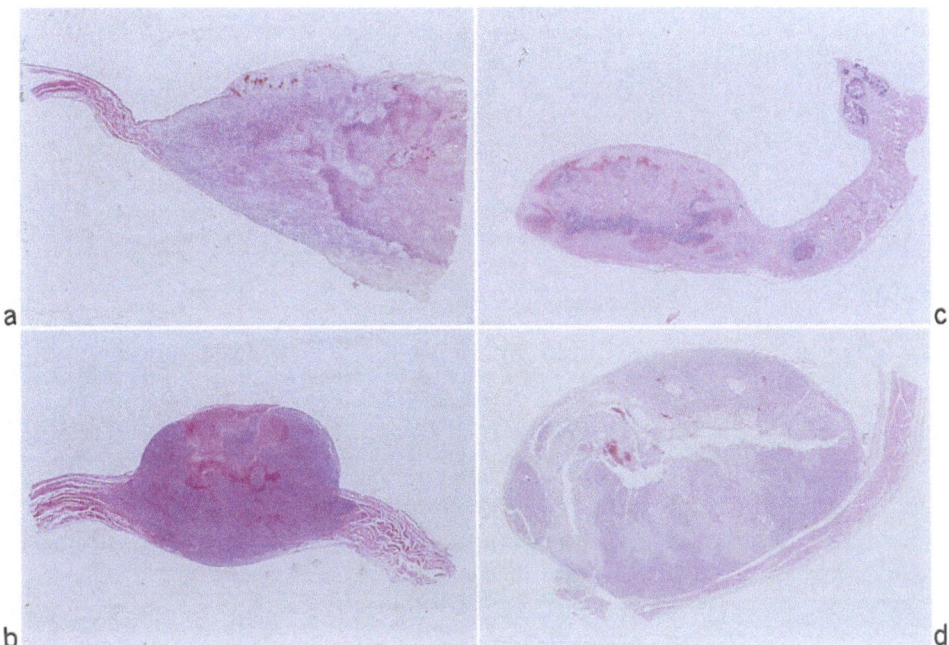

Fig. 9.49a–d. Disseminated metastasis. Metastatic foci in the diaphragm. HE, × 1

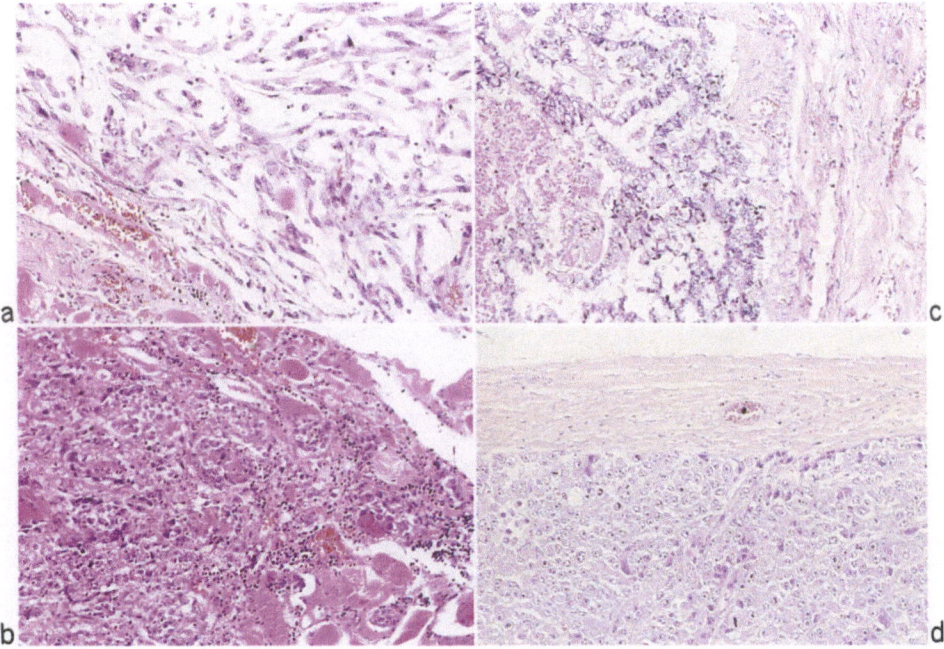

Fig. 9.50a–d. Disseminated metastasis in the diaphragm. **a** Sarcomatous HCC; **b** Solid HCC. HE, × 50

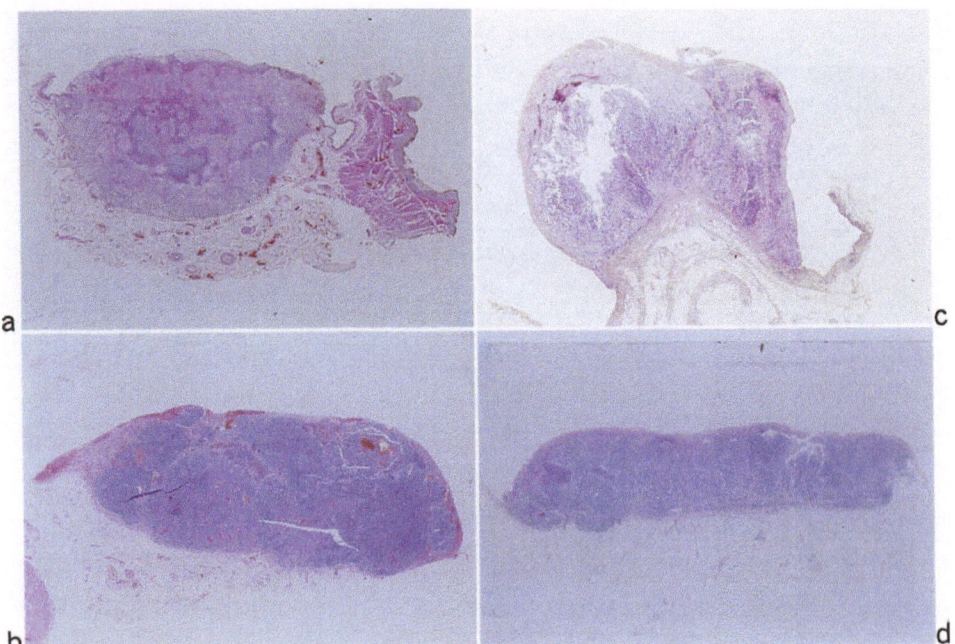

Fig. 9.51a–d. Disseminated metastasis in Douglas' cavity. HE, × 1

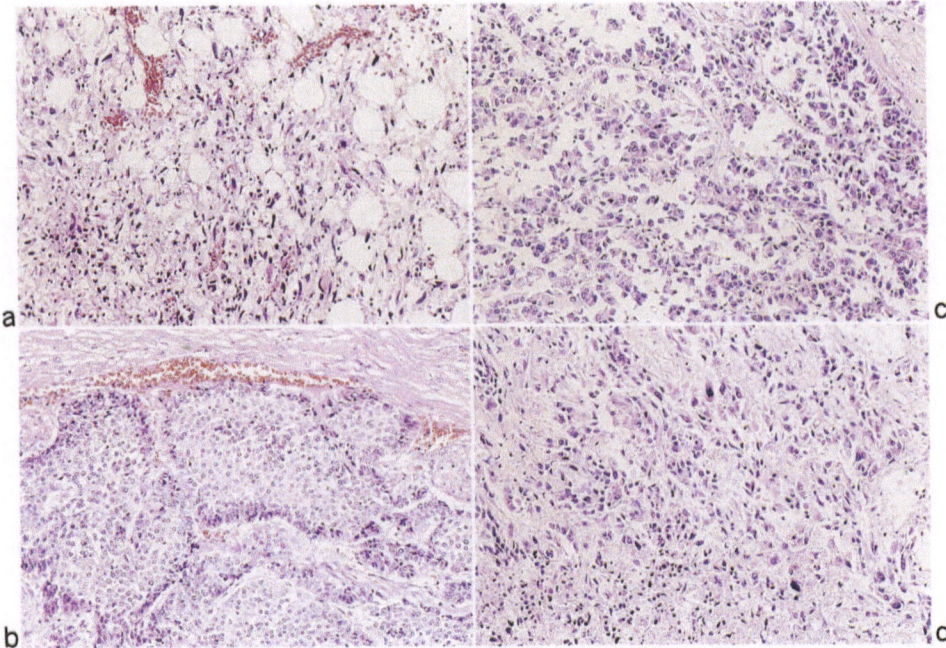

Fig. 9.52a–d. Disseminated metastasis in Douglas' cavity. **a, d** Sarcomatous HCC; **b** Trabecular HCC; **c** Pseudoglandular HCC. HE, × 50

Chapter 10
Hepatocellular Carcinoma
and Liver Cirrhosis

Hepatocellular carcinoma is usually associated with some variety of liver cirrhosis. The frequency varies, however, among reports and geographical regions.

Frequency of Associated Liver Cirrhosis

Eggel [6] stated that 86.4% of HCC arise in cirrhotic liver. Yamagiwa [7] gave a figure of 74.7%, Kika [131] 88.4%, Tull [155] 75.5%, Gustafson [128] 64.1%, Greene [177] 87%, Edmondson and Steiner [9] 89.2%, Mori [40] 76.9%, MacDonald [130] 76.9% MacSween [178], 75%, Inde et al. [179] 69%, Shikata [180] 85.5%, Jim [181] 86%, and Lin et al. [182] 80%. The figure in our series is 80%.

Shikata [180] questioned the accuracy of reports indicating lower incidences of associated liver cirrhosis in HCC, correctly pointing out that many reports of an incidence of only 65%–75% may have been based on material that did not convincingly exclude cholangiocarcinoma. Peters [66] agreed with Shikata and stated that in regions with a low incidence of HCC, cholangiocarcinoma may make up a larger proportion of the cases of total primary liver cancer, and since cholangiocarcinoma is less frequently superimposed on a cirrhotic liver, grouping cholangiocarcinoma and HCC together would be misleading. The association of liver cirrhosis is low among certain African blacks with high incidence of HCC.

Types of Liver Cirrhosis Associated with HCC

The association of liver cirrhosis with HCC varies in frequency depending on the etiology of the cirrhosis [183, 184]. Viral hepatitis, various toxications, alcohol abuse, and malnutrition are among the more common etiological factors. Some cases of cirrhosis result from hepatic injuries secondary to bile stasis, congestion, and parasites. Cryptogenic cirrhosis includes five classes: precirrhotic liver, posthepatitic cirrhosis, postnecrotic cirrhosis, nutritional cirrhosis, and toxic cirrhosis.

Posthepatitic cirrhosis
Posthepatitic cirrhosis (Figs. 10.1–6) was encountered in as many as 69.2% of the 439 autopsy cases of HCC in our series.

Viral hepatitis or toxication may cause necrosis of hepatic cells and lead to scarring. Regeneration following liver cell damage results in nodularity. The morphological pattern may vary depending on the degree of pathological change, the duration of the injuries, and involvement of immunological mechanisms. Histologi-cally, the occurrence of pseudolobules composed of several lobules is markedly increased, and massive elastic fibers are noted in the stroma. Macroscopically, this type corresponds to macronodular cirrhosis. Serum HBs antigen (HBs Ag) was demonstrated in 36.5% of the cases of posthepatitic cirrhosis associated with HCC in our series. The rate was reported as 40% by Nishioka [185].

Postnecrotic cirrhosis

Postnecrotic cirrhosis (Figs. 10.7, 8) occurs mainly following viral hepatitis or toxication. After extensive necrosis, scarring occurs in the necrotic area. Regenera-tive nodules, consisting of unaffected liver tissue and regenerated liver cells, are separated by a broad stromal band. Macroscopically, pseudolobules of varying size and a broad fibrotic band are noted. Cirrhosis of this type is seldom found in asso-ciation with HCC. In our series it was found in 1.8% of cases, in 42.8% of which HBs Ag was positive.

Alcoholic cirrhosis

Alcoholic cirrhosis (Figs. 10.9–12) may follow hepatic injury resulting from alco-hol abuse or malabsorption. This corresponds to nutritional cirrhosis in a catego-rization by Gall [183]. Mori [186] compared liver cirrhosis and HCC in the Tokyo area with that in Cincinnati. In Tokyo, HCC was encountered in about 23% of cirrhosis cases, in contrast with only 7% in Cincinnati. Despite this remarkable difference, the occurrence of liver cirrhosis in HCC was 70% and 60%, respectively, essentially the same. Mori mentioned that the proportion of liver cirrhosis made up by nutritional cirrhosis is far higher in the United States than in Japan and that HCC seldom occurs in association with nutritional liver cirrhosis. Alcohol abuse has been increasing recently in Japan, but the histological features of liver cirrhosis associated with alcohol abuse in Japan differ from those in the United States [187]. Nonomura et al. [188] described that HCC was frequently associated with mac-ronodular cirrhosis, regardless of the presence or absence of alcohol abuse of HBV infection, but rare in micronodular cirrhosis. Hepatic disease resulting from alco-hol abuse will increase in future in Japan; monitoring of hepatic histology by biopsy after alcohol intake may help to elucidate of correlation between alcohol abuse and HCC. Typical alcoholic liver cirrhosis in association with HCC was found in only three (0.7%) of our series of 439 cases. However, the superimposition of nonalcoholic hepatic changes on alcoholic cirrhosis with HCC was noted in 10.9%.

Precirrhotic liver

Precirrhotic liver (Fig. 10.13) precedes posthepatitic cirrhosis. The histological fea-tures include the extension of fibrous bands from Glisson's capsule. The fibrous tissue tends to form an intervening zone, but the formation of the fibrous band which encloses lobules completely to form pseudolobules in posthepatitic cirrhosis is incomplete. Lesions of this type, which change into posthepatitic cirrhosis sooner or later, were noted in only 3.4% of our 439 cases of HCC.

Congestive liver cirrhosis

In 1911, Yamagiwa [7] described four cases of congestive liver cirrhosis bearing HCC among a total of 27 HCC cases. Simson [189] found 47 cases of HCC among

101 cases of congestive hepatic fibrosis due to membranous obstruction of the inferior vena cava and stressed a close correlation between these two diseases in South Africa. In our series, HCC was found in one case of congestive liver cirrhosis resulting from tumor thrombus of the inferior vena cava and in one case of congestive hepatic fibrosis due to insufficiency of the aortic valve (Figs. 10.14–16).

Primary hemochromatosis

The association of HCC and primary hemochromatosis (Figs. 10.17–20) has been a subject of inconclusive debate for a long time. HCC was found in 9% of primary hemochromatosis by Rosenthal [190], in 7.3% by Berk and Lieber [191], in 18.9% by Warren and Drake [192], and in 13% by Edmondson and Steiner [9]. In our HCC series, primary hemochromatosis was noted only once, in a case of small liver cancer.

Parasitic cirrhosis due to *Schistosoma japonicum*

HCC has been reported to have a geographical prevalence similar to that of schistosomiasis, but the existence of an etiological relation between these two diseases has long been controversial [193–196]. We studied the association of HCC and chronic schistosomiasis japonica among 4886 adult autopsy cases in our institute (Figs. 10.21–24). HCC was present in 59 (25.7%) of the 229 cases of chronic schistosomiasis. Among cases without schistosomiasis, 399 (8.5%) had HCC. The incidence of HCC in patients with chronic schistosomiasis japonica was significantly higher than that in other autopsy cases ($P < 0.01$). HBs Ag was positive in 26.7% of 35 HCC cases with schistosomiasis examined for hepatitis B virus markers. Anti-HBs and/or anti-HBc were positive in 10 of the 12 HBs Ag-negative cases associated with schistosomiasis. Thus, most HCC victims with schistosomiasis probably had HBV infection at one time. Morphological examination revealed varying degrees of nonschistosomal hepatic change, including macronodular or mixed macro- and micronodular cirrhosis superimposed on schistosomal fibrosis in about two-thirds of the cases of HCC associated with schistosomiasis.

Although no conclusive evidence as to whether or not schistosomal infection plays a direct role in hepatocarcinogenesis could be obtained, we believe that the additional nonschistosomal factors, particularly HBV infection, may play a synergistic role.

Clonorchis sinensis

Clonorchis sinensis is prevalent in most areas in Japan, but very few cases of liver cirrhosis due to *Clonorchis sinensis* have been reported in man. Gibson [197] reported that the occurrence of HCC did not differ significantly between controls and clonorchiasis cases, but the occurrence of cholangiocarcinoma was higher with clonorchiasis, in agreement with the results of Hou [198] and Liang and Tung [199]. In our 439 HCC cases, cirrhosis and fibrosis due to *Clonorchis sinensis* were seen in one case each (Figs. 10.25–28).

Thorotrast

Thorotrast (Fig. 10.29–32), a stabilized 25% colloidal solution of thorium dioxide, was utilized in many countries in the 1930s and 1940s as a contrast medium for various roentgenographic examinations. Although the possible carcinogenicity of Thorotrast, particularly in the liver, had been warned against, Thorotrast was increasingly used because it lacked acute toxicity and provided excellent radiographic results. Since MacMahon et al. [200] first reported the occurrence of Thorotrast-induced hepatic angiosarcoma, numerous cases of Thorotrast-related hepatic tumors have been reported worldwide [201–205].

We studied 127 livers with Thorotrast deposition collected from various institutes in Japan and found hepatic fibrosis of varying degrees in most of them. Cholangiocarcinoma was found in 43 cases, angiosarcoma in 32 cases, and HCC in 18 cases. Thus, in Thorotrast cases the occurrence of HCC is relatively infrequent, although it is the commonest hepatic tumor.

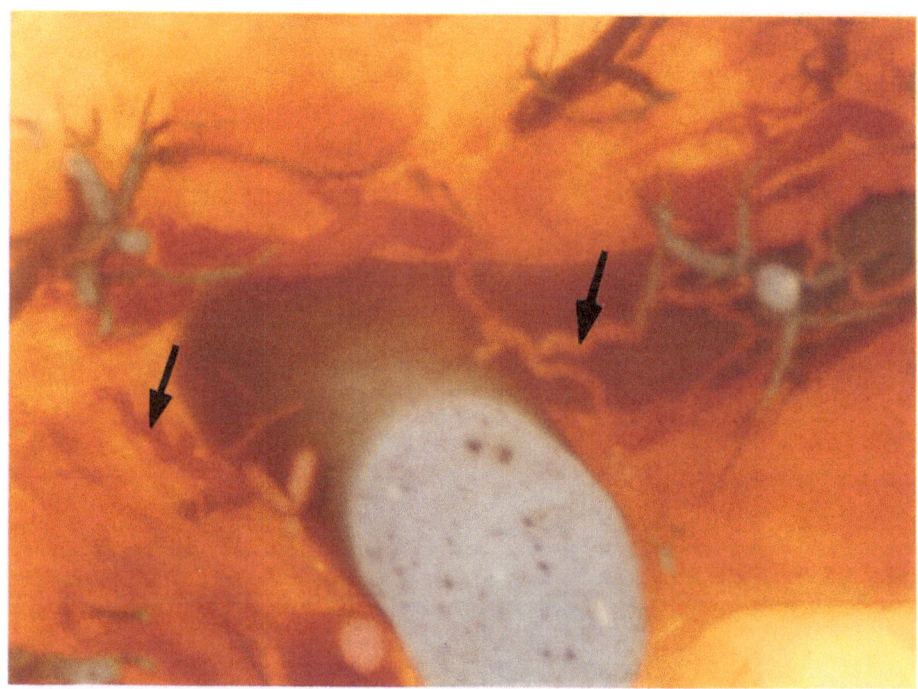

Fig. 10.1. Angioarchitecture of mixed macro- and micronodular cirrhosis. The hepatic arteries have a "corkscrew" appearance (*arrows*). Transparent preparation: *red*, artery; *blue*, portal vein

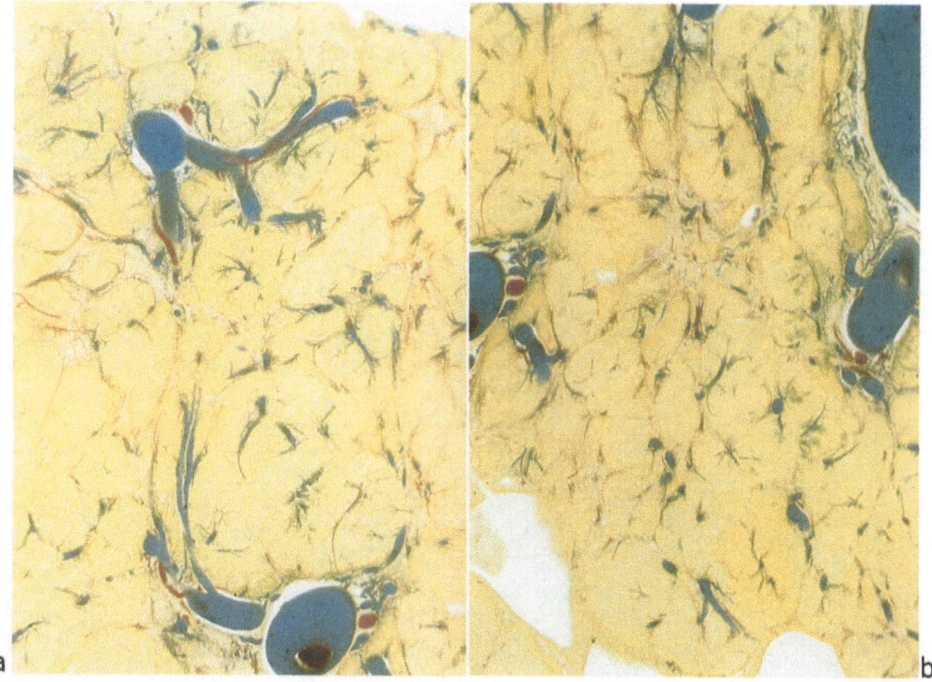

Fig. 10.2a, b. Angioarchitecture of mixed macro- and micronodular cirrhosis. The arterial beds are increased. Transparent preparation: *red*, artery; *blue*, portal vein

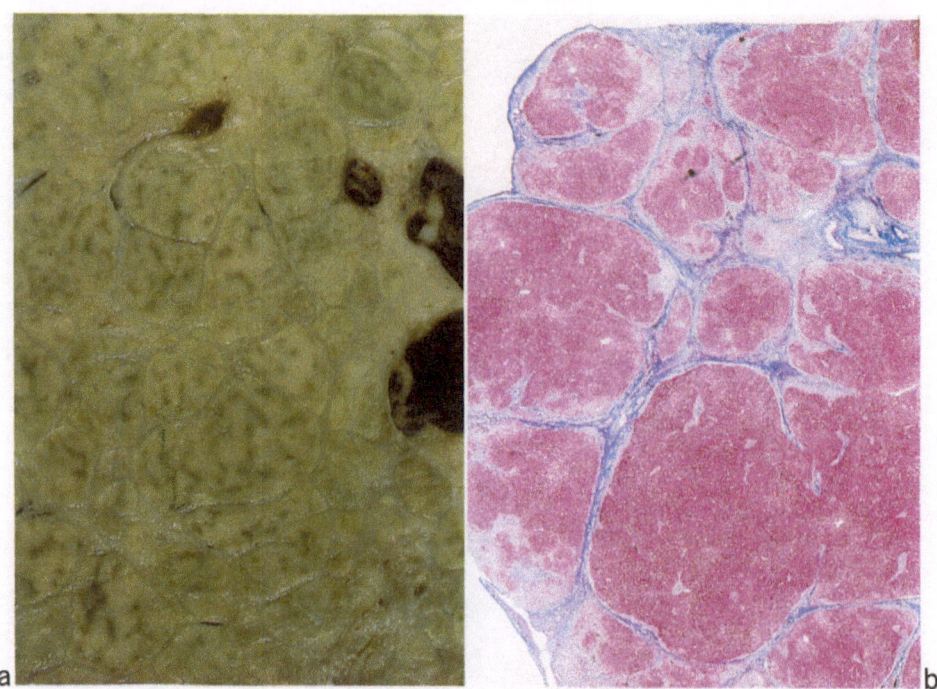

Fig. 10.3a, b. Mixed macro- and micronodular cirrhosis. **a** Gross features; **b** Azan-Mallory, × 1
Cirrhotic nodules are separated by thin fibrous bands

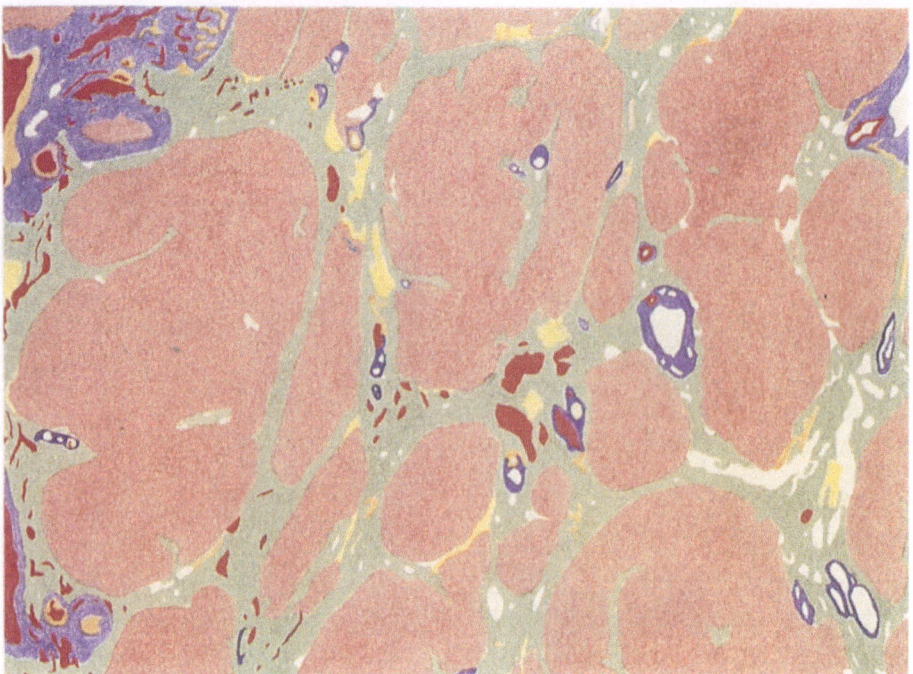

Fig. 10.4. Schema of mixed macro- and micronodular cirrhosis

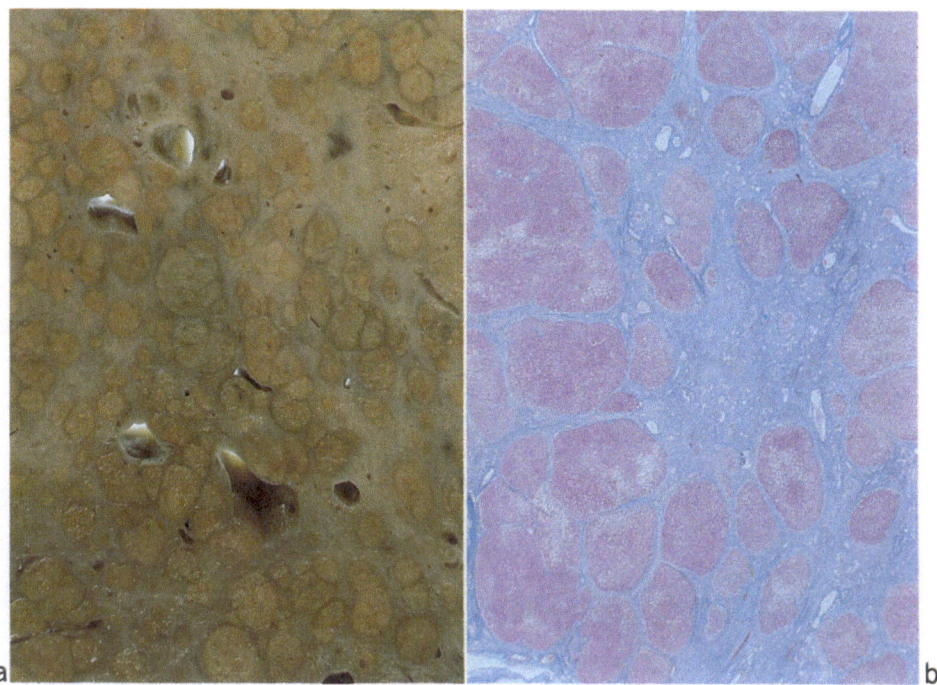

Fig. 10.5a, b. Mixed macro- and micronodular cirrhosis with thick fibrous septa. **a** Gross features; **b** Azan- Mallory, × 1. Cirrhotic nodules are separated by irregular thick fibrous bands

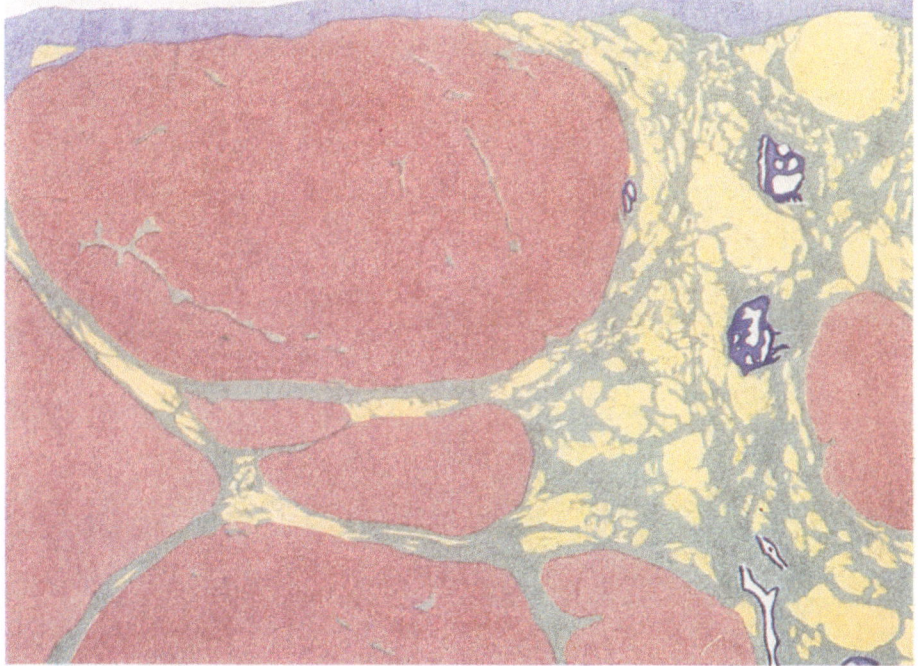

Fig. 10.6. Schema of mixed macro- and micronodular cirrhosis with thick fibrous septa

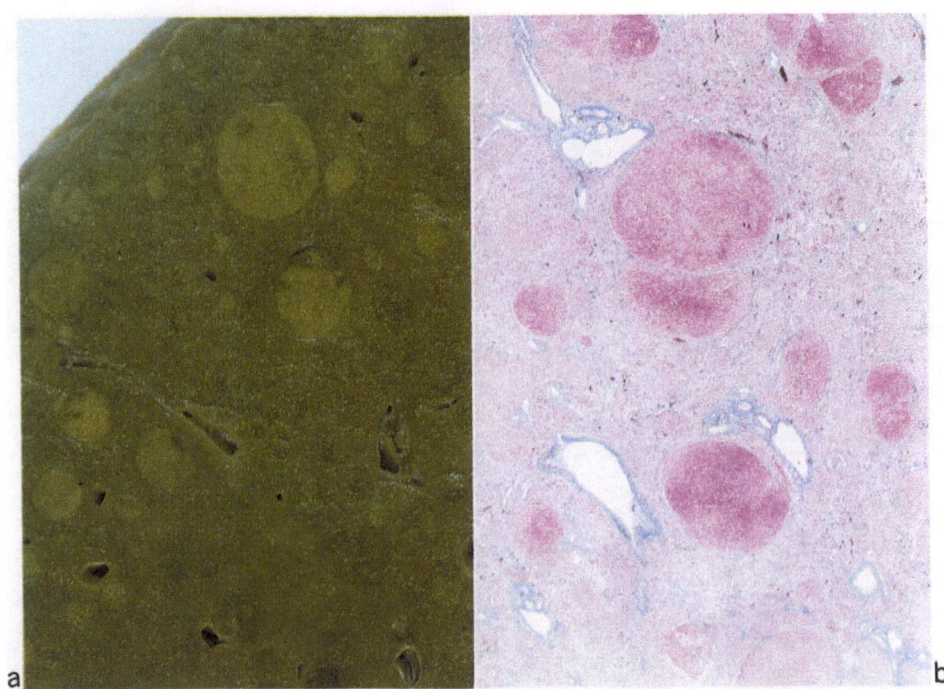

Fig. 10.7a, b. Micronodular cirrhosis. Small cirrhotic nodules are separated by thick fibrous septa.
a Gross features; **b** Azan-Mallory, × 1

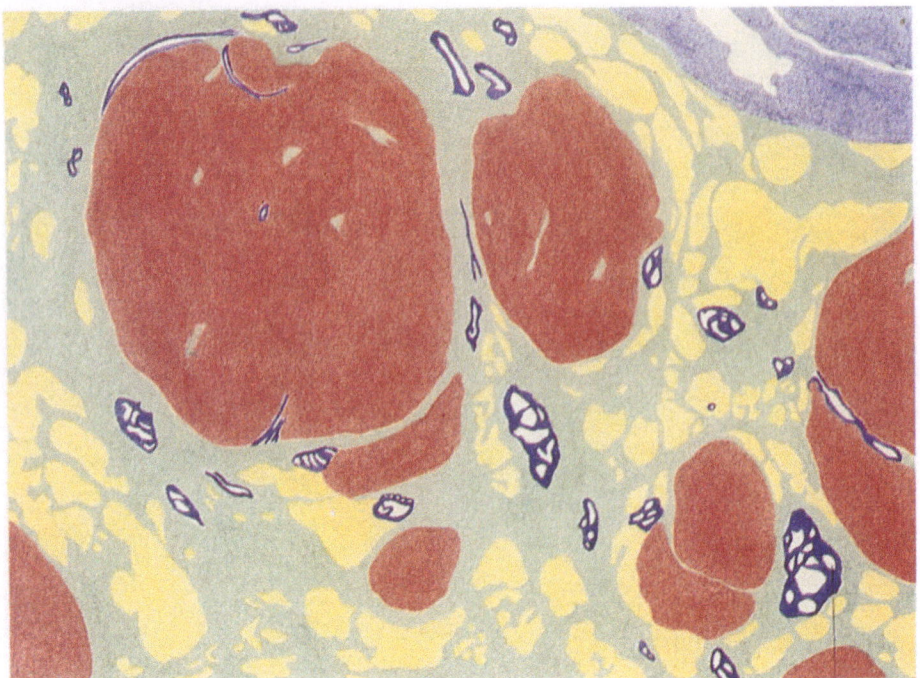

Fig. 10.8. Schema of micronodular cirrhosis

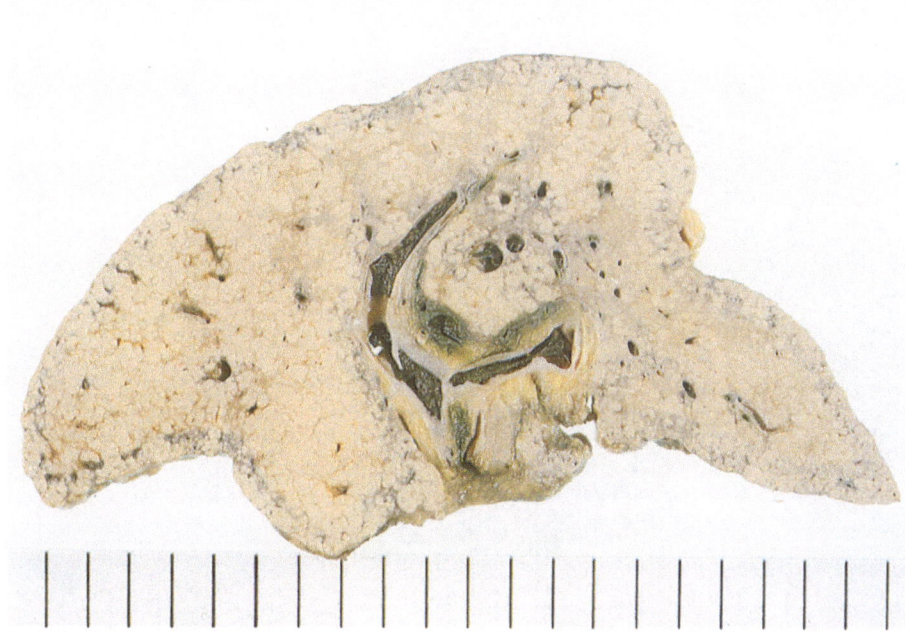

Fig. 10.9. Alcoholic liver cirrhosis

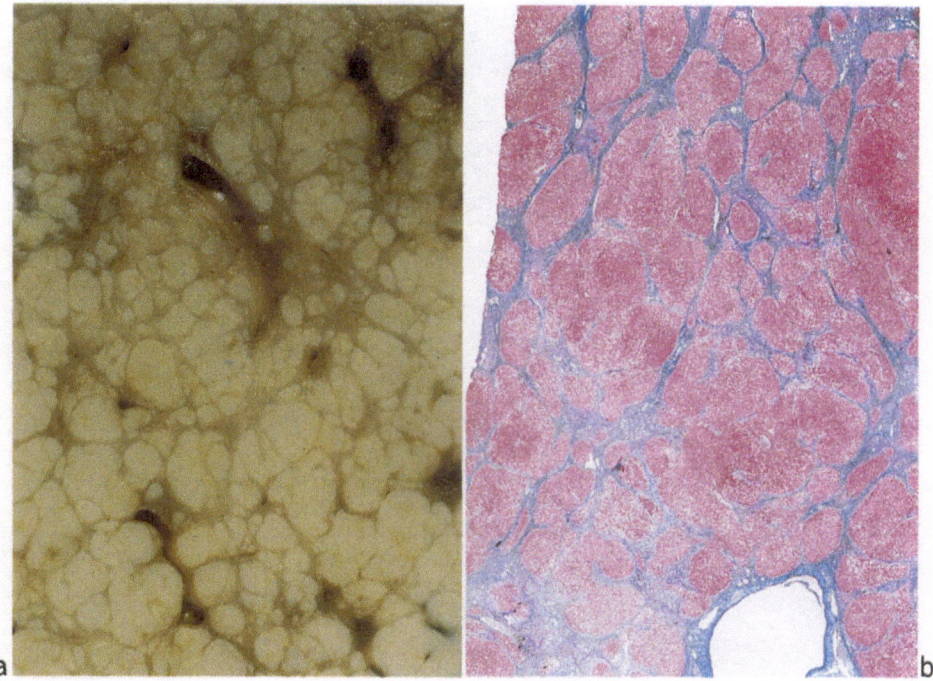

Fig. 10.10a, b. Same case. Cirrhotic nodules vary in size. **a** Gross features; **b** Azan-Mallory, × 1

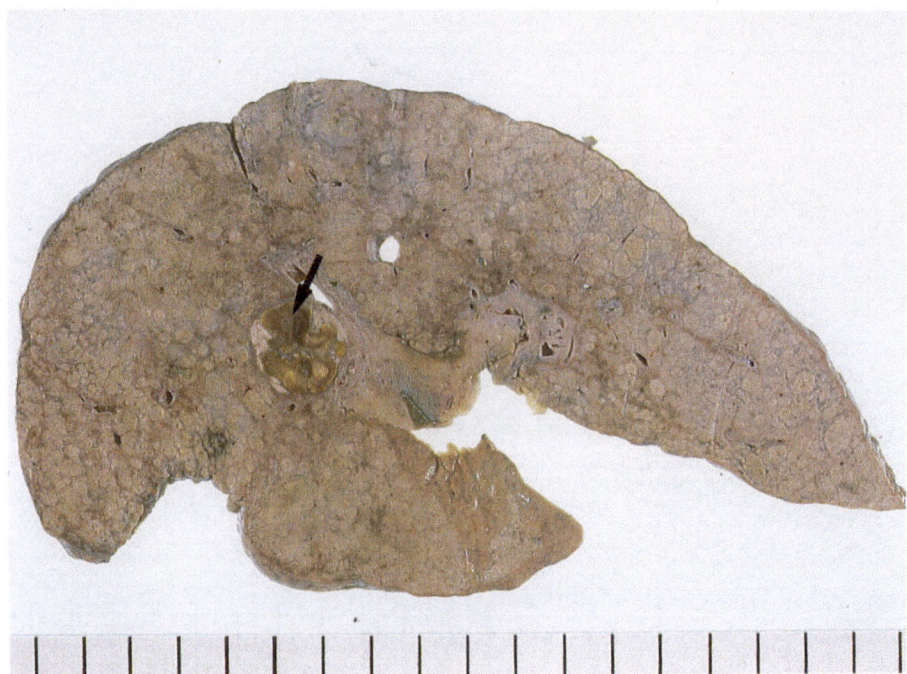

Fig. 10.11. Alcoholic liver cirrhosis with small liver cancer (*arrow*)

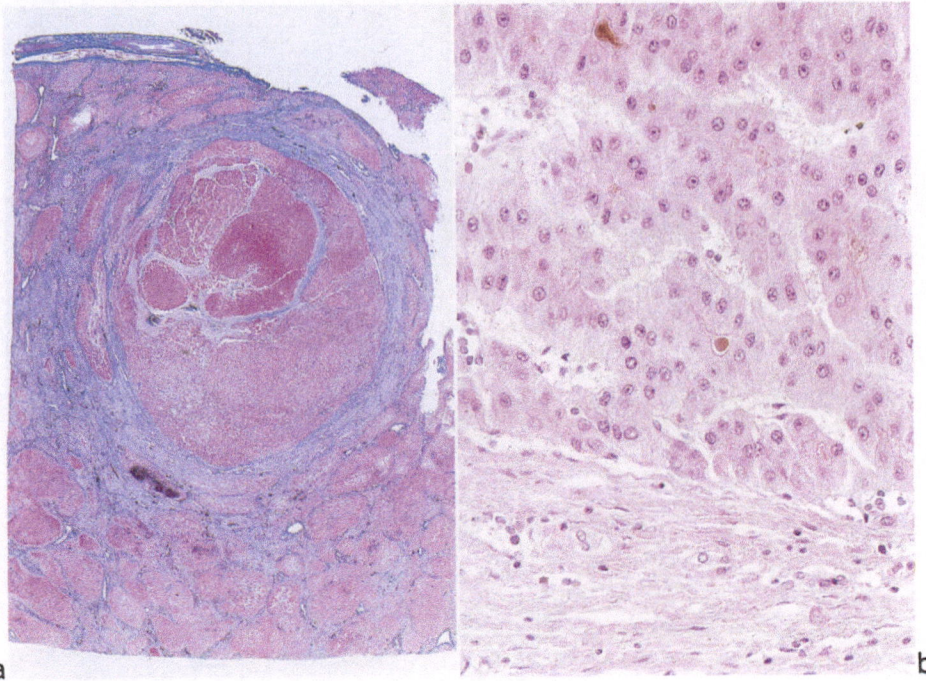

Fig. 10.12a, b. Same case. The small liver cancer is encapsulated and well-differentiated. **a** Azan-Mallory, × 1; **b** HE, × 200

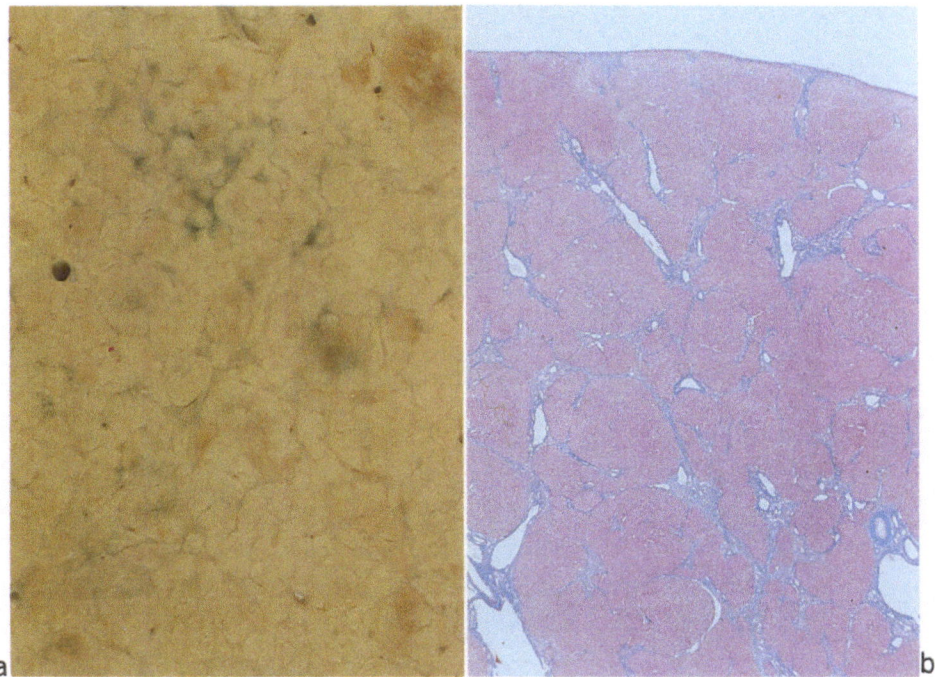

Fig. 10.13a, b. Precirrhotic liver. Formation of cirrhotic nodules is incomplete. **a** Gross features; **b** Azan-Mallory, × 1

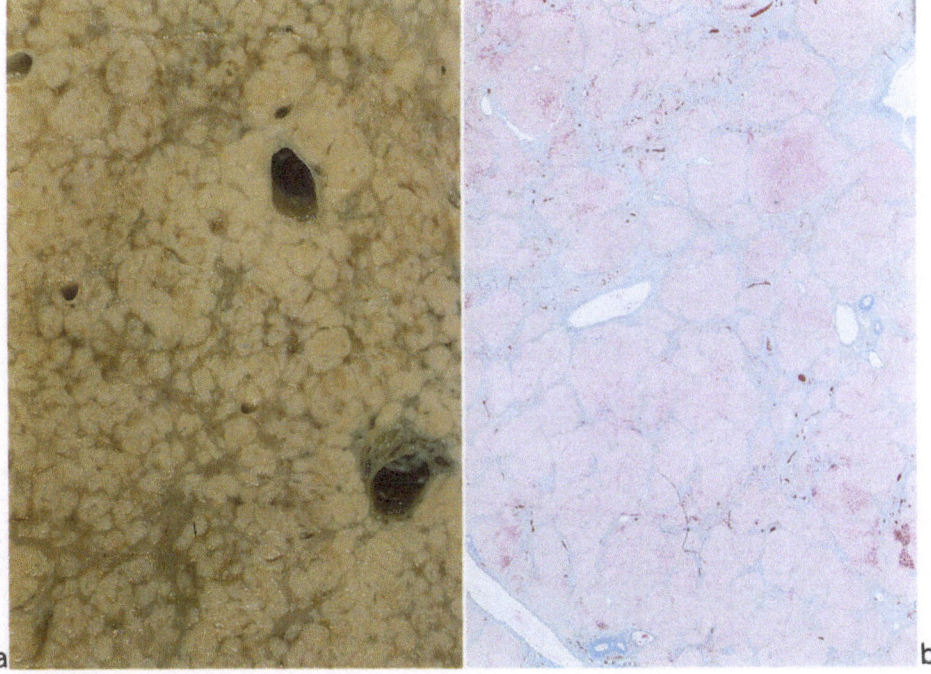

Fig. 10.14a, b. Congestive liver cirrhosis. The hepatic veins are dilated. **a** Gross features; **b** Azan-Mallory, × 1

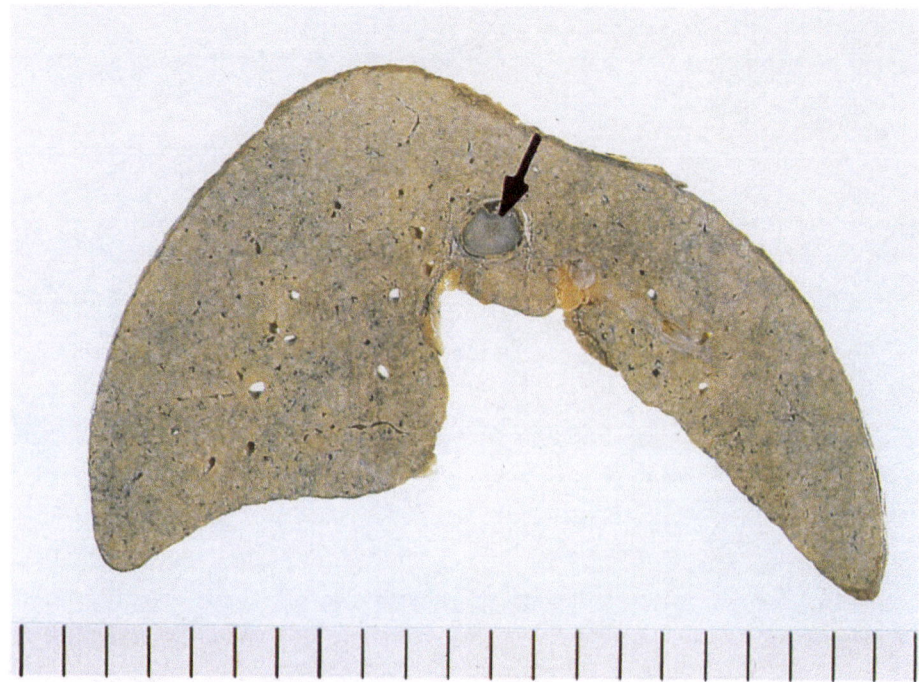

Fig. 10.15. Congestive liver cirrhosis with small liver cancer (*arrow*)

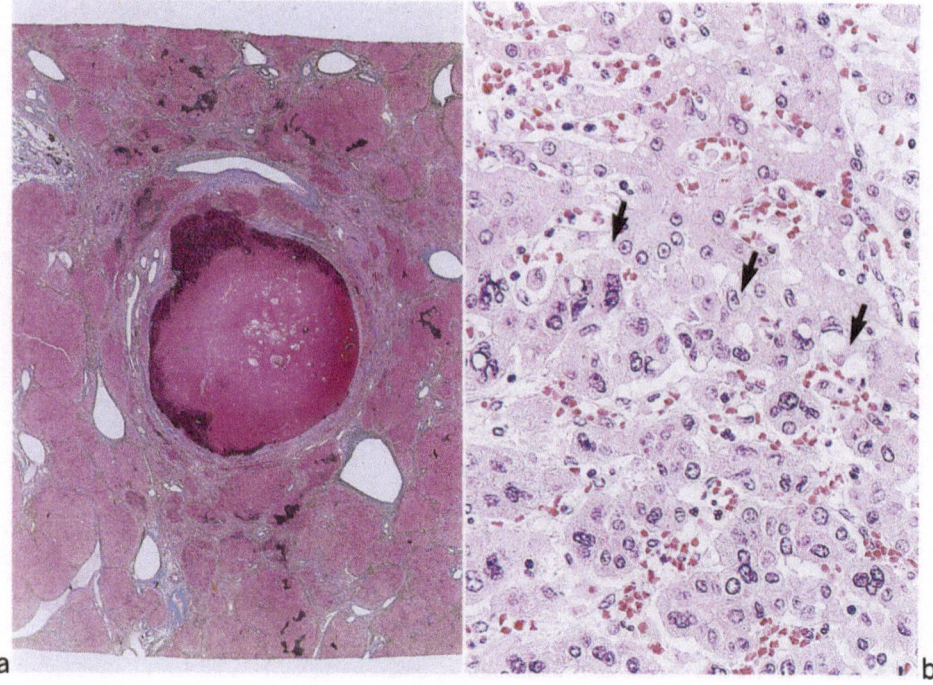

Fig. 10.16a, b. Same case. **a** The small liver cancer is encapsulated and necrotic. **b** Replacing growth (*arrows*) of extracapsular HCC cells. **a** Azan-Mallory, × 1; **b** HE, × 200

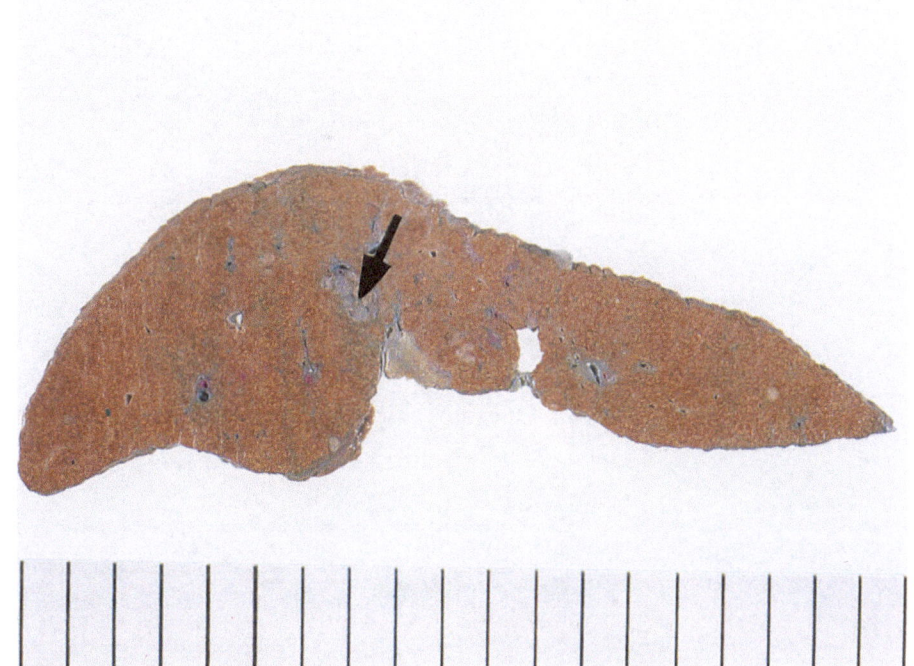

Fig. 10.17. Liver cirrhosis due to hemochromatosis. Grossly, the liver shows a brownish color due to excessive hemosiderin deposition. Small liver cancer is associated (*arrow*).

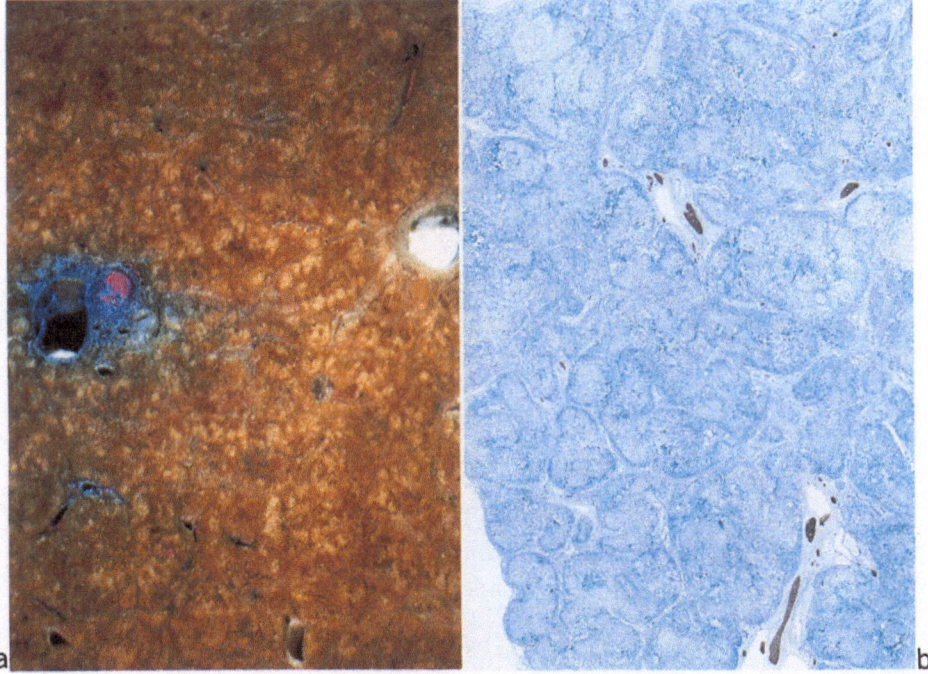

Fig. 10.18a, b. Same case. **a** Close-up view. **b** Excessive hemosiderin deposition. Berlin blue, × 1

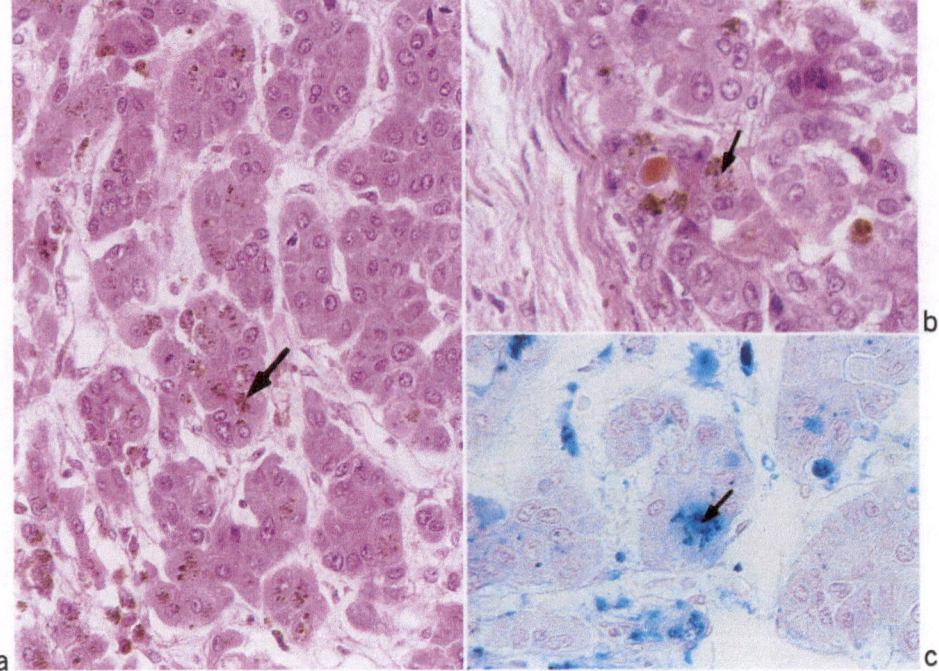

Fig. 10.19a, b. Same case. **a** Intrahepatic metastasis of HCC (*arrow*). Hemosiderin deposits in the noncancerous area. **b** Hemosiderin deposits in cirrhotic nodules. HE; **a** × 20, **b** × 50

Fig. 10.20a–c. Same case. **a, b** Hepatocyte with hemosiderin deposition (*arrow*) retained in HCC tissue. HE; **a** × 100, **b** × 200. **c** Hemosiderin deposition in hepatocytes (*arrow*). Berlin blue, × 200

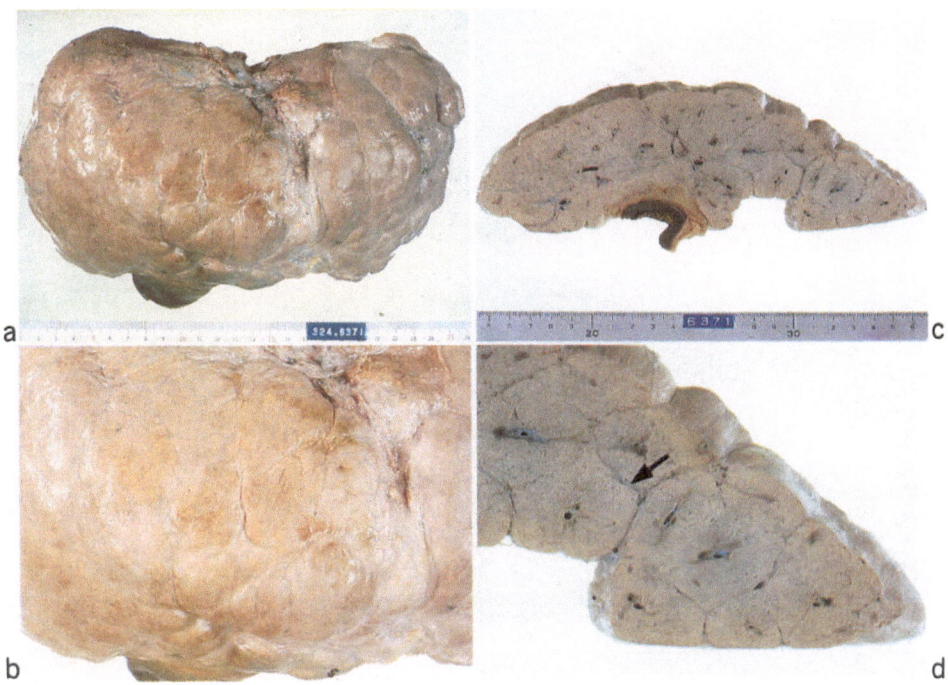

Fig. 10.21a–d. Liver cirrhosis due to *Schistosoma japonicum*. **a, b** The liver shows a coarse nodular surface, the "tortoise-shell" appearance. **c, d** Thin septa (*arrow*) forming deep furrows

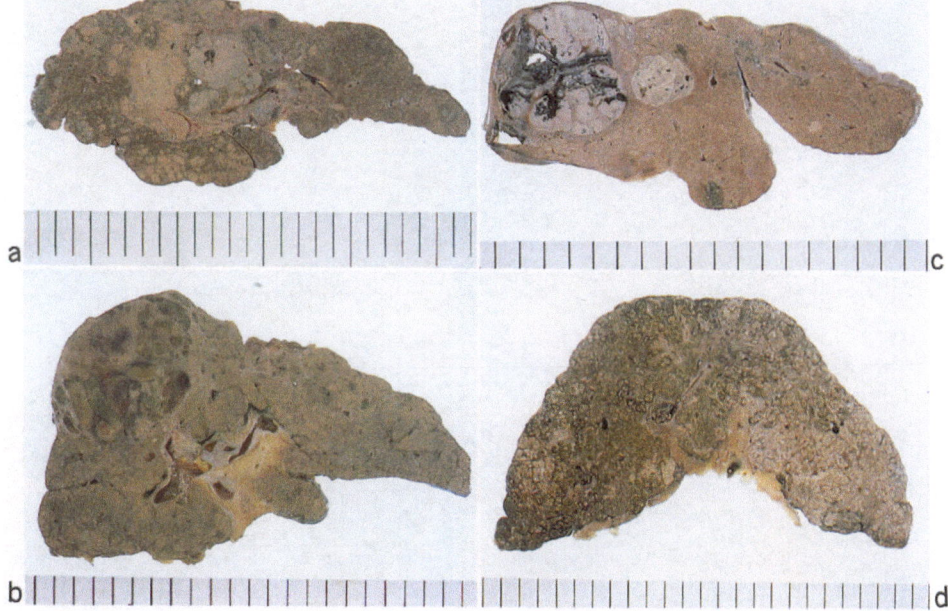

Fig. 10.22a–d. Liver cirrhosis due to *Schistosoma japonicum* bearing HCC. Non-schistosomal hepatic changes are superimposed in all cases

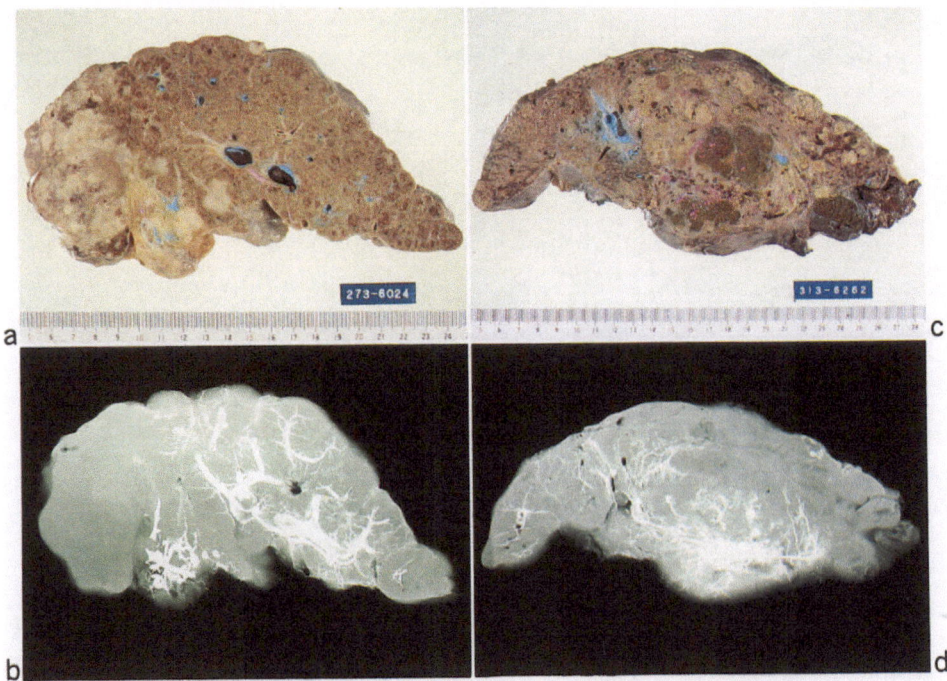

Fig. 10.23a–d. Liver cirrhosis due to *Schistosoma japonicum* bearing HCC. **a, c** Non-schistosomal hepatic changes are superimposed. **b, d** Soft X-ray findings

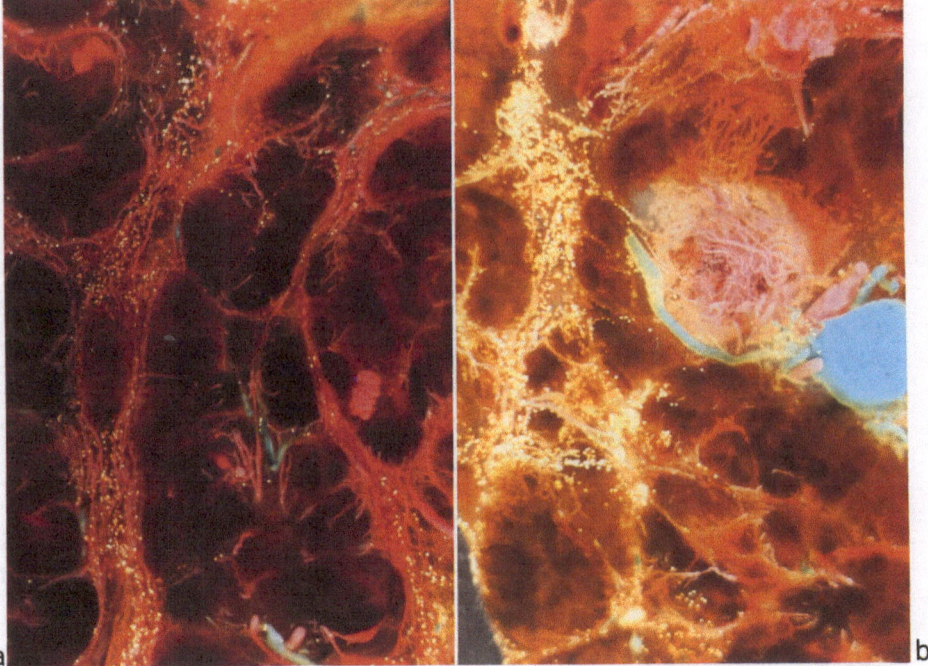

Fig. 10.24a, b. Angioarchitecture of schistosomal liver bearing HCC. **a** Collapse of the portal vein branches in the noncancerous area. **b** The small HCC is nourished solely by arterial tumor vessels. Numerous yellowish granules (eggs) in noncancerous area. Transparent preparation: *red*, artery; *blue*, portal vein

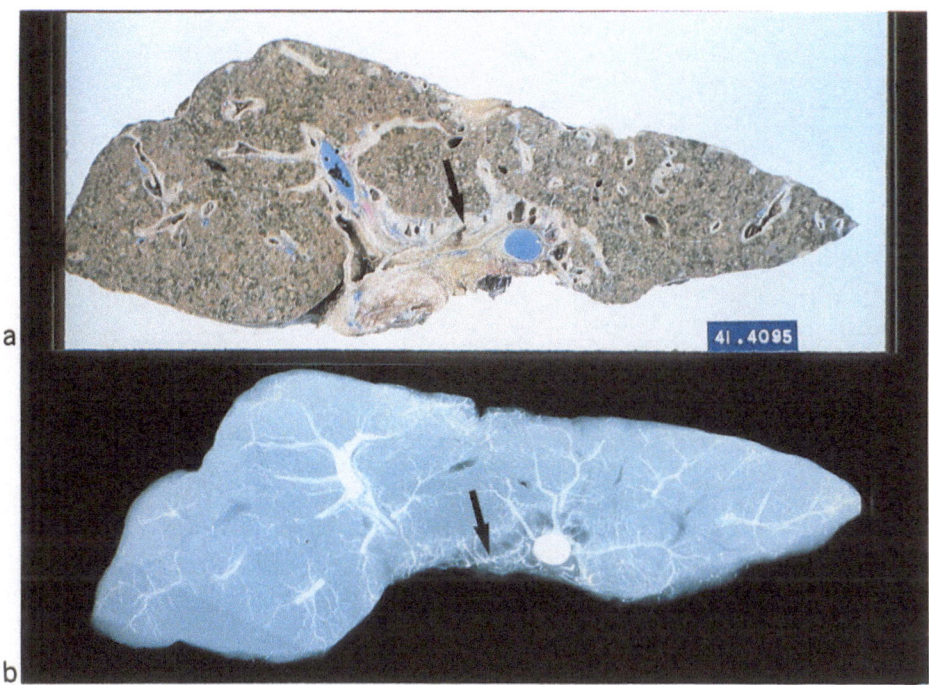

Fig. 10.25a, b. Liver cirrhosis due to *Clonorchis sinensis*. **a** The bile ducts are dilated (*arrow*). **b** Soft X-ray finding. The dilated bile ducts seen as transparent channels (*arrow*)

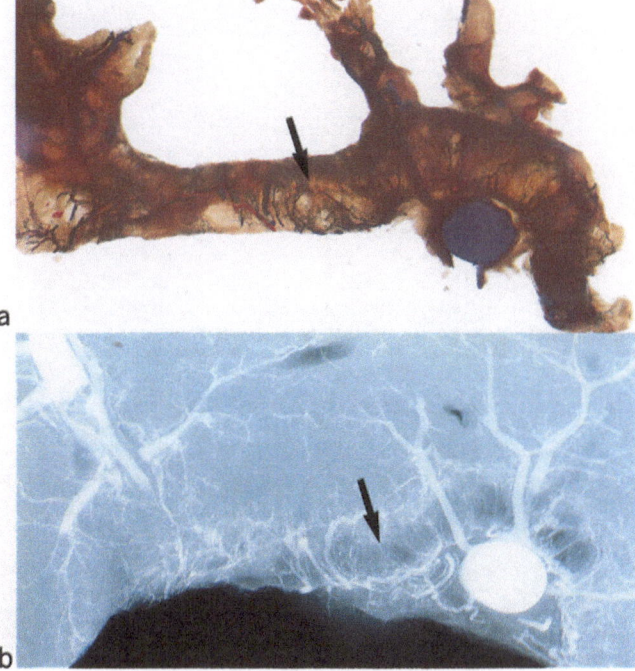

Fig. 10.26a, b. Same case. **a** Markedly dilated bile duct. Increased arterial and portal vein branches surround the bile duct (*arrow*). **b** Soft X-ray view of the same bile duct (*arrow*)

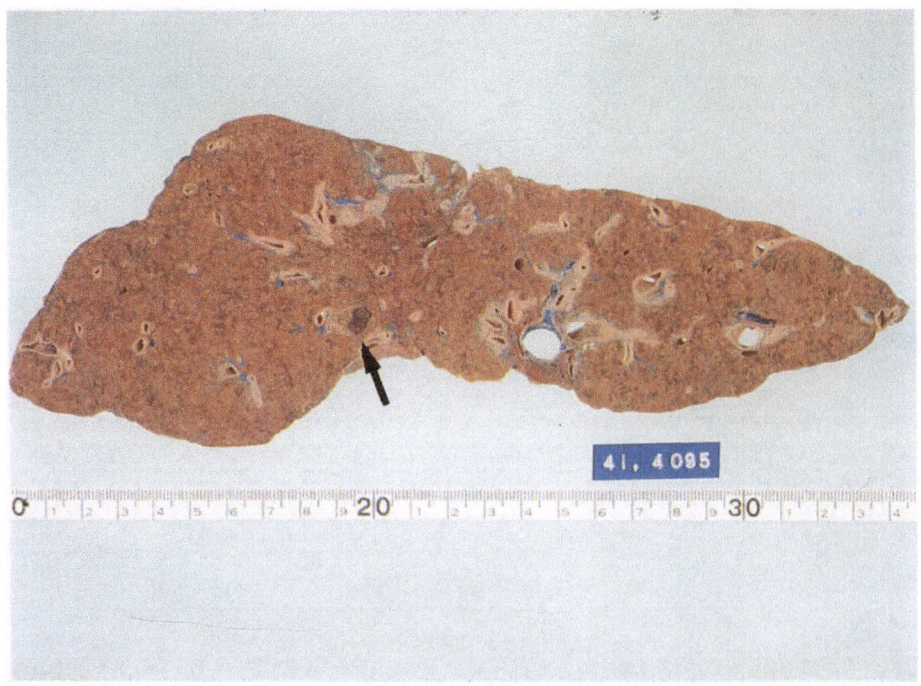

Fig. 10.27. Liver cirrhosis due to *Clonorchis sinensis* bearing small liver cancer (*arrow*)

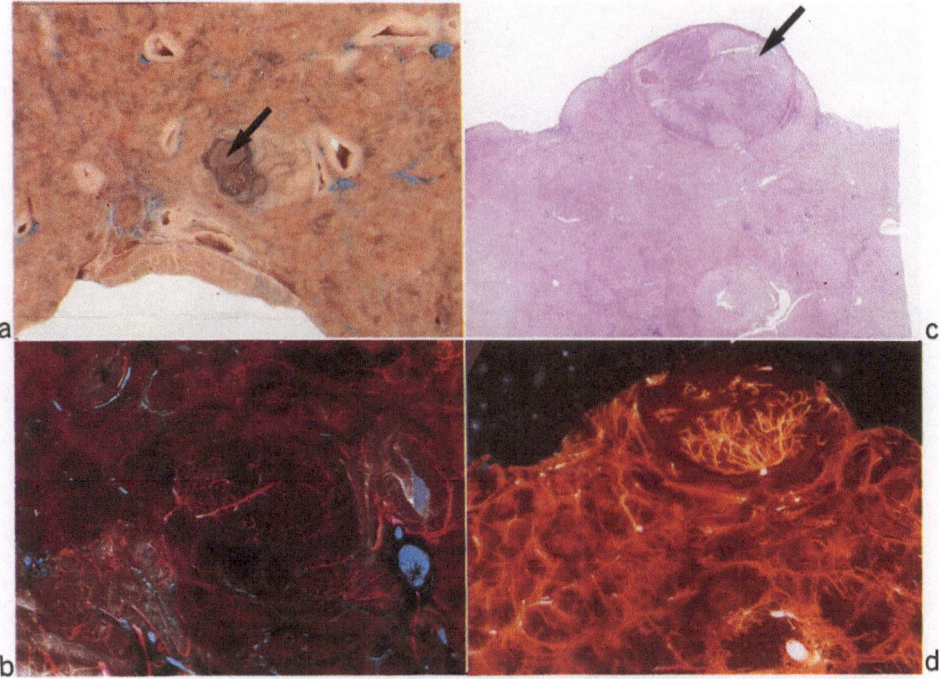

Fig. 10.28a–d. Liver cirrhosis due to *Clonorchis sinensis* bearing small liver cancer. **a** The associated small liver cancer displays remarkable necrosis in part (*arrow*). **b** The necrotic area of the small liver cancer is avascular. **c** Small liver cancer occurring beneath the capsule of the cirrhotic liver (*arrow*). **d** The small liver cancer is hypervascular. **b, d** Transparent preparations

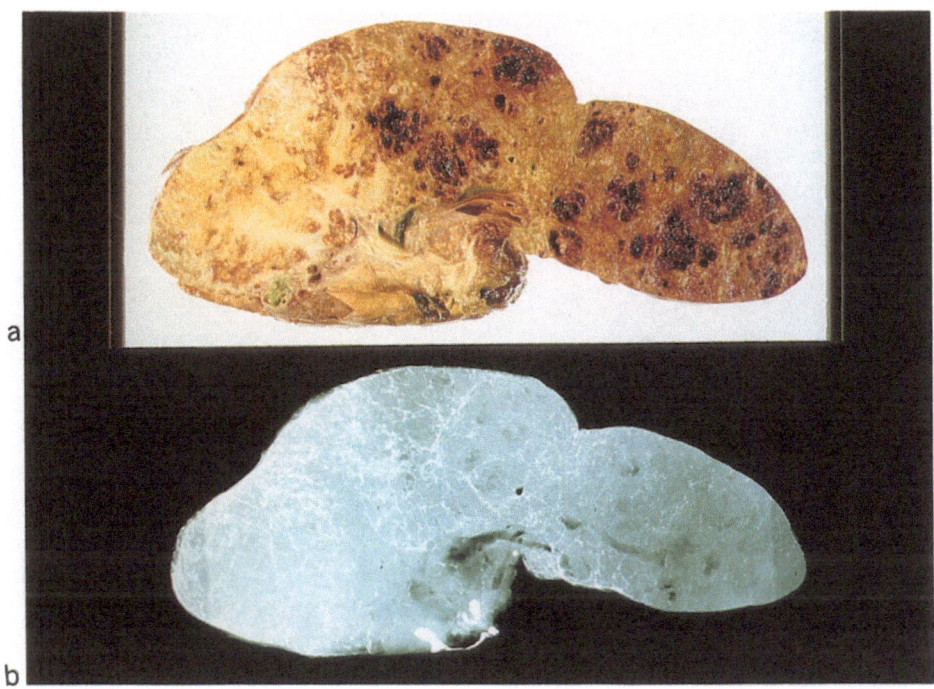

Fig. 10.29. a Thorotrast liver with coexisting HCC, angiosarcoma and cholangiocarcinoma. **b** Soft X-ray finding. The Thorotrast depositions are seen as reticular shadows

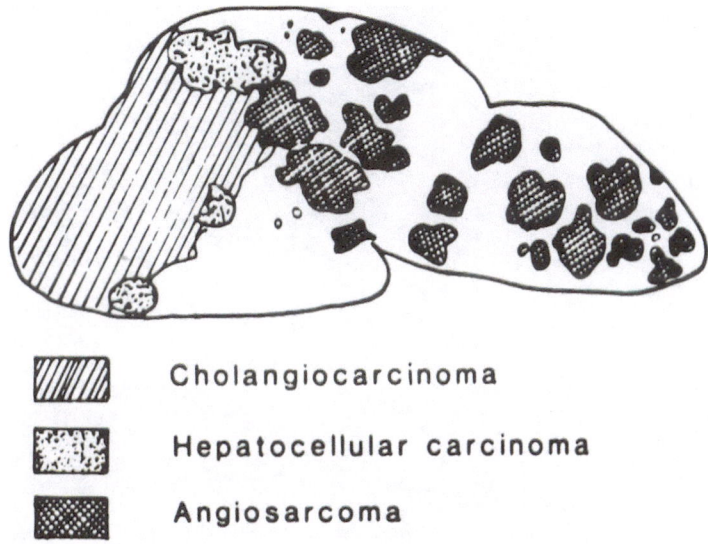

Cholangiocarcinoma

Hepatocellular carcinoma

Angiosarcoma

Fig. 10.30. Same case. Schema of the distribution of each type of tumor

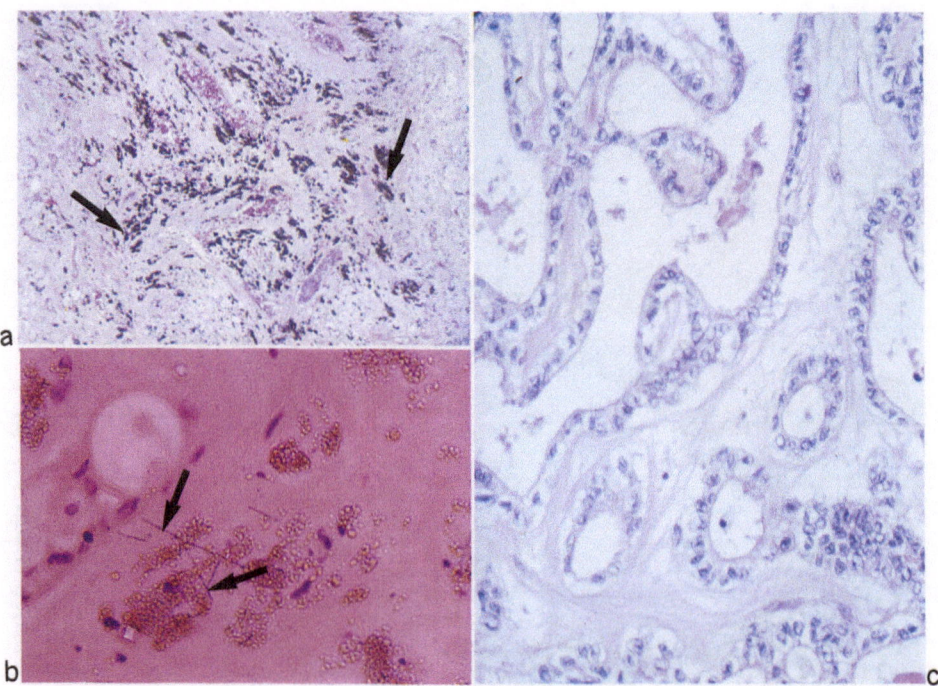

Fig. 10.31a–c. Thorotrast liver. **a** Thorotrast depositions (*arrows*). HE, × 20. **b** α-ray tracks (*arrows*) from Thorotrast depositions. Autoradiogram, × 200. **c** Cholangiocarcinoma. HE, × 200

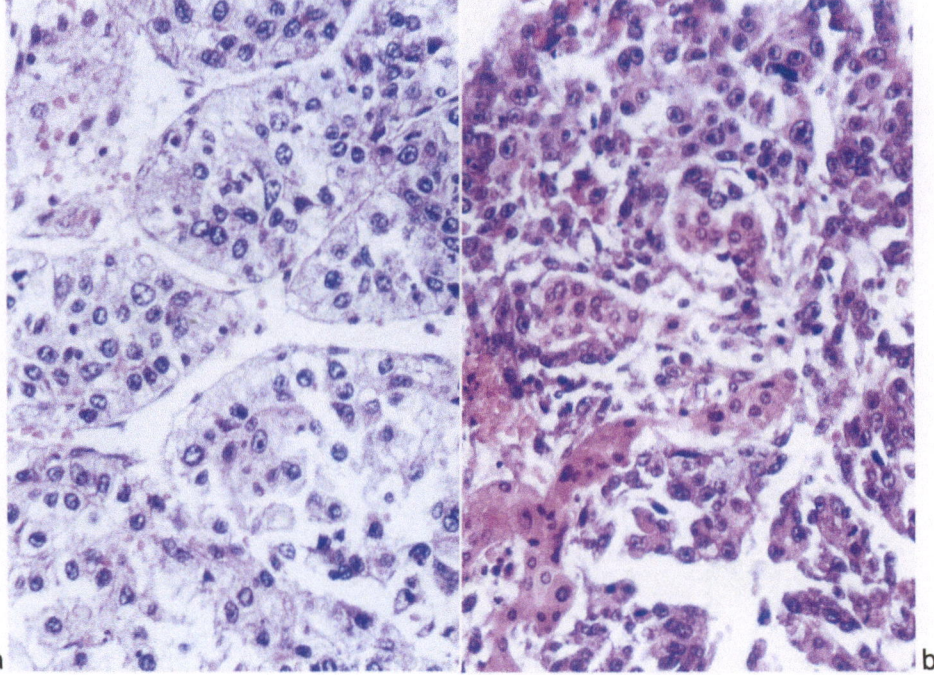

Fig. 10.32a, b. Trabecular HCC (**a**) and angiosarcoma (**b**) in Thorotrast liver. HE, × 200

Chapter 11
Hepatitis B Virus
and Hepatocellular Carcinoma

Serum HBs Ag and HCC

It is well known that HBs Ag in serum is more frequently positive in patients with HCC than in controls in any given area. The incidence of HBV markers in serum is five- to ten-fold higher in patients with HCC than in controls. Viral hepatitis may lead to liver cirrhosis through the chronic phase and go on to HCC. This process has been closely related to healthy carriers of HBs Ag in epidemiological studies.

HBs Ag in serum and tissue
The positive rate of HBs Ag in the serum in healthy people varies widely from country to country. The rate has been reported to be 2.6% in Japan, 4.5% in China, 12.2% in Hong Kong, and 16.1% in the Philippines [206]. The positive rate among HCC patients also varies markedly in different countries. Serum HBs Ag was positive in 5.8% of HCC cases in the United States [207] and in 62% in South Africa [208], In Taiwan, the rate is remarkably high at 80% (44 of 55 cases) [209, 210]. Both serum and hepatic tissue were examined for HBs Ag in 240 cases of our series. HBs Ag was positive in the serum of 81 (33.7%) cases and positive in the hepatic tissue of 65 (27.0%) cases. The difference between the two rates may be attributed to the uneven distribution of the antigen in the liver.The rate in hepatic tissue is higher than any reported by others, possibly because we examined a slice of the whole liver.

Distribution of HBs Ag in hepatic tissue and histological features of liver
HBs Ag in the liver tissue is positive in 3.5% of 28 cases of HCC without histological evidence of liver cirrhosis and fibrotic changes, in 21.1% of HCC in association with hepatic fibrosis, in 9.0% of HCC arising in precirrhotic liver, in 30.4% of HCC associated with posthepatitic cirrhosis, and in 42.8% of HCC with postnecrotic cirrhosis. These results suggest a close correlation of posthepatitic cirrhosis and postnecrotic cirrhosis with viral B hepatitis.

Distribution of HBs Ag in liver tissue
In 240 autopsy cases of HCC, specimens of the liver were examined for HBs Ag by orcein stain and/or immunoperoxidase method (Figs. 11.1–8). HBs Ag was found to be positive in 65 (27.0%) cases. According to Sakurai and Miyaji [211], intrahepatic distribution of HBs Ag can be roughly divided into two types—massive distribution and spotty distribution—and intracellular distribution into three types—diffuse type, inclusion-body type, and mixed type. The diffuse type of intracellular

distribution tends to be coupled with intrahepatic distribution of the massive type, and the inclusion-body type with spotty distribution. In our series of HCC, in cases associated with posthepatitic cirrhosis, the intracellular distribution of HBs Ag is of inclusion-body or mixed type, and in case in association with postnecrotic cirrhosis or hepatic fibrosis, the intracellular distribution of HBs Ag tends to be diffuse. The intrahepatic distribution of HBs Ag-positive cells, as estimated by a reconstruction method, varies widely. The positive cells may be distributed throughout the pseudo-lobules in various manners, such as spotty distribution and massive distribution. Therefore, it is quite difficult to describe quantitatively the precise distribution of HBs Ag-positive cells in the hepatic lobules.

HCC and viral hepatitis

Epidemiological and other evidence strongly suggests a possible etiological relationship between HBV infection and HCC. Exposure to HBV can be followed by acute and chronic hepatitis. In addition, it has been noted that there is a significantly high incidence HCC in HBs Ag carriers. Recent progress in molecular biology has provided another approach to investigating the relationship between HCC and HBV.

Demonstration of HBs Ag in the HCC cell line, and integration of HBV DNA into DNA of HCC cells have been reported by various authors [30–34]. In addition, when replication of the virus is partly suppressed, the whole genome of the virus or a part of the genome which is responsible for tumorigenesis is incorporated into chromatin DNA during cell division of hepatic cells, and protein synthesized according to the abnormal DNA may alter normal cells into tumor cells through some mechanism. Thus, there is striking progress in this field. Integration of HBV DNA into HCC DNA has also been identified in serum HBs Ag-negative cases.

Distribution of HBs Ag-positive cells in tumor tissue of HCC

Bartok et al. [212], who examined the localization of HBs Ag in liver tissue using orcein stain, did not observe HBs Ag in any HCC cells. According to Cohen et al. [213], the cytoplasm of cancer cells revealed an orcein-positive reaction in 3 (6%) of 50 cases of HCC. Hsu et al. [214] found HBs Ag-positive tumor cells in 27 (21.1%) of 223 cases of HCC. In our autopsy series of HCC, HBs Ag-positive cells are demonstrated in the tumor tissue in ten cases [215]. The growth pattern of HCC tissue at the tumor-nontumor boundary is of either the sinusoidal or the replacing type in most of the ten cases. HBs Ag-positive cells are frequently located near the boundary in nine cases. Such HBs Ag-positive cells are estimated to be HBs Ag-positive hepatocytes left behind in the tumor tissue on the extension of HCC. In the remaining one case, of the encapsulated type, the HBs Ag-positive cells are identified in the center of the cancer nodule, and the possibility that they are cancer cells cannot be excluded (Fig. 11.6). No HBs Ag-positive cells can be demonstrated in the tumor thrombus of the portal vein or in metastatic foci. This also suggests that there is a strong possibility that HBs Ag-positive cancer cells are hardly detectable at the immunohistochemical level.

Liver Cell Dysplasia

Anthony [216] defined liver cell dysplasia (LCD) as cellular enlargement, nuclear pleomorphism, and multinucleation of liver cells occuring in groups or occupying whole cirrhotic lobules and considered it precancerous change. Since he reported LCD as a premalignant condition, its significance has been discussed, but no conclusion has been reached [217–220]. The reported incidence of LCD ranges from 25% to 65.7%, but it is present in cirrhotic liver bearing HCC in all reports. Furthermore, a close relationship with HBs Ag is suggested. In our series, LCD was found in 30% of the cases, but most dysplastic hepatocytes were found to be negative for HBs Ag (Figs. 11.7, 8).

According to the evidence that most minute HCCs consist of extremely well-differentiated tumor cells, as described in Chap. 2, the authors do not regard LCD as a premalignant condition but as an associated feature secondary to the occurrence of HCC.

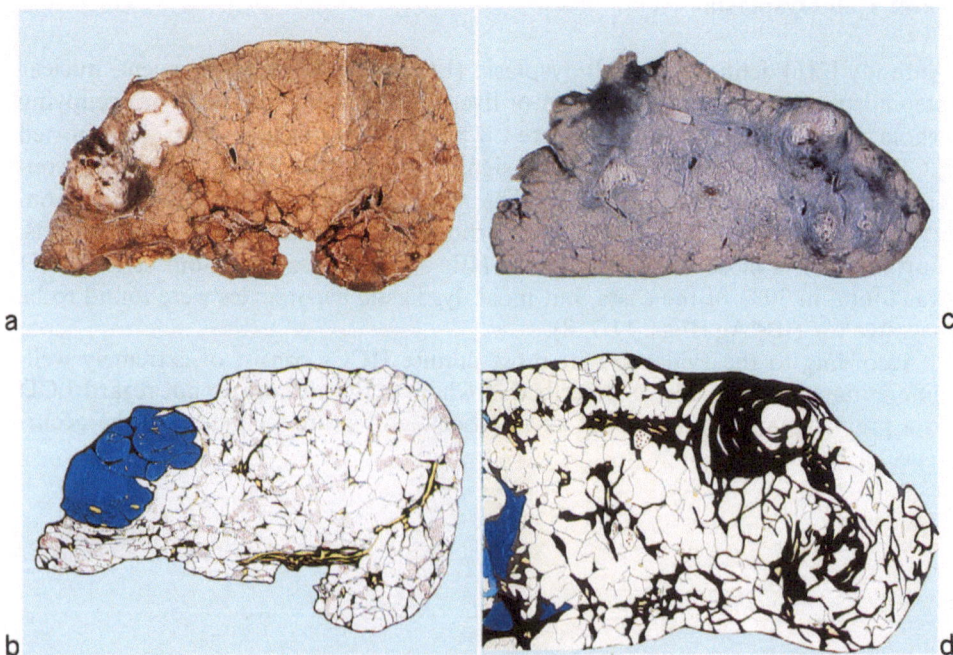

Fig. 11.1a–d. Distribution of HBs Ag-positive cells in mixed macro- and micronodular cirrhosis. The distribution of positive cells is not uniform. *Red dots*, positive cells

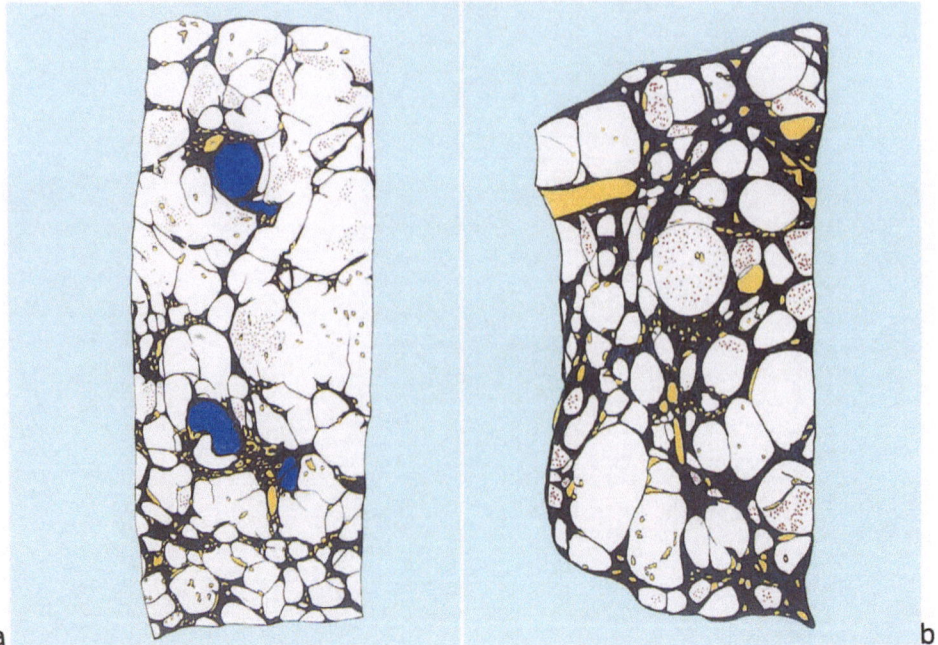

Fig. 11.2a, b. Distribution of HBs Ag-positive cells in liver cirrhosis. **a** Mixed macro- and micro-nudular cirrhosis bearing HCC. **b** Mixed macro- and micronodular cirrhosis with thick fibrous septa bearing HCC. The distribution of the positive cells is not uniform. *Red dots*, positive cells

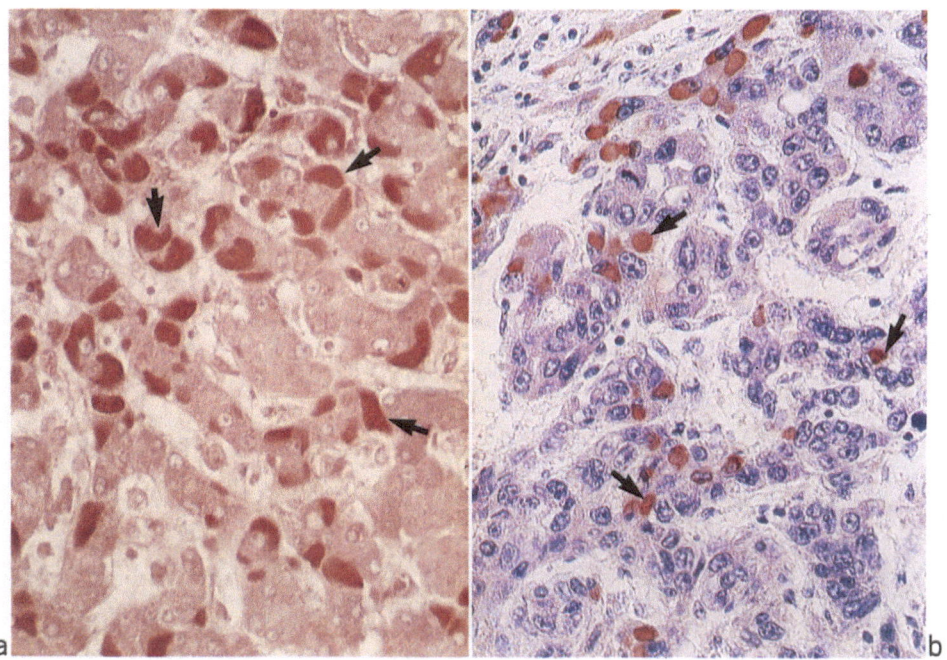

Fig. 11.3a, b. Distribution of HBs Ag-positive cells in the liver. **a** Orcein-positive hepatocytes (*arrows*) in macronodular cirrhosis. Orcein, × 200. **b** HBs Ag-positive cells (*arrows*) in HCC tissue. Immunoperoxidase, × 200

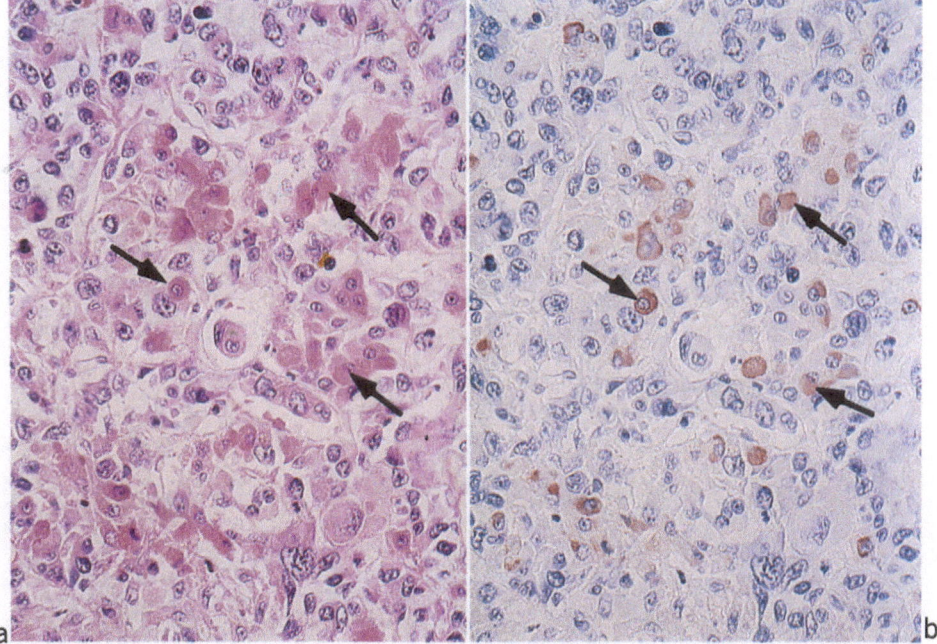

Fig. 11.4a, b. Distribution of HBs Ag-positive cells. **a** Hepatocytes retained in HCC tissue (*arrows*). HE, × 200. **b** Immunoperoxidase method in same specimen. HBs Ag-positive cells (*arrows*) correspond to retained hepatocytes. × 200

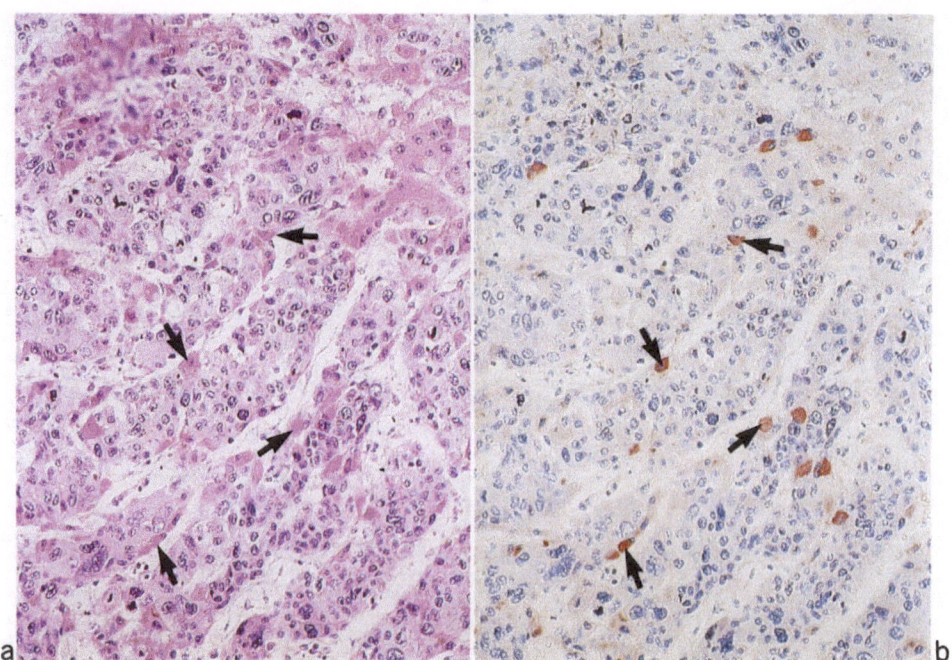

Fig. 11.5a, b. Distribution of HBs Ag-positive cells. **a** Entangled hepatocytes (*arrows*) in trabecular HCC showing a replacing growth pattern. HE, × 100. **b** Immunoperoxidase method in same specimen. HBs Ag-positive cells (*arrows*) correspond to retained hepatocytes in HCC tissue. × 100

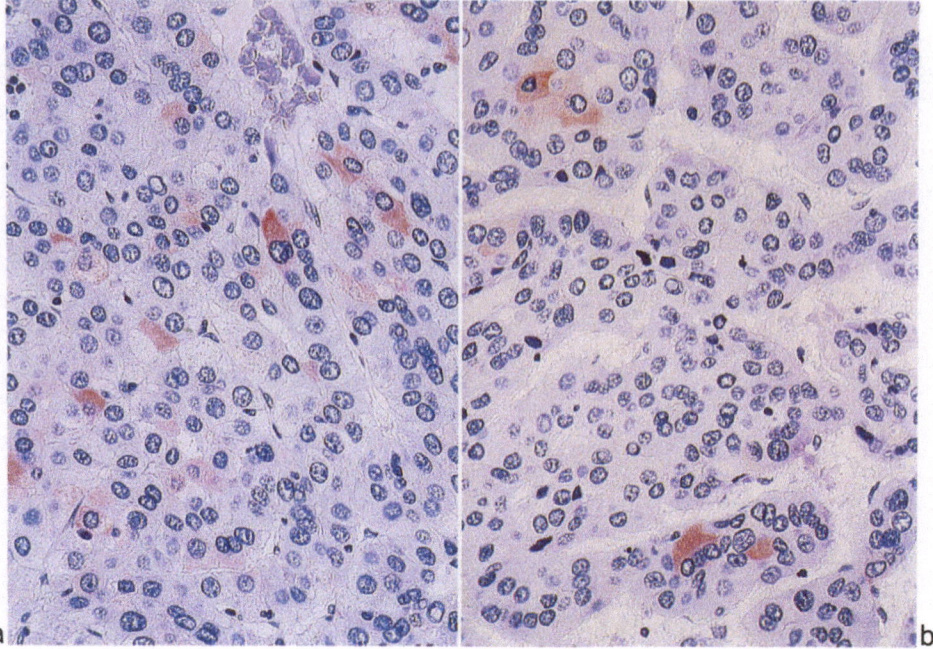

Fig. 11.6a, b. Distribution of HBs Ag-positive cells. HBs Ag-positive cancer cells in the center of encapsulated HCC

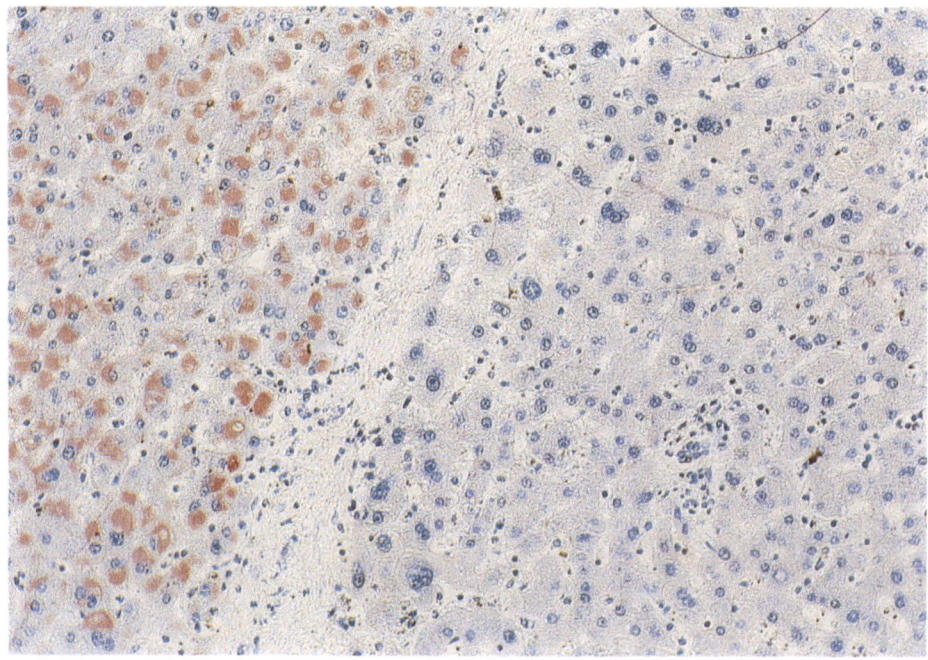

Fig. 11.7 Liver cell dysplasia and HBs Ag. Dysplastic hepatocytes are found to be negative for HBs Ag, but many non-dysplastic hepatocytes in the neighboring pseudolobule are positive. Immunoperoxidase, × 100

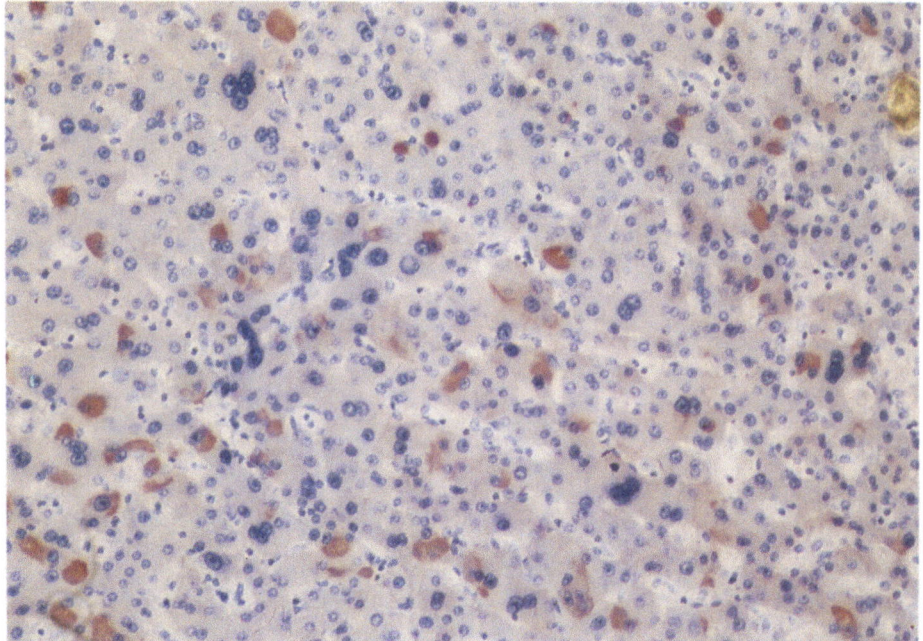

Fig. 11.8. Liver cell dysplasia and HBs Ag. Most of the dysplastic hepatocytes are negative for HBs Ag. Immunoperoxidase, × 100

Chapter 12
Hepatocellular Carcinoma and Multiple Cancer

The incidence of HCC combined with other malignancies arising in organs other than the liver has risen continuously in recent years. As diagnostic techniques for malignant lesions have advanced and effective therapies have been introduced, the resulting early diagnosis and increased survival rate are probably reflected in the steady increase in incidence.

Total Incidence of Multiple Cancer

A total of 100 352 autopsy cases of cancer are listed in the Annual of the Pathological Autopsy Cases in Japan from 1967 to 1974, and multiple cancer was found in 3213 (3.2%) of the these cases [221]. Of 53 353 autopsy cases during the first 4 years, 870 (1.63%) had multiple cancer; the 46 999 autopsy cases for the last 4 years included 2343 (4.98%) multiple cancer cases. The latter figure is about three times higher than the former. The first cancers in the 3213 multiple cancer cases included, in decreasing order of frequency, 918 (0.15%) cases of gastric cancer, 563 (0.13%) of lung cancer, 370 (0.20%) thyroid cancer, 250 (0.14%) of uterine cancer, 205 (0.11%) of colon cancer, 199 (0.11%) HCC, 194 (0.10%) of prostatic cancer, 171 (0.09%) of esophageal cancer, 164 (0.09%) of rectal cancer, 65 (0.2%) of pancreatic cancer, and 114 of other types. Multiple cancer involving HCC accounted for 0.11% of all multiple cases. In our series, the incidence of multiple cancer among autopsy cases of cancer was O.55% (31 of 5545 cases).

In the Annual of the Pathological Autopsy Cases in Japan [221] from 1967 to 1974, of a total of 2292 cases of HCC for the first 4-year period, 49 (2.23%) accompanied other malignant lesions, and 150 (5.09%) multiple cases were found among 2842 HCC cases during the latter 4 years; the rate had doubled. In our series, multiple cancer was found in 8 (5.83%) of 137 HCC cases during the first 7 years and in 23 (8.33%) of 276 HCC cases during the latter 7 years. The rate tended to increase, but the difference was not significant.

Average Age of Patients

In our series of HCC cases, the average ages for males and females were 58.3 ± 10.4 years and 58.3 ± 13.4 years, respectively. The average ages for multiple cancer cases were 64.8 ± 9.5 years and 56.4 ± 18.9 years for males and females, respectively. The difference is significant only in males ($P < 0.01$).

Associated Liver Cirrhosis

Liver cirrhosis was present in 81.2% of HCC cases with other malignancies in our series.

Frequency of Associated Malignancies

In our series, gastric cancer was noted in 6 (18.7%) of 32 cases of HCC associated with other malignancies, followed by large bowel, thyroid, and lung cancer in four (12.5%) cases each, esophageal, pancreatic, laryngeal, and renal cancer in two (6.2%) cases each, and myeloma, cancer of the tongue, malignant lymphoma, Bowen's disease, prostatic cancer, and rectal cancer in one case each. Of the 32 cases, 18 (56.2%) involved cancers arising in the gastrointestinal tract. This result was to be expected, as cancers of the gastrointestinal tract are the most common kind in Japan.

According to Nakamura and Aizawa [222], HCC associated with gastric cancer was found in 39 (6%) of 1129 multiple cases. It occurred more frequently in males; the high incidence in males is characteristic of this combination. In our series, all six such multiple cases occurred in men.

Metastasis in HCC with Other Cancers

In our series, extrahepatic metastases were seen in 63.3% of the total 439 HCC cases and in 56.2% of the 32 cases associated with other forms of cancer (Figs. 12.1–8). There is no significant difference between the two figures. Malignant tumors combined with HCC very seldom metastasize (21.8%). The rate is still as low as 24.4% even if five cases of occult cancer of the thyroid and prostate are excluded. Of the 32 cases of HCC with other kinds of cancer, three cases—one each of renal cancer, lymphoma (Figs. 11.3, 4) and esophageal cancer—showed metastasis to the liver, and histological and macroscopic examination of a whole liver slice in each case demonstrated a metastasis within the HCC lesion only in the case of the renal cancer (Figs. 11.1, 2). In one case of HCC coupled with esophageal cancer, the esophageal cancer formed a tumor thrombus of the portal vein but had no contact with the HCC lesion (Figs. 11.5–8). In addition, histological study revealed that the esophageal cancer cells in the liver extended into the sinusoid in a manner entirely different from the replacing growth pattern of HCC cells.

HCC Associated with Sarcoma

A few cases of HCC associated with sarcoma have been reported [223, 224]. It is quite characteristic of HCC for the histological pattern to vary widely among cases and even within a single case or single focus. Occasionally, HCC appears sarcomatous in addition to these typical characteristics. In such lesions, cells of spindle-shaped or free-cell type proliferate into the sinusoid in the sarcomatous area, while those typical of HCC proliferate in a replacing fashion. Some of these lesions are indistinguishable from true sarcomas due to the sarcomatous changes. The incidence of sarcomatous cases has increased in cases of survival with advances in chemotherapy for HCC, which suggests that such therapy may alter the histological pattern of HCC.

Triple Cancer

In our series, triple cancer was found in 3 (9.37%) of the 32 cases of HCC and multiple cancer.

The combinations of associated malignancies in triple cancer were as follows: HCC, cancer of the tongue, and gastric cancer; HCC, lung cancer, and rectal cancer; HCC, lung cancer, and colon cancer. In the first case, widespread metastasis of the tongue cancer to the liver was prominent but there was no metastasis of the gastric cancer to the liver. In the second case, hematogenous metastases of the lung cancer were found bilaterally in the kidneys and skin and there was infiltrative extension to the aortic arch, but there was no metastasis of the HCC or the rectal cancer. In the third case, there was no metastasis of any of the three cancers.

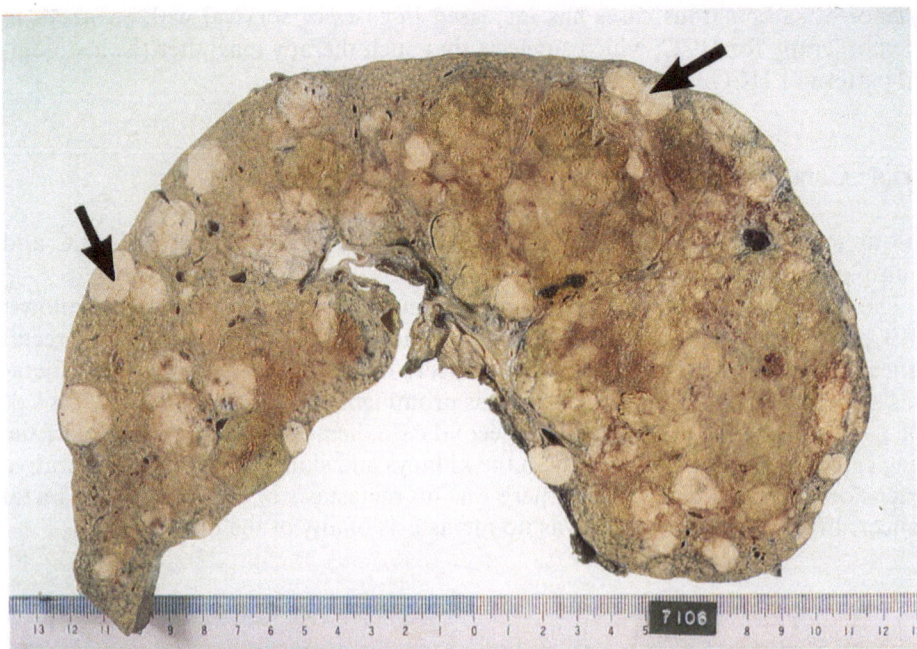

Fig. 12.1. HCC coupled with renal cell carcinoma. Many whitish-gray metastatic nodules of renal cell carcinoma (*arrows*) are distinguishable from the HCC nodules

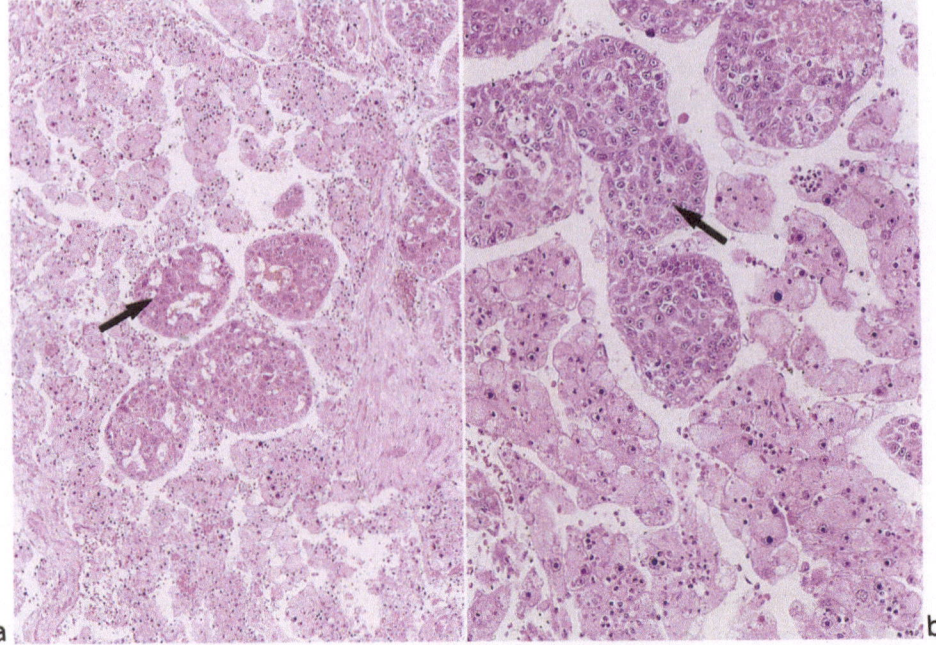

Fig. 12.2a, b. Same case. **a** HCC tumor nests (*arrow*) in metastasized renal cell carcinoma. **b** Coexistence of HCC tumor nest (*arrow*) and renal cell carcinoma. HE; **a** × 50, **b** × 100

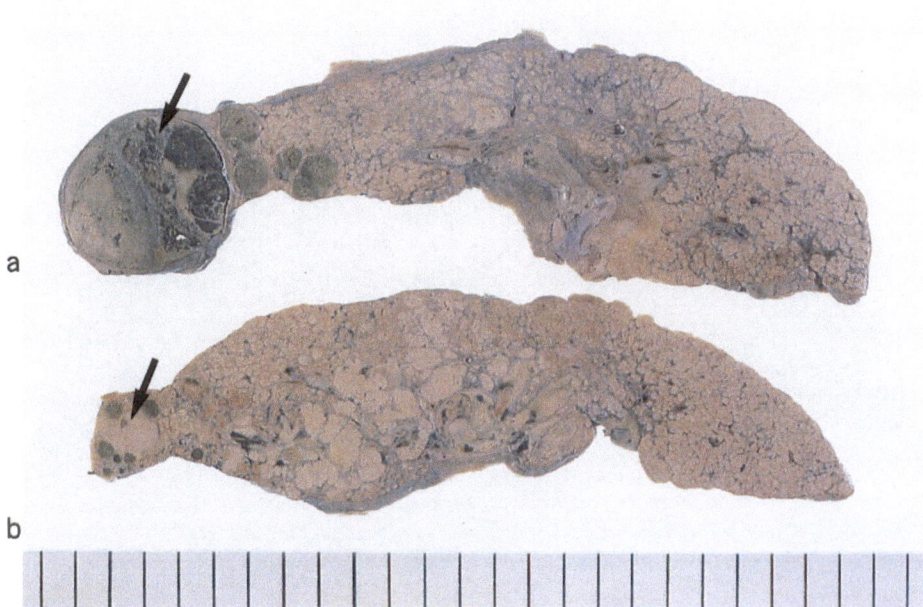

Fig. 12.3a, b. HCC coupled with malignant lymphoma. **a** The HCC tumor is encapsulated (*arrow*) and is greenish in color due to bile production. **b** Small HCC nodules showing a greenish color are observed beside the malignant lymphoma (*arrow*)

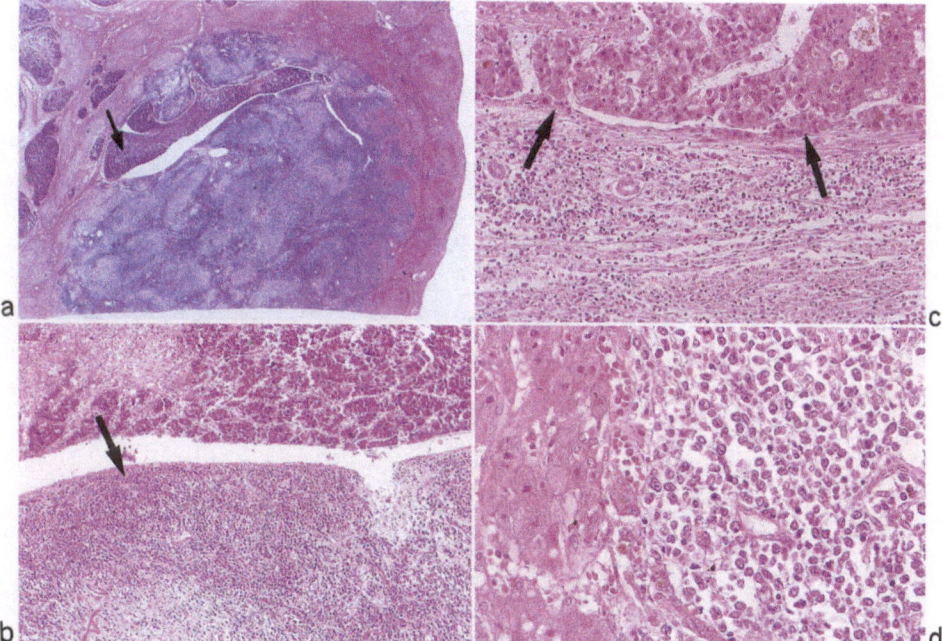

Fig. 12.4a–d. Same case. **a** Tumor thrombus of HCC in the portal vein (*arrow*) entangled in lymphoma focus. **b** Malignant lymphoma (*arrow*) and trabecular HCC (*upper half*) are not mixed. **c** The HCC is enclosed by a thin fibrous capsule (*arrows*). **d** Non-Hodgkin's lymphoma cells are proliferating in a sinusoidal growth fashion. HE; **a** × 10, **b** × 20, **c** × 50, **d** × 100

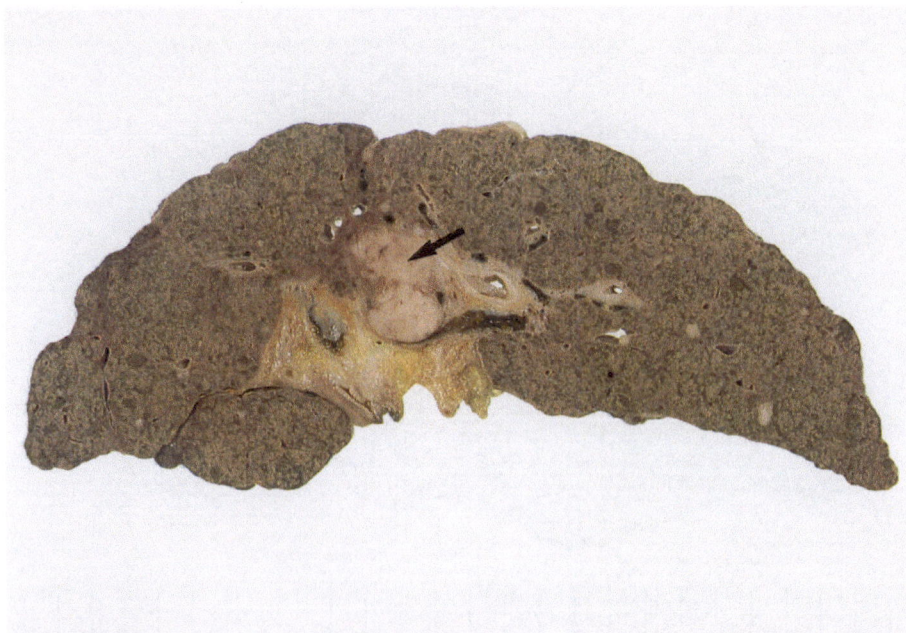

Fig. 12.5. Combined hepatocellular and cholangiocarcinoma coupled with esophageal cancer. There are metastatic nodules of esophageal cancer (*arrow*) in the hepatic hilum. Liver cancer is seen as small greenish nodules

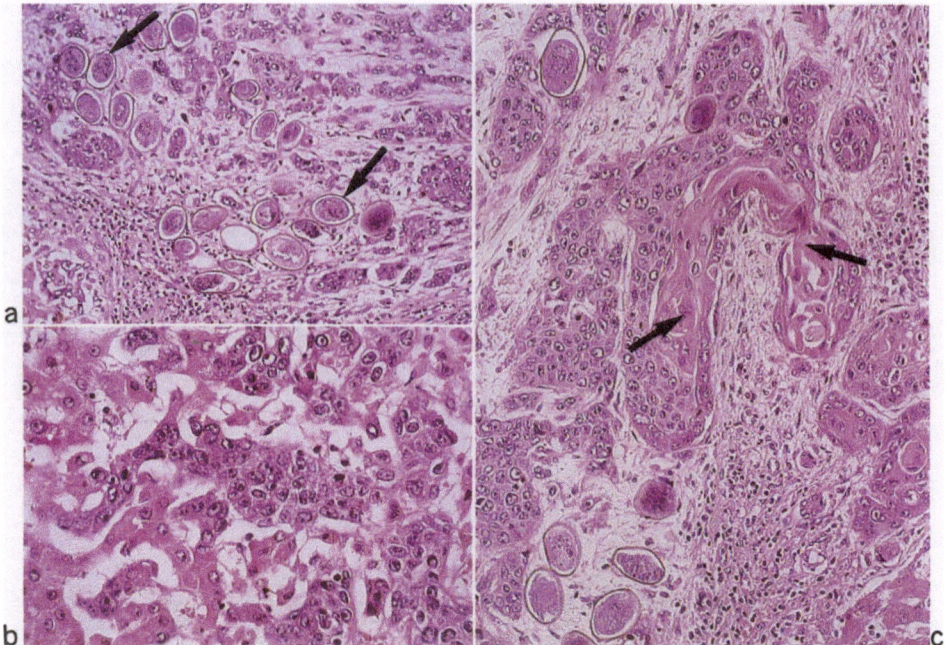

Fig. 12.6a–c. Same case. **a** Calcified eggs of *Schistosoma japonicum* (*arrows*). **b** Esophageal cancer (squamous cell carcinoma) is infiltrating into the sinusoids. **c** Metastasized esophageal cancer showing marked keratinization (*arrows*). HE; **a** × 50, **b**, **c** × 100

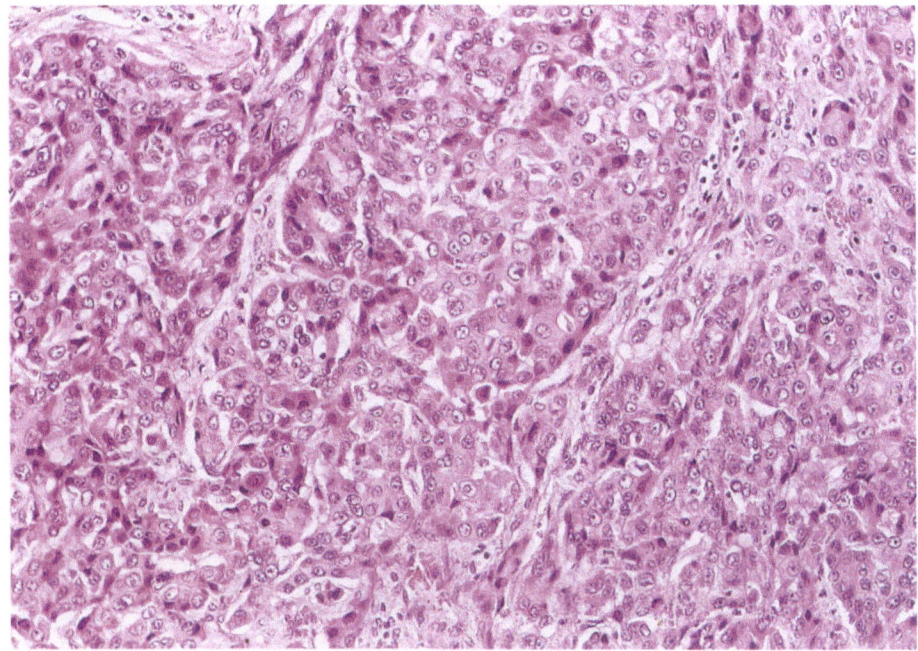

Fig. 12.7. Same case. Part of HCC showing a trabecular structure. HE, × 200

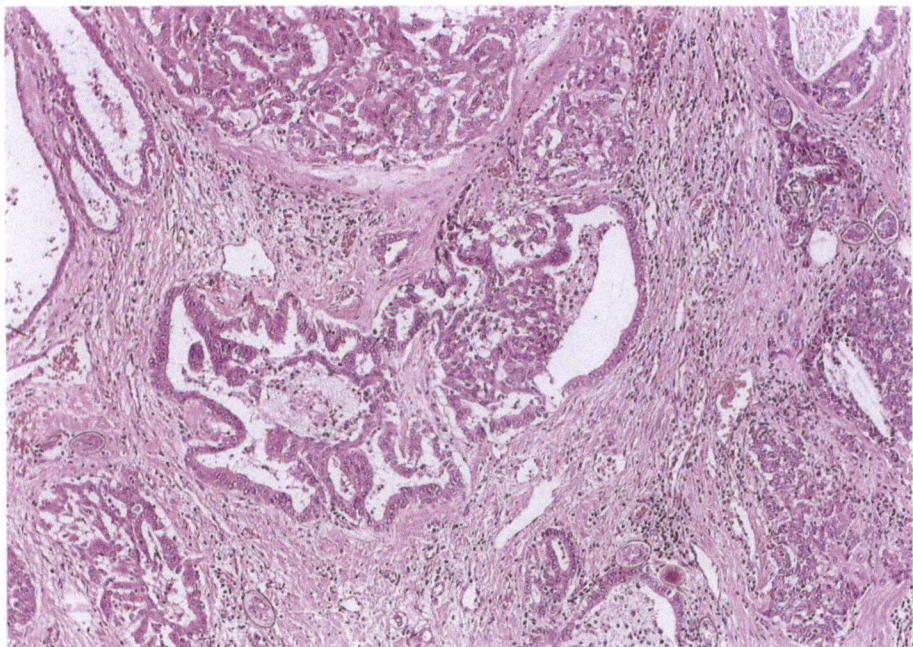

Fig. 12.8. Same case. Part of transition between HCC and cholangiocarcinoma. HE, × 100

Chapter 13
Histological Changes in Hepatocellular Carcinoma Associated with Transcatheter Arterial Embolization Therapy

It has recently been reported that transcatheter arterial embolization (TAE) [114, 115] is effective as a conservative therapy for inoperable HCC. The histological changes in HCC after treatment largely remain to be elucidated.

Effects of TAE and One-Shot Injection in HCC

The therapeutic effects of TAE on encapsulated HCC differ markedly from those on HCC without a capsule [61, 225].

Non-encapsulated HCC
In non-encapsulated HCC, the survival times and the proportion of the cancerous tissue taken up by the necrotic area in cancerous tissue do not differ significantly between patients receiving TAE therapy and those patients receiving a one-shot injection of anticancer agents.

Encapsulated HCC
No significant differences have been demonstrated between the survival times after treatment with TAE and those after a one-shot injection of anticancer agents, but the proportion of the cancerous tissue occupied by the necrotic area after TAE is significantly higher than that after one-shot injection.

Histological Features of HCC Treated with TAE

The effects of TAE on the tumor tissue (Figs. 13.1–8) are closely related to the growth patterns of HCC.

It is relatively rare for one of the three types of HCC—replacing, sinusoidal, pseudocapsular—to occur singly. In most cases, the sinusoidal type occurs in combination with either the replacing or the pseudocapsular type. TAE therapy is effective in HCC of the pseudocapsular type, in which the tumor foci receive only the arterial tumor vessels but cannot induce necrosis at the front of tumor growth in HCC of the replacing type, because such tumor lesions seem to be nourished by both arterial blood from the arterial tumor vessels and portal vein blood via the sinusoids. The tissue left alive continues to grow.

In HCC of the sinusoidal type, tumor foci continue to grow by virtue of receiving portal blood from the sinusoids. Therefore, TAE alone is not effective against lesions of this type. Fortunately, there are extremely few cases of HCC where growth follows an exclusively sinusoidal pattern.

Problems to Be Solved in TAE Therapy

TAE is not satisfactorily effective against HCC of the sinusoidal type. In HCC of the replacing type, it is only partly effective because the tumor tissue at the tumor-nontumor boundary does not undergo necrosis. These difficulties remain to be solved. Remarkable changes in the histological features of HCC, such as degeneration of the cancer cells and sarcomatous changes, suggesting growth of another clone of cancer cells and change of phenotype of cancer cells, have occasionally been found in cases of HCC in which TAE produced long-term survival. These two points may affect the prognosis remarkably. The changes in cancer cells due to anticancer therapy should be clarified by both in vitro and in vivo studies, using techniques such as tissue culture and heterotransplantation of tumor to nude mice.

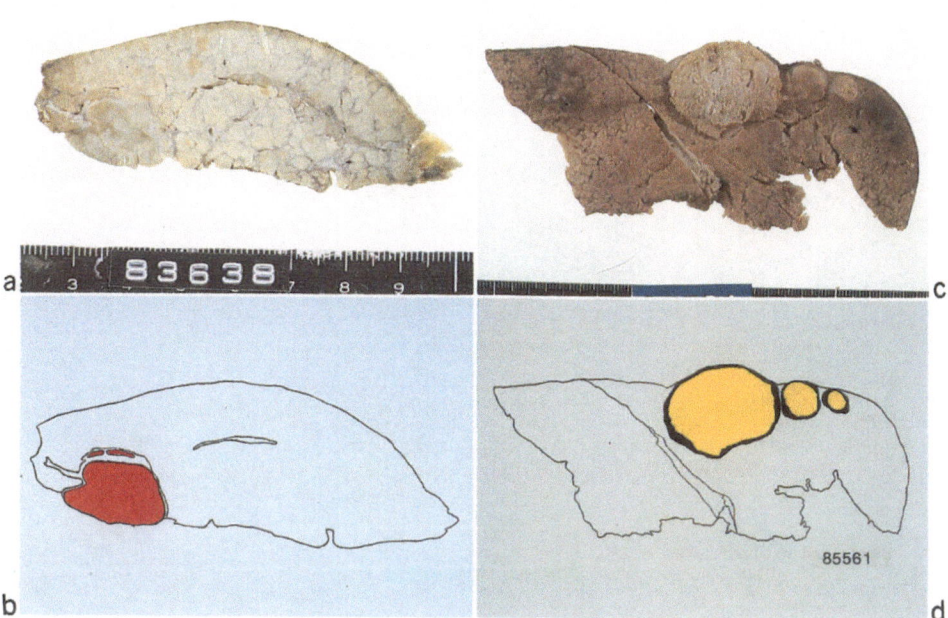

Fig. 13.1a, b Resected HCC without TAE therapy. Tumor shows no degeneration. **c, d** Resected HCC treated with TAE. Tumors are completely necrotized. *red*, viable tissue; *yellow*, necrosis

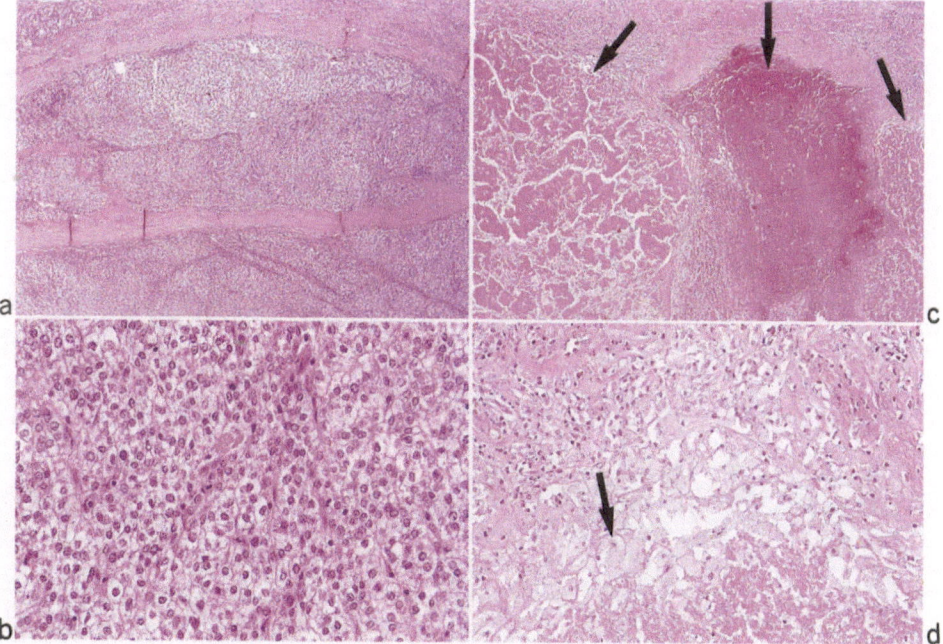

Fig. 13.2a–d. Same cases. **a, b** Nontreated case. HCC tissue shows no degeneration. **c,** Treated case. HCC tissue shows coagulative necrosis (*arrows*). **d** Accumulation of foamy histiocytes (*arrow*) around necrotized HCC. HE; **a, c** × 20, **b** × 100, **d** × 50

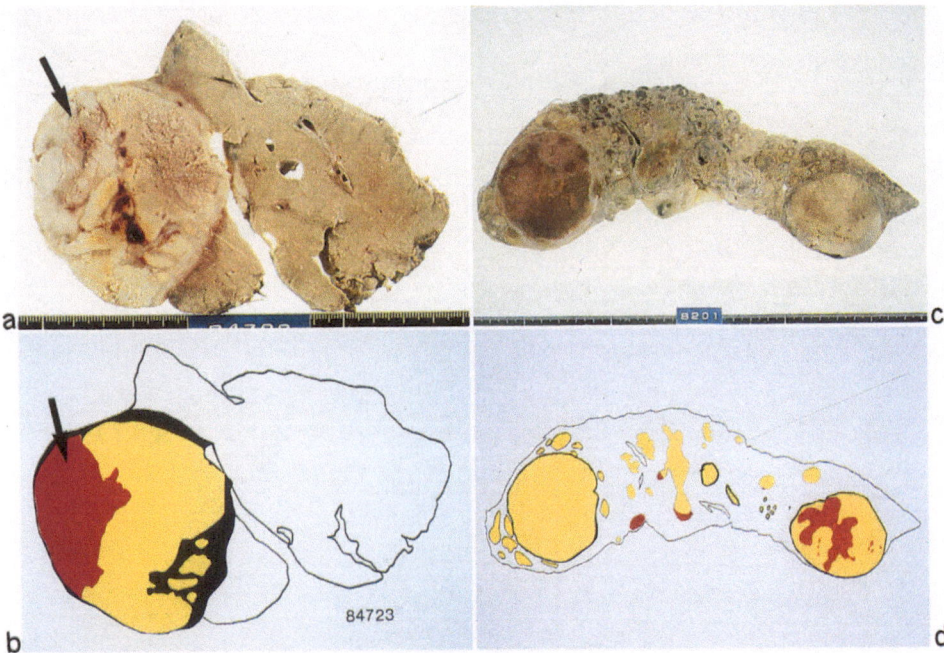

Fig. 13.3a–d. Resected HCC treated by TAE. **a, b** Part of the HCC tumor is nourished by the subphrenic artery and is viable (*arrows*). **c, d** Case treated by TAE. The tumors and the tumor thrombi of the portal veins are mostly necrotized. *red*, viable area; *yellow*, necrosis

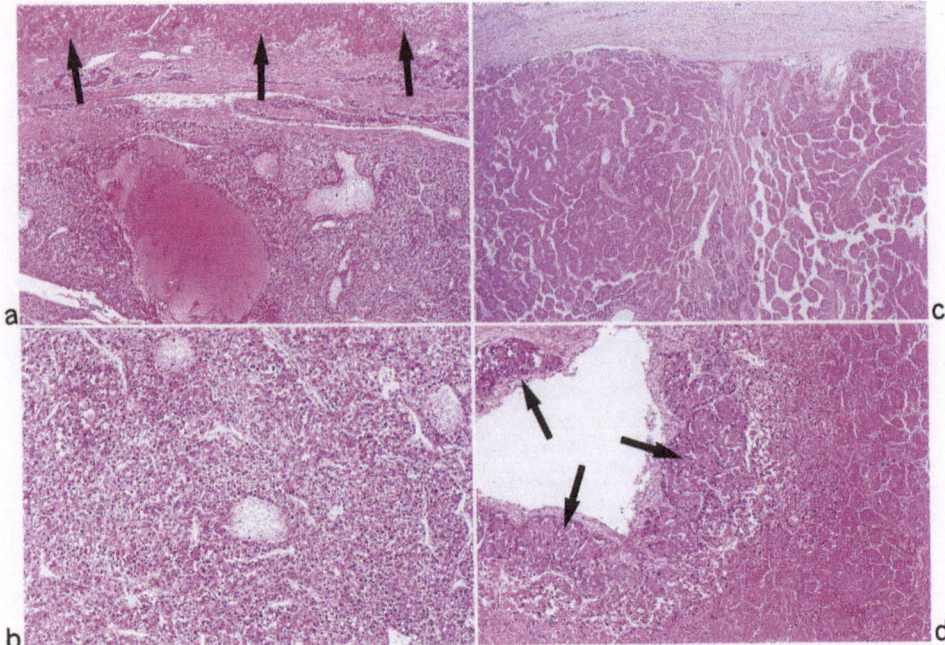

Fig. 13.4a–d. Same cases. **a** The HCC tissue nourished by the hepatic artery is completely necrotized (*arrows*). **b, c** The area nourished by the subphrenic artery is viable. **d** Only perivascular areas (*arrows*) are viable in most part of the tumor. HE; **a, c** × 10, **b, d** × 20

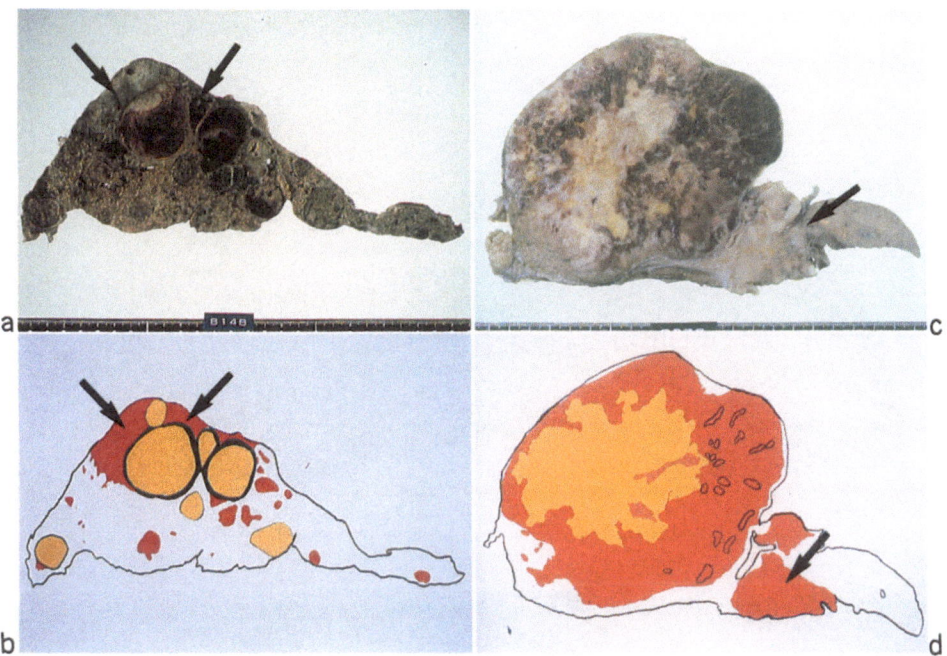

Fig. 13.5. a, b Mixed infiltrative and expansive HCC with TAE. The tumors infiltrating around encapsulated tumors are viable (*arrows*), but the encapsulated tumors are completely necrotized. **c, d** Infiltrative HCC with TAE. The periphery and infiltrating tumor (*arrows*) are viable. *red*, viable area; *yellow*, necrosis

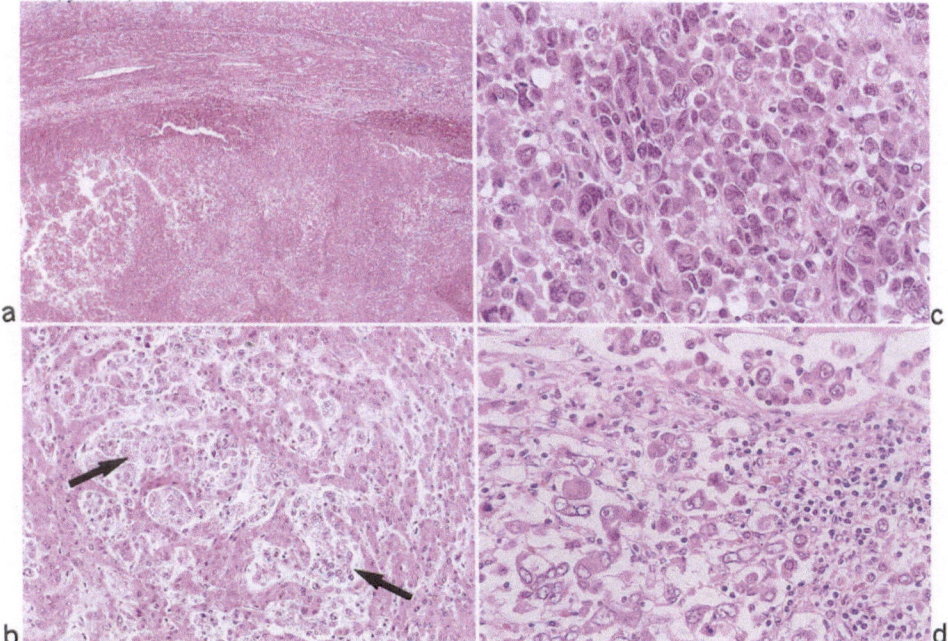

Fig. 13.6a–d. Same case. **a, b** The viable HCC tissue is of the free-cell type and shows a sinusoidal growth pattern (*arrows*). **c, d** Free-cell type HCC has metastatized to the lymph node. HE; **a** × 20, **b** × 50, **c** × 200, **d** × 100

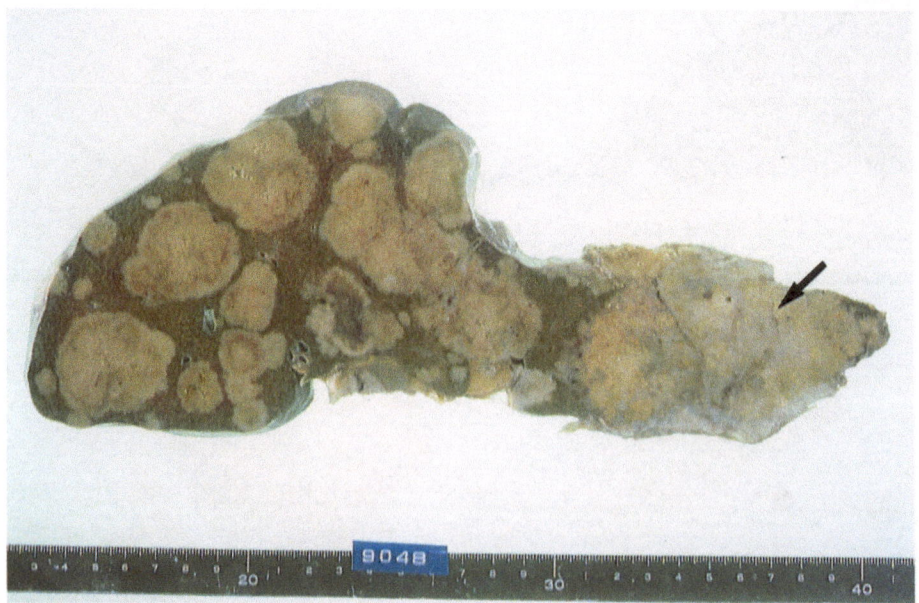

Fig. 13.7. HCC treated by TAE. The primary focus is hyalinized (*arrow*). This case resembles metastatic liver cancer

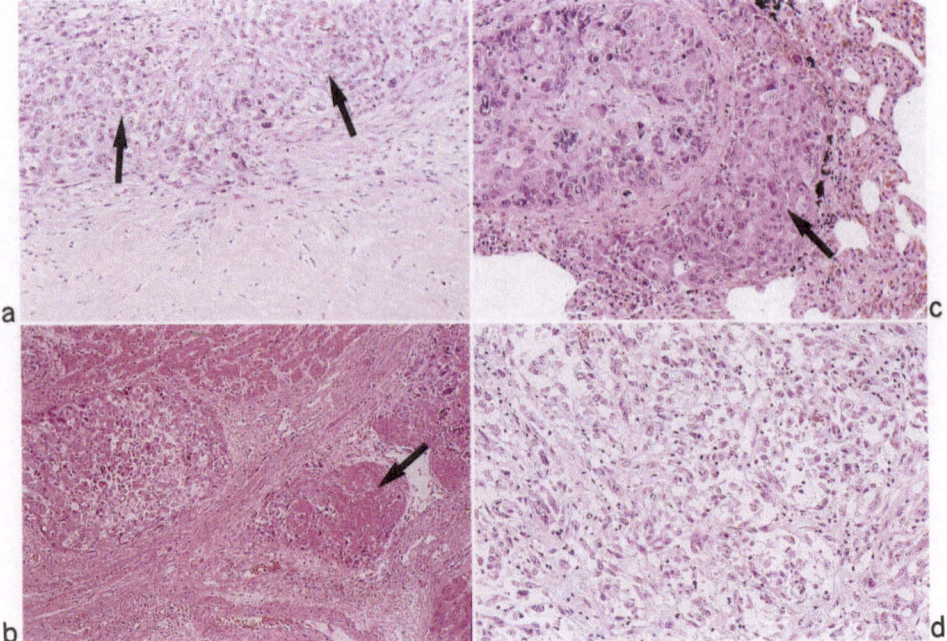

Fig. 13.8a–d. Same case. **a** The viable tumor cells (*arrows*) around the hyalinized area are of the free-cell type. **b** Highly necrotic tumor thrombus (*arrow*) of the portal vein. **c** Lung metastasis (*arrow*). **d** A part of the HCC showing sarcomatous change. HE; **a, c, d** × 50, **b** × 20

Chapter 14
Tissue Culture of Hepatocellular Carcinoma Cells and Hetero-Transplantation to the Nude Mouse

Establishment of Human HCC Cell Lines

Tissue culture techniques provide the most powerful means for studying the function and biological characteristics of human cancer cells. A considerable number of human HCC cell lines has been established [27, 29, 226–230], but the number is still insufficient.

HBs Ag-producing HCC cell lines, including the HCC cell line PLC/PRF/5 established by Alexander et al. [27], have provided an experimental system useful for studies on the correlation between hepatitis B virus and HCC. HCC cancer cells possess various functions, such as protein synthesis and various antigenicities. Because of these profiles, HCC cells will be increasingly used in cancer studies in the future. It is now necessary that more cancer cell lines of different types be established. Recent progress in HCC therapy, however, has made it difficult for us to obtain tissue for culture, since in patients treated by new therapeutic procedures, such as arterial injection or arterial embolization, cancer cells usually undergo degeneration and necrosis. The establishment of new cell lines is also difficult because HCC is difficult to culture.

HCC Cell Line KIM-1 and its Hetero-Transplantation to the Nude Mouse

In addition to a cell line system, nude mice provide an excellent experimental model for basic studies on human cancer and the assessment of therapeutic effects. Cancer cells obtained from 14 surgical cases of human HCC were transplanted to nude mice by Kuwahara [231]. Six of the fourteen transplants were successful, but serial transplantation was achieved in only one case. Thus, the rate of successful transplantation is still low. According to Sasaki [232], however, an HCC cancer cell line was easily established using tissue which had been successively cultured in nude mice. In establishing cell lines, it seems far better to use cells first cultured in nude mice than to use tissue obtained directly from man. In our laboratory, KIM-1 cells [233] which were first implanted in nude mice were successfully cultured in vitro; the success was attributed to the extreme freshness of the tissue and the minimal presence of intervening connective tissue.

KIM-1 cell line
The cultured cells adhere to each other, forming trabecular or island-like nests (Fig. 14.6) reminiscent of the original cancer (Figs. 14.1, 2). Light-microscopically, the

individual cells are polygonal and large with fine granules and distinct nuclei (Fig. 14.5). Electron-microscopically, junctional complexes, a bile canaliculus-like structure, and a filament-like structure, as noted in the original tumor, are observed (Figs. 14.3, 4, 7). These profiles indicate that the cultured cells are quite similar to the original cancer. Tumors growing in nude mice, like the original tumors, are primarily of the trabecular type and the trabeculae are covered with a single layer of endothelial cells (Fig. 14.10). The presence of abundant rough endoplasmic reticulum suggests active protein synthesis (Figs. 14.15, 16).

Tumors growing in nude mice, however, include less stromal connective tissue than the original tumors and partly have tissue in solid patterns. As only HCC cells have been implanted to nude mice, the endothelial cells constituting the blood spaces or stroma surrounding the trabeculae of HCC may derive from the nude mice. It is interesting that cells from a different species constitute part of the tumor in the host. Not only the morphological features of HCC cells are well preserved in tumors growing in nude mice; intracellular filament-like structures and inclusion bodies encircled with a limiting membrane, as seen in the original cancer cells, are also demonstrated by electron microscopy (Fig. 14.16b).

Protein Synthesis in HCC Cell Lines

Hepatic cancers are known to possess the ability to synthesize various kinds of serum proteins, like hepatocytes [235]. In KIM-1 cells, various proteins, including beta-2-microglobulin (BMG), ferritin, and albumin, are produced and their intracellular localization has been demonstrated in cultured cells using the immunofluorescent technique.

When KIM-1 cells are cultured for 48 h the cell population in the culture approximately corresponds to the alpha-fetoprotein (AFP) and BMG levels in the culture medium. BMG continues to increase for a while after the steady state is established, but AFP decreases rapidly. The BMG concentration for 10^5 cells is constant throughout the cultivation period, but the AFP levels reach a maximum in the middle of the log phase when the proliferation is most active, suggesting that the activity of AFP synthesis or secretion is more closely related to cell proliferation. In addition, it is possible that AFP and BMG are synthesized and secreted by different mechanisms.

Presence and Distribution of Albumin, AFP, and Alpha-1-Antitrypsin in Tumor Tissue Implanted into Nude Mice

It can be demonstrated immunohistochemically that HCC cells contain albumin to various degrees (Fig. 14.11). The authors [235] reported that albumin-positive cells are observed diffusely in moderately and well-differentiated HCC and in a localized or sparse pattern in poorly differentiated HCC. In agreement with this result, albumin-positive cells are observed in a diffuse pattern in tumors presenting the histological features of relatively well-differentiated HCC.

Alpha-1-antitrypsin (Fig. 14.12) is a major constituent of proteinase inhibitor and is a glycoprotein with a molecular weight of 54 000. Its relationship to HCC and other liver diseases has recently been investigated.

AFP and BMG in Nude Mouse Serum and Ascites

Relatively high levels of AFP and BMG have been determined in KIM-1 culture medium. In nude mice into which KIM-1 cells were subcutaneously transplanted, serum levels of AFP and BMG increased markedly, from 10 000 to 26 300 ng/ml and from 220 to 980 mg/l, respectively. The secretory function is well preserved even if KIM-1 is transplanted into nude mice. In mice receiving KIM-1 cells intraperitioneally, a remarkable elevation of AFP concentration was observed in the ascites, but the elevation in serum AFP levels was lower than that in nude mice receiving KIM-1 cells subcutaneously. However, according to Motoyama and Watanabe [236], who carried out a similar experiment using a gastric cancer cell line in mice, carcinoembryonic antigen (CEA) levels in the serum were, interestingly, higher than in a transplanted tumor. As HCC is rich in blood spaces, AFP secreted from the tumor cells might rapidly enter the blood circulation or the peritoneal cavity.

Establishment of Cell Line of Combined Hepatocellular and Cholangiocarcinoma (KMCH-1)

There have been a number of discussions about the pathological features and histogenesis of combined hepatocellular and cholangiocarcinoma (CHC) [238, 239]. Cell culture and hetero-transplantation approaches may be useful in the investigation of the histogenesis of CHC, but there have been only two reports of CHC tumors transplanted into nude mice, and neither study employed an established cell line. Murakami et al. [237], in our department, established a cell line (KMCH-1) from surgically resected tumor which was AFP-negative and had a CEA level of 4.2 ng/ml. The resected tumor consisted of HCC with a trabecular arrangement and cholangiocarcinoma exhibiting a glandular structure and a solid pattern with abundant fibrous stroma (Figs. 14.17, 18). KMCH-1 cells have a large, round nucleus containing serveral nucleoli. They have abundant cytoplasm and proliferate in a paving-stone arrangement. Electron-microscopically, a number of desmosomes and tight junctions are observed between tumor cells, and the mutual contact between the cells is tight. Abundant microfilaments are observed in the cytoplasm and some of the cells exhibit intracytoplasmic lumina, resembling adenocarcinoma cells (Figs. 14.19, 22).

Histological study of the subcutaneously transplanted tumors in nude mice shows tumor cells with round nuclei, two to three nucleoli, and abundant cytoplasm in most areas. The cells grew in solid nests, with only rare foci of gland formation. Fine collagen is present between the tumor nests, resembling the pattern exhibited in the solid, scirrhous area of the original tumor. Some glands contain mucicarmin-positive materials. Electron-microscopically, the transplanted tumor shows remarkable gland structures with microvilli and a basement membrane (Figs. 14.23–28).

There are three possible explanations of these findings: (1) Culture favored initial isolation of cells having the character of cholangiocarcinoma; (2) Culture isolated a cell capable of HCC or cholangiocarcinoma differentiation, but the latter pattern was favored; (3) Both HCC and cholangiocarcinoma cells grew initially during culture, but cholangiocarcinoma cells proliferated preferentially in vitro.

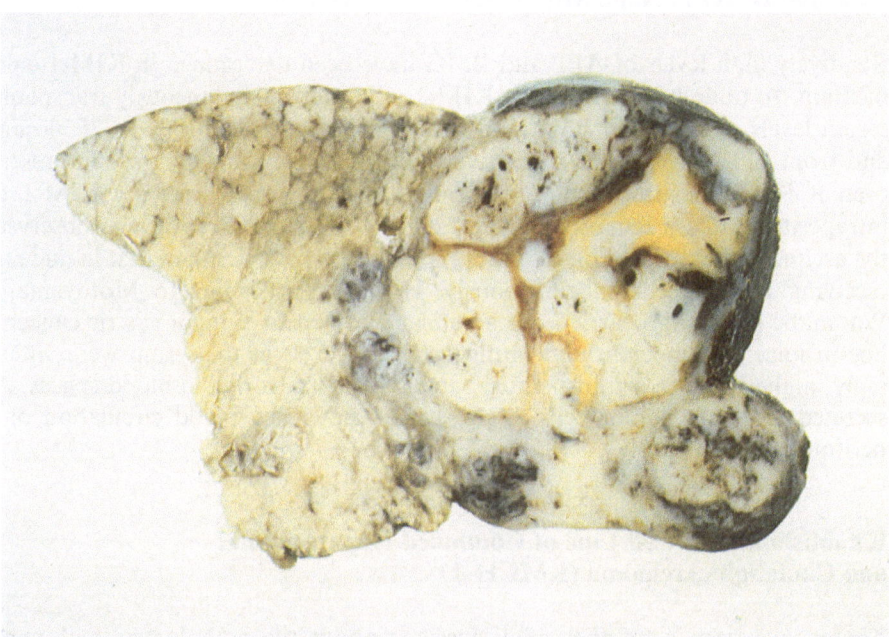

Fig. 14.1. Resected original tumor of KIM-1 cells. The tumor is well encapsulated and a daughter nodule is observed. The noncancerous area displays macronodular liver cirrhosis

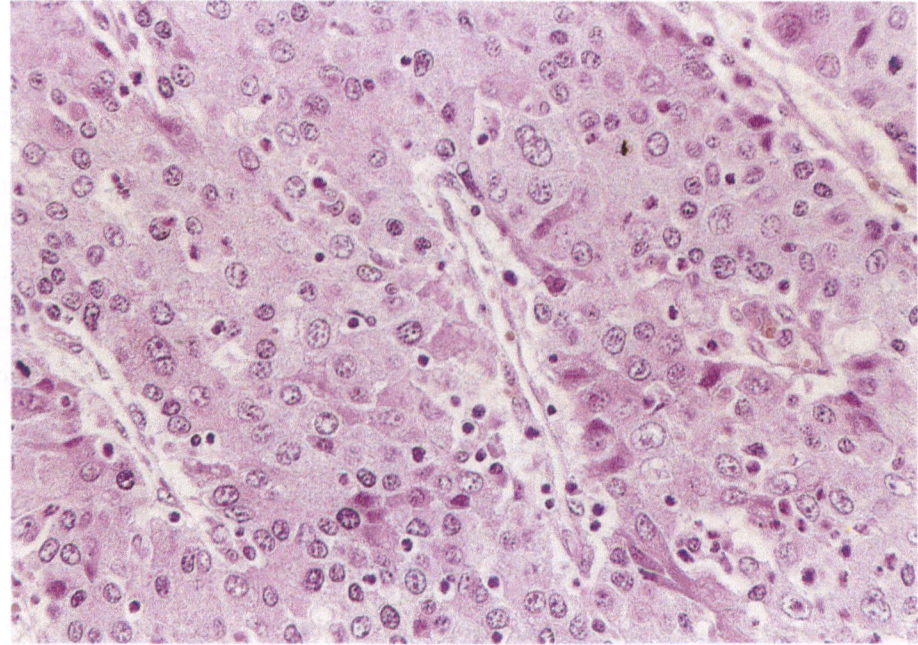

Fig. 14.2. Histological features of the original tumor of KIM-1 cells. The tumor is moderately differentiated and display a thick trabecular arrangement. HE, × 200

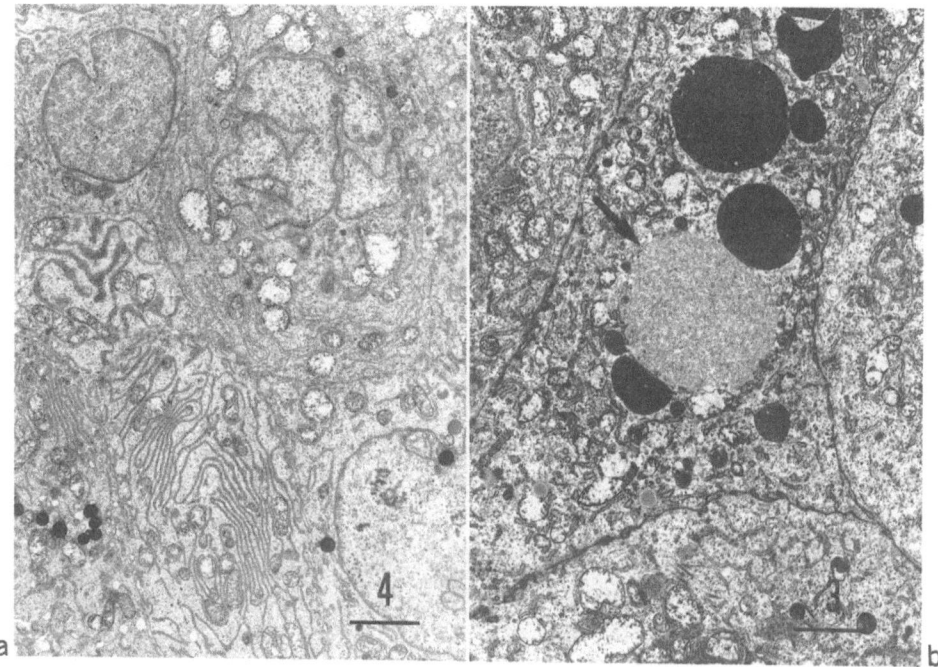

Fig. 14.3a, b. Ultrastructure of the original tumor (KIM-1 cells). **a** The HCC cells show a good mutual adhesion and well-developed cytoplasmic organelles. **b** Inclusion body-like substance (*arrow*) is seen in the cytoplasm

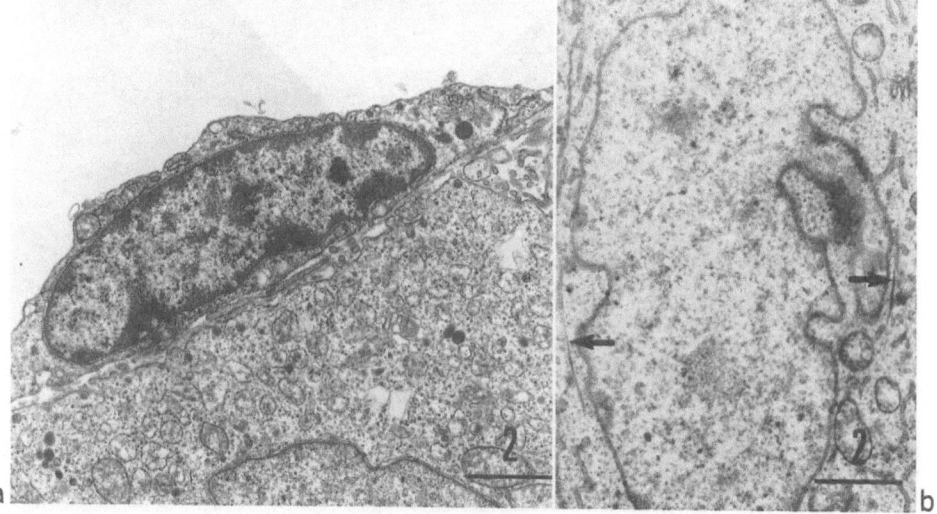

Fig. 14.4a, b. Ultrastructure of the original tumor (KIM-1 cells). **a** Endothelial cell covering blood space of HCC. **b** Filament-like structure (*arrow*) seen in the cytoplasm of the HCC cell

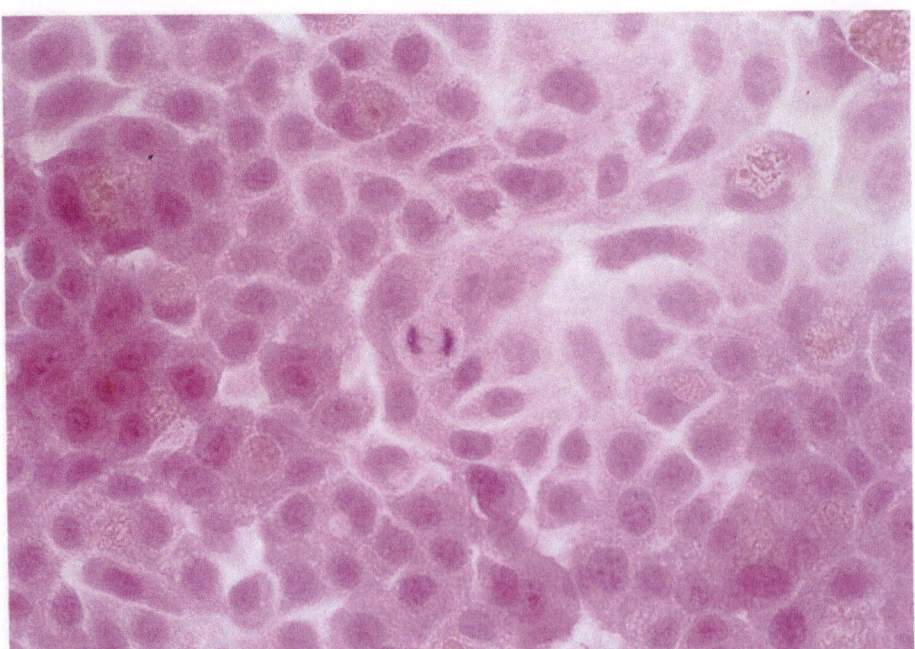

Fig. 14.5. KIM-1 cells. The cultured cells have eosinophilic cytoplasm and round to oval nuclei with one to a few nucleoli. They adhere to each other forming a paving-stone arrangement. HE, × 400

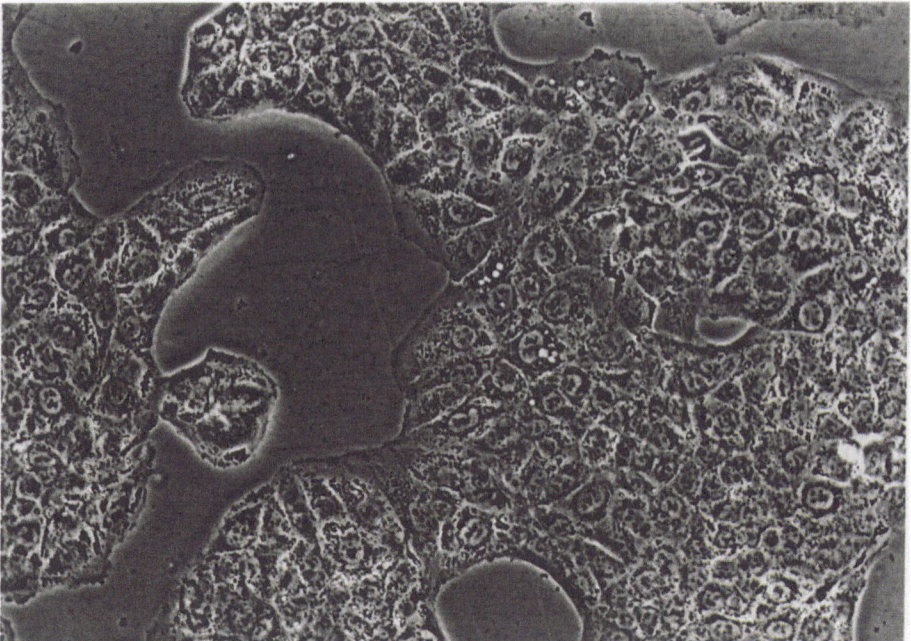

Fig. 14.6. Phase contrast-microscopic features of KIM-1 cells. The KIM-1 cells are polygonal and have large nuclei and distinct nucleoli. × 400

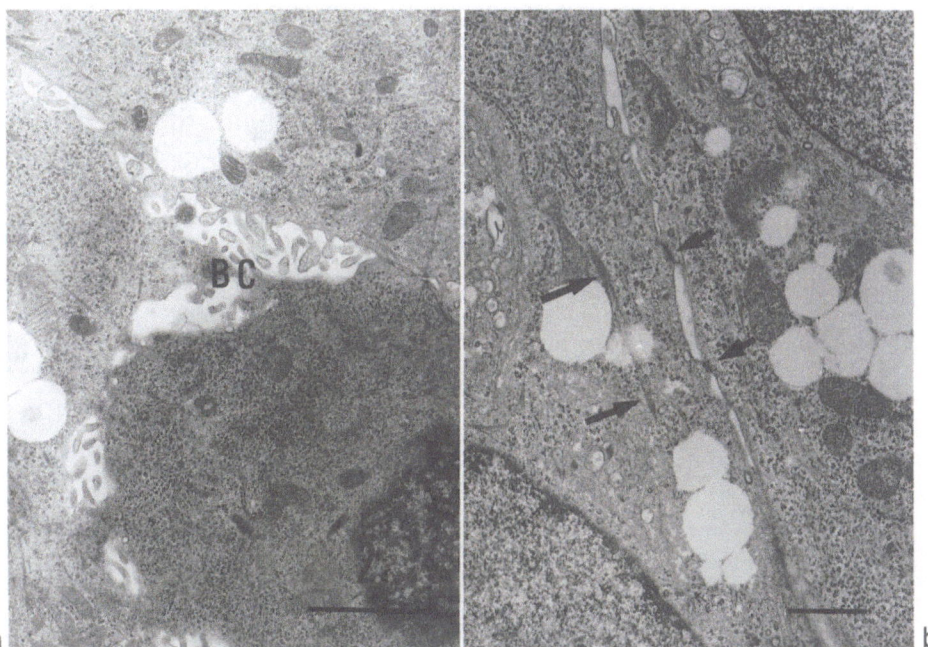

Fig. 14.7a, b. Ultrastructure of KIM-1 cells. **a** Bile canaliculi-like structure (*BC*) between tumor cells. **b** Well-developed junctional complexes (*short arrows*) and microfilaments (*long arrows*)

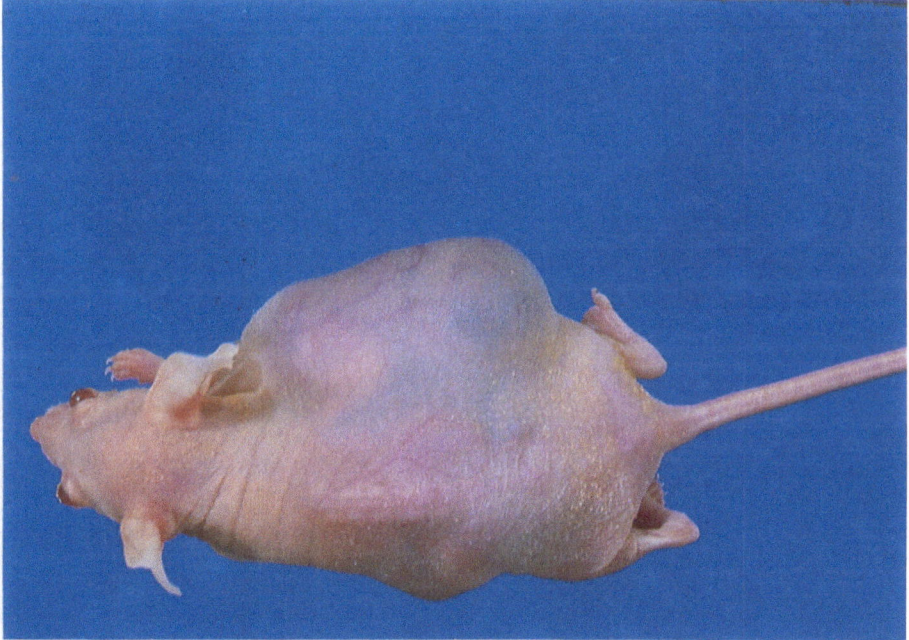

Fig. 14.8. Transplanted tumor in nude mouse (KIM-1 cells)

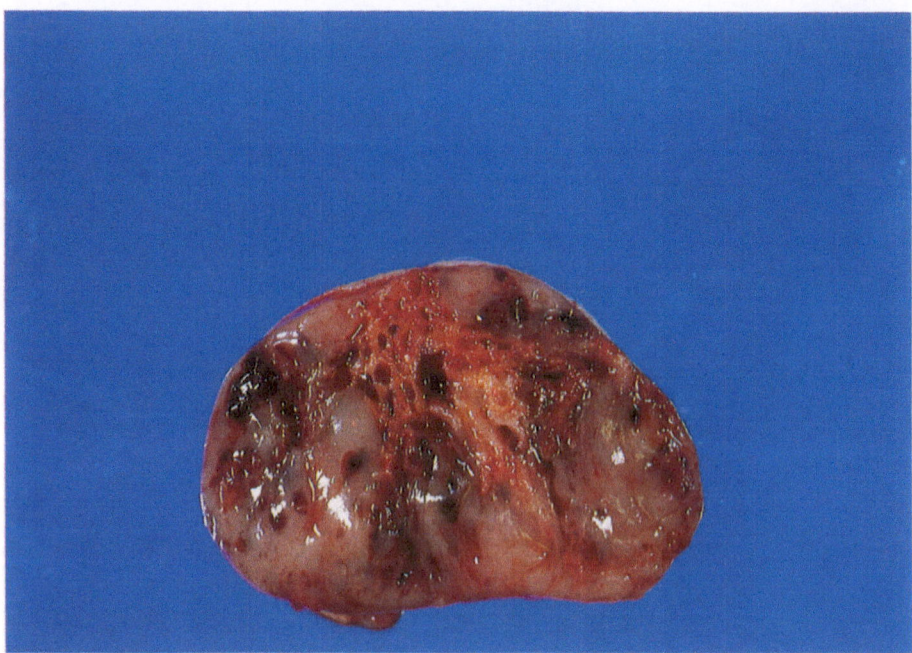

Fig. 14.9. Cut surface of transplanted tumor (KIM-1 cells). The tumor is solid and shows hemorrhage in parts

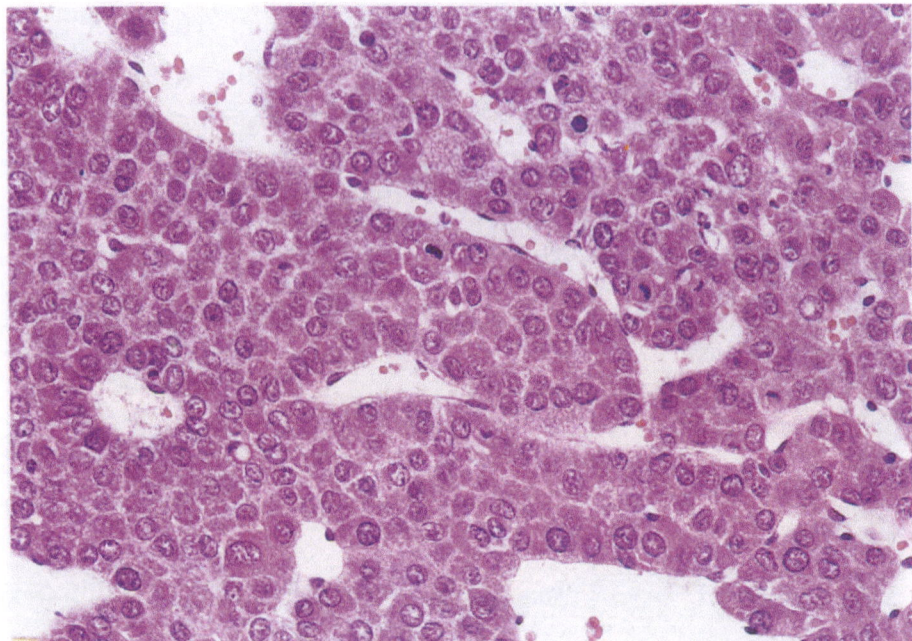

Fig. 14.10. Transplanted tumor in nude mouse (KIM-1 cells). The tumor shows a trabecular arrangement, and endothelial cells derived from the nude mouse cover the trabeculae of HCC. HE, × 200

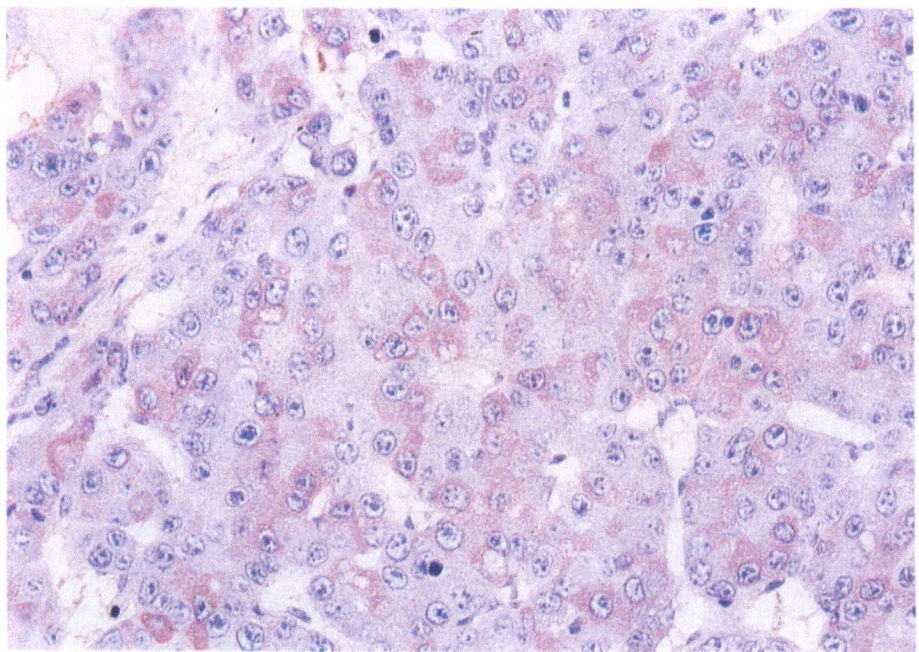

Fig. 14.11. Albumin-positive cells in transplanted tumor in nude mouse (KIM-1 cells). The albumin-positive cells are seen in a mosaic pattern in the tumor. Immunoperoxidase, × 200

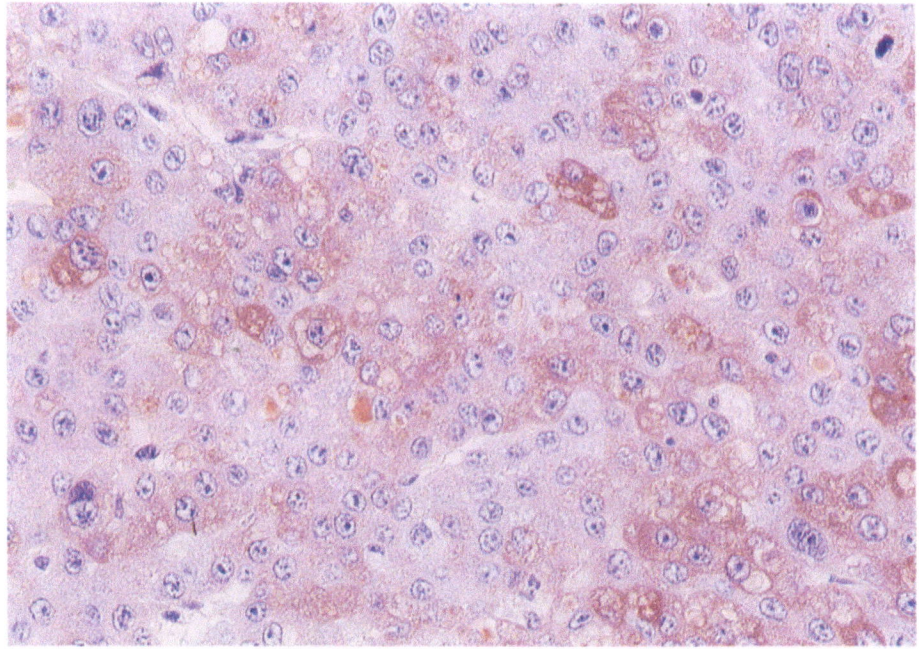

Fig. 14.12. Alpha-1-antitrypsin-positive cells in the same tumor. Immunoperoxidase, × 200

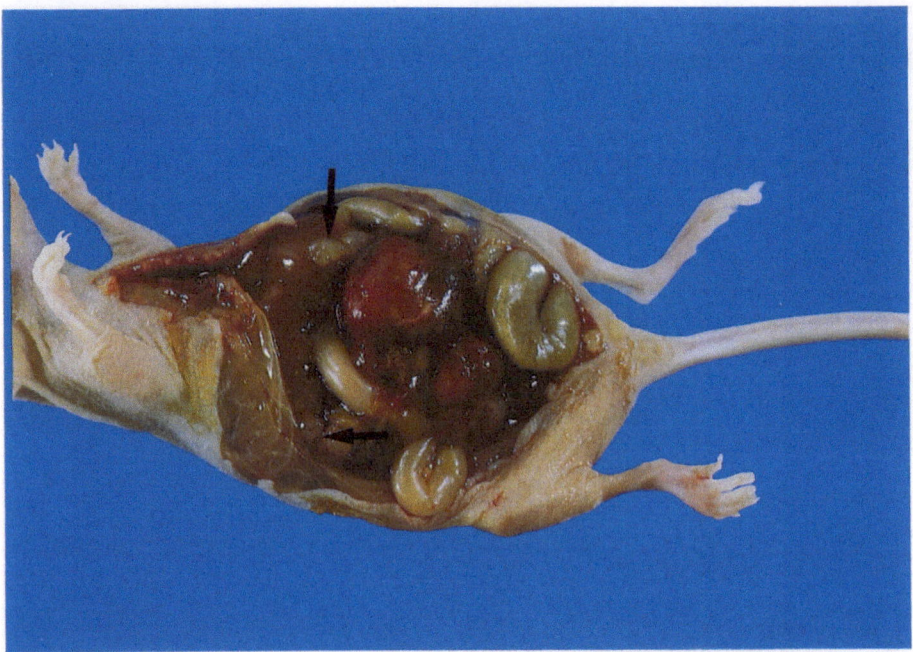

Fig. 14.13. Tumor formation (*arrows*) in the abdominal cavity of a nude mouse after intraperitoneal transplantation of KIM-1 cells

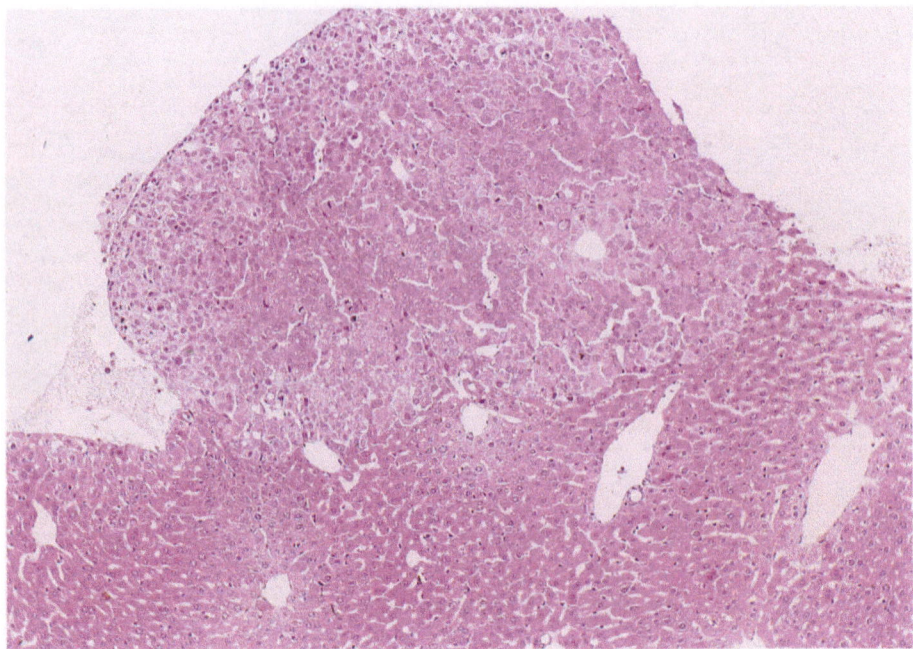

Fig. 14.14. Tumor formed in the liver after intraperitoneal transplantation of KIM-1 cells. HCC cells are proliferating in the sinusoids. HE, × 50

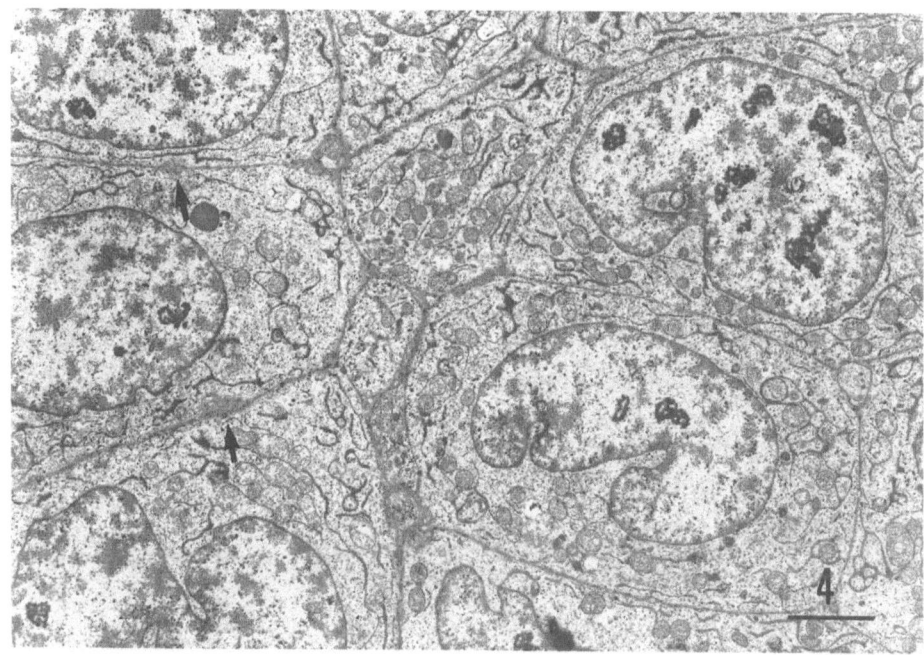

Fig. 14.15. Ultrastructure of subcutaneously transplanted tumor in a nude mouse (KIM-1 cells). Bile canaliculi and junctional complexes (*arrows*) are observed between the tumor cells

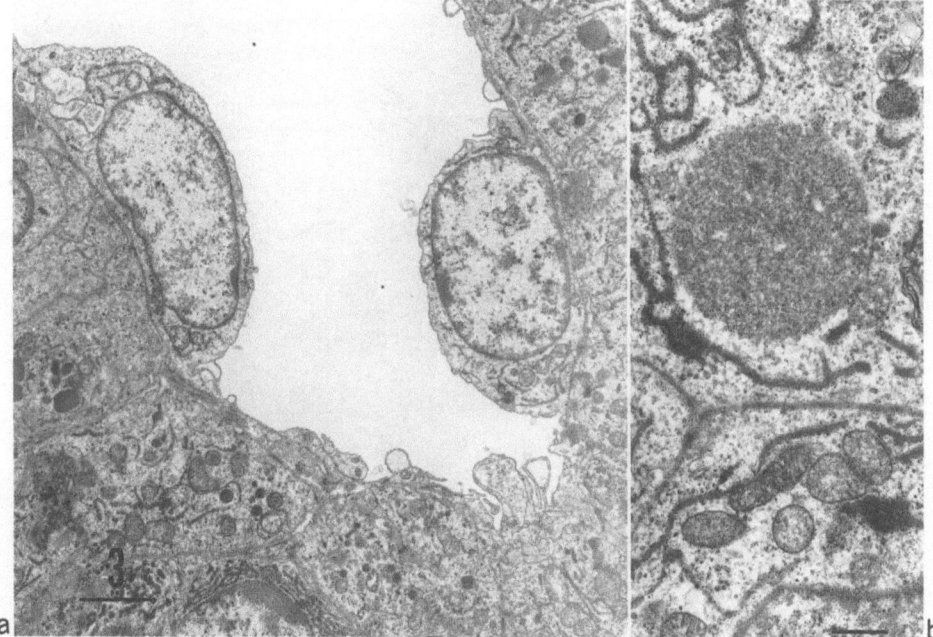

Fig. 14.16a, b. Ultrastructure of subcutaneously transplanted tumor in a nude mouse (KIM-1 cells). **a** Swollen endothelial cells covering blood space of HCC tissue. **b** Inclusion body-like structure seen in the cytoplasm of the HCC cell

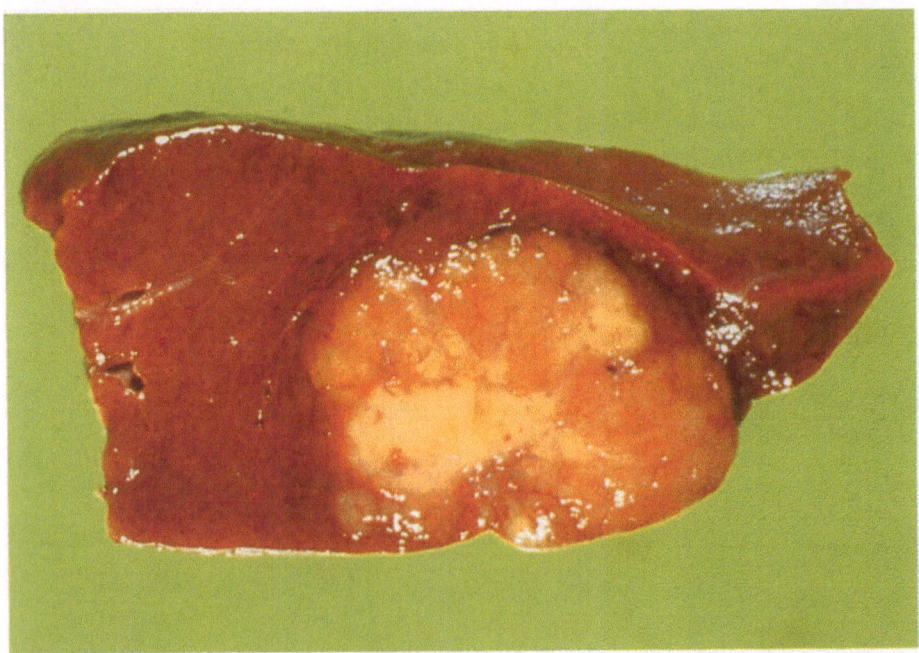

Fig. 14.17. Resected original tumor of KMCH-1 cells. The whitish-yellow tumor is not encapsulated and is 6.6 × 4.5 cm in size. There is no associated liver cirrhosis

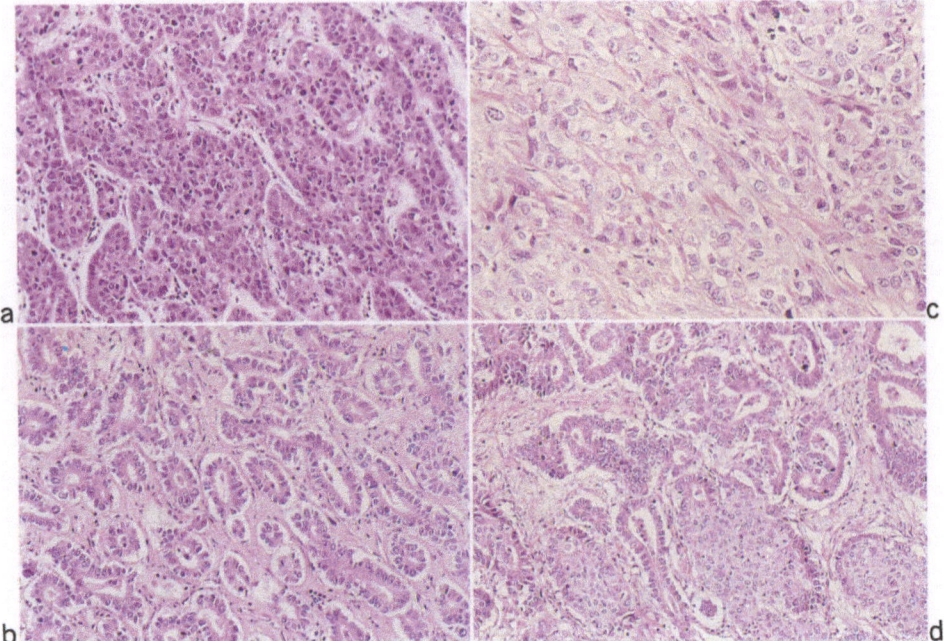

Fig. 14.18a–d. Histological features of the original tumor (KMCH-1 cells). **a** Part of trabecular HCC. **b** Part of well-differentiated cholangiocarcinoma. **c** Part of poorly differentiated cholangio-carcinoma. **d** Part of transition between HCC and cholangiocarcinoma. HE; **a, b, d** × 100, **c** × 200

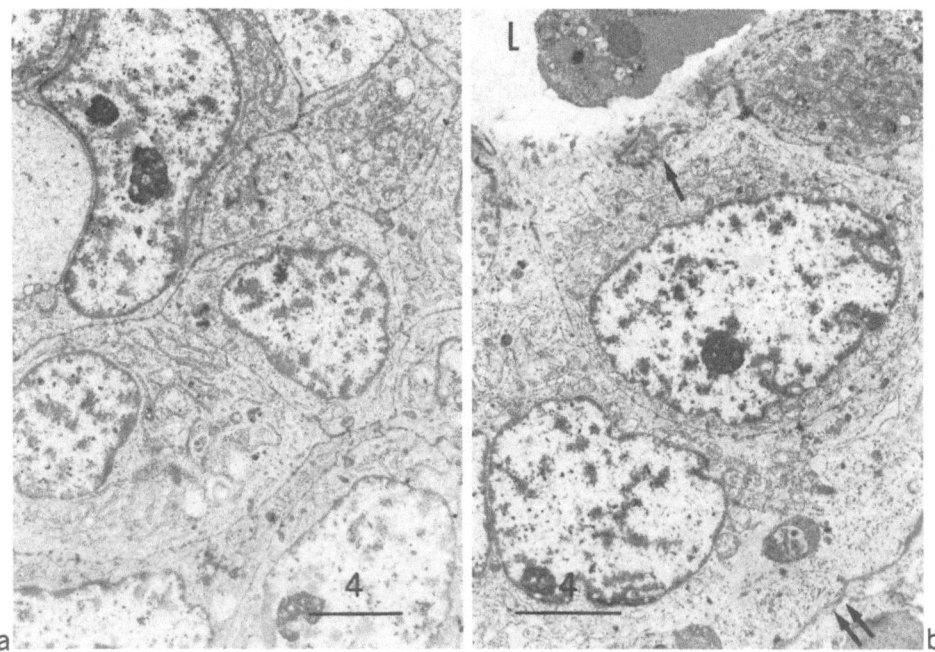

Fig. 14.19a, b. Ultrastructure of original tumor of KMCH-1 cells. **a** Tumor cells with well-developed organelles characteristic of HCC cells. **b** Part of cholangiocarcinoma has glandular structure. Microvilli (*top arrow*) in luminal side and basement membrane (*bottom arrows*) surrounds tumor cells

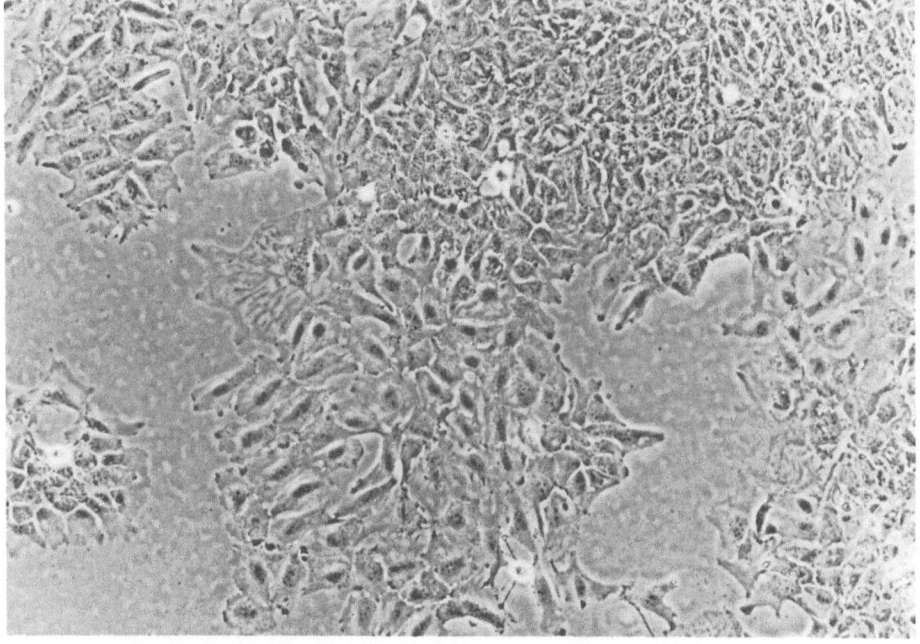

Fig. 14.20. Phase contrast-microscopic finding of KMCH-1 cells. The cultured cells show a paving-stone arrangement. × 200

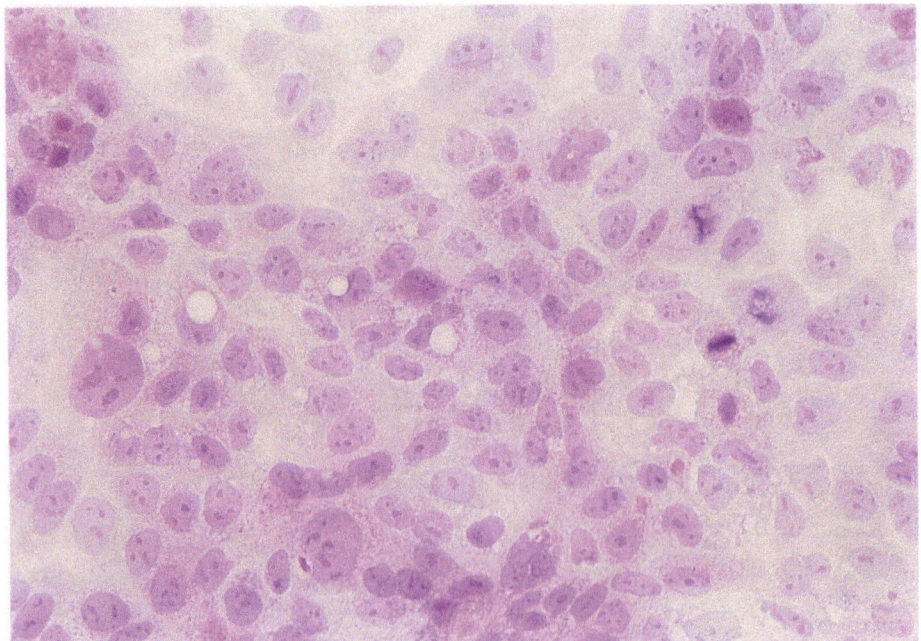

Fig. 14.21. KMCH-1 cells. The cultured cells have pale cytoplasm and oval-shaped nuclei with one to several nucleoli. HE, × 400

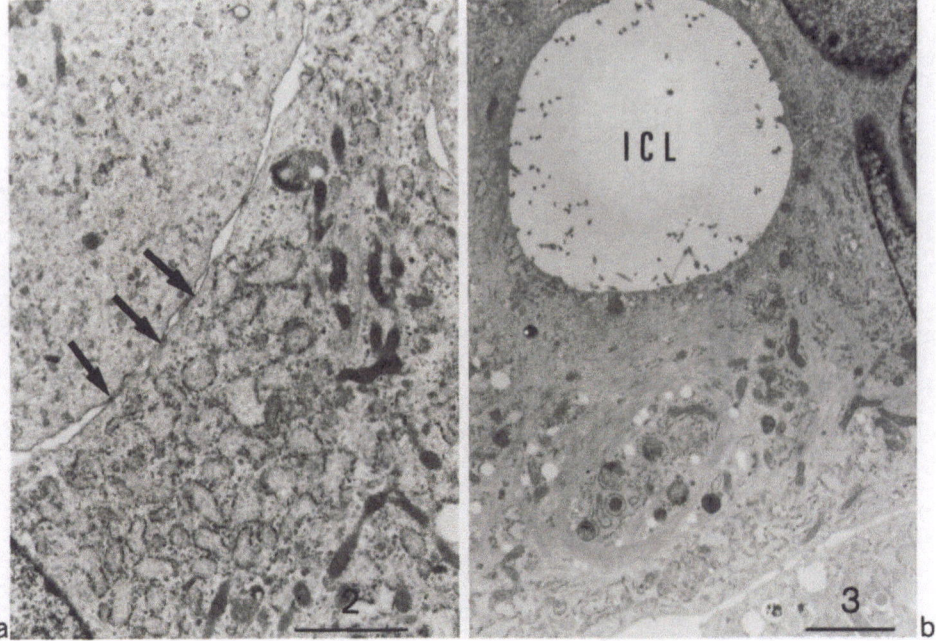

Fig. 14.22a, b. Ultrastructure of KMCH-1 cells. **a** Well-developed junctional complexes (*arrows*) between tumor cells. **b** An intracytoplasmic lumen (*ICL*) is seen in some cells

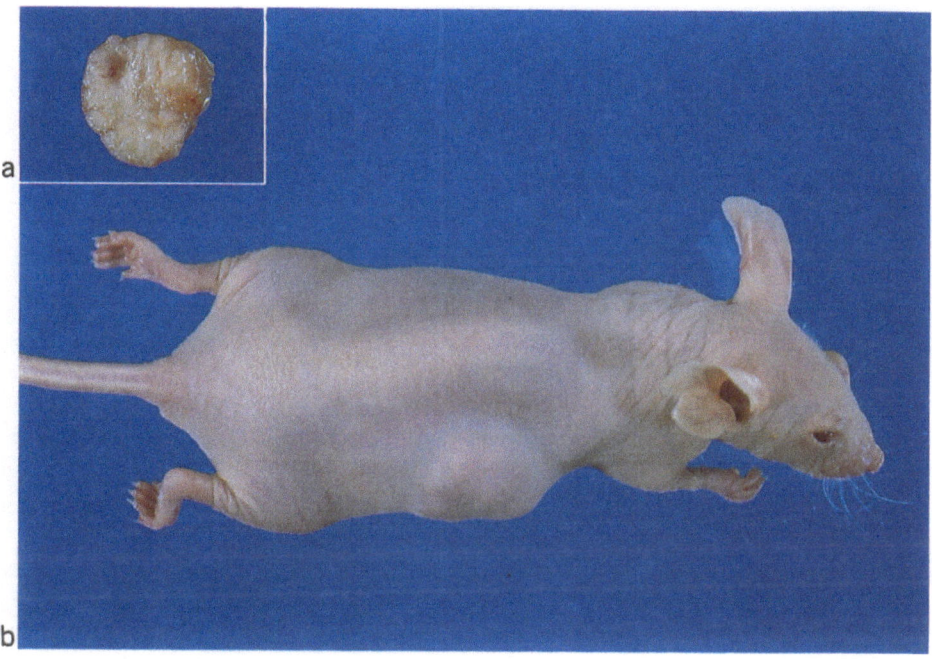

Fig. 14.23. a Cut surface of transplanted tumor. The tumor is solid and relatively hard. **b** Transplanted tumor in a nude mouse (KMCH-1 cells)

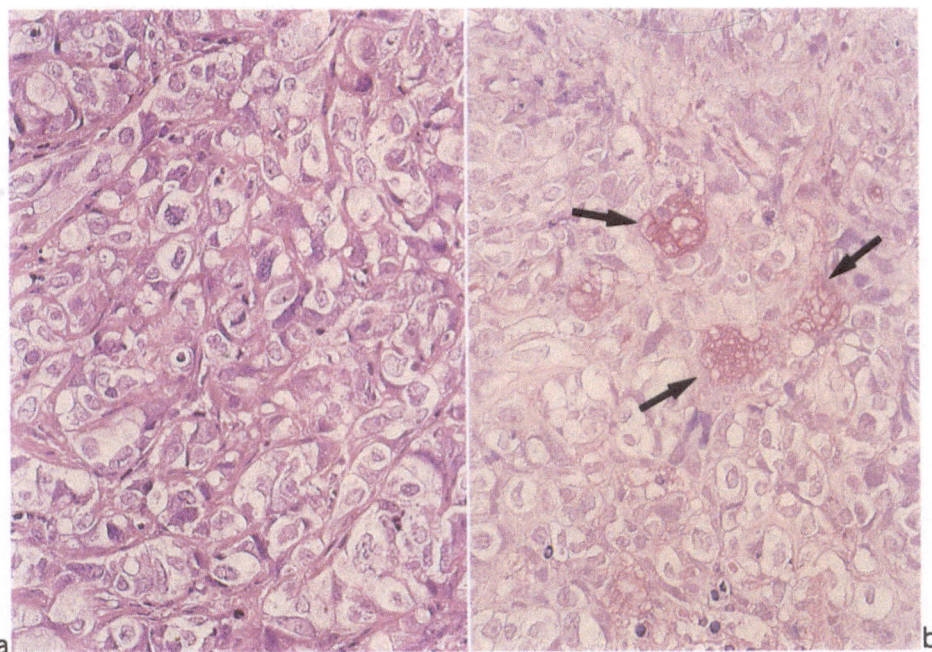

Fig. 14.24a, b. Histology of transplanted tumor in a nude mouse (KMCH-1 cells). **a** The tumor cells are proliferating in a solid pattern with fine fibrous stroma. **b** Mucin production (*arrows*) is observed in some tumor cells. **a** HE, × 200. **b** Mayer's mucicarmin, × 200

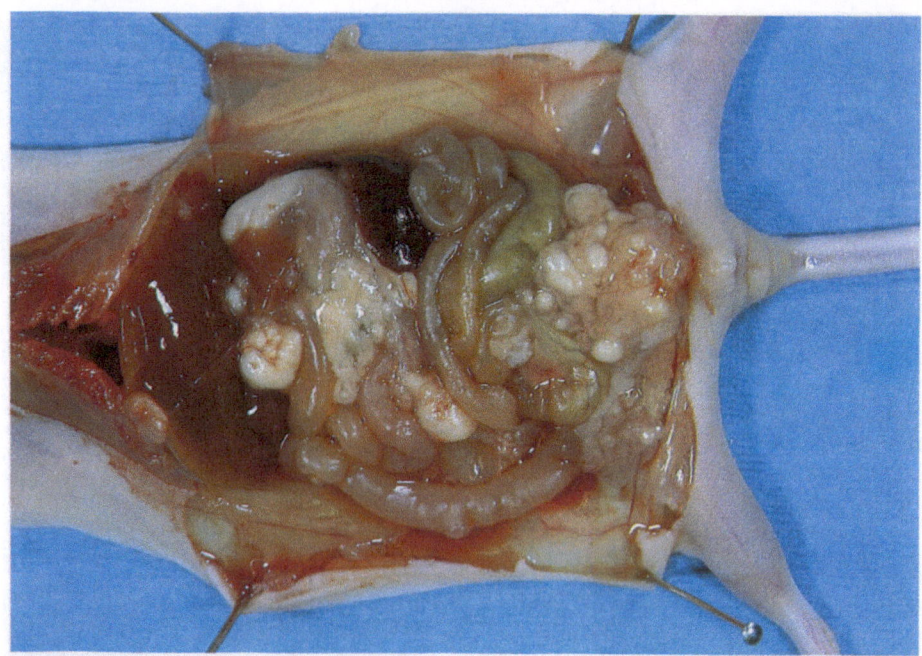

Fig. 14.25. Formation of tumors of varying size in the abdominal cavity of a nude mouse after intraperitoneal transplantation of KMCH-1 cells

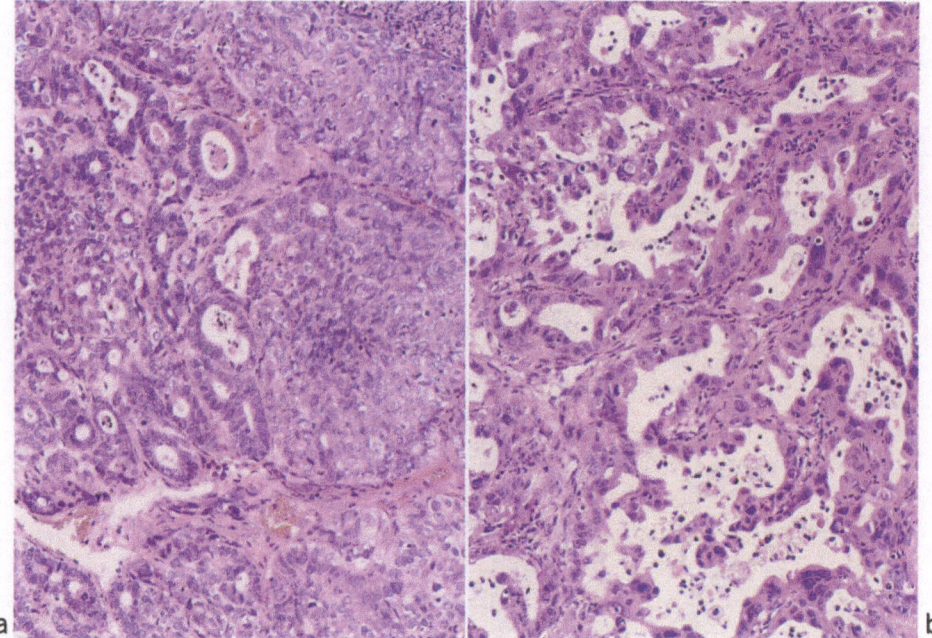

Fig. 14.26a, b. Histological features of peritoneal tumors (KMCH-1 cells). **a** Part of tumor showing both solid and glandular patterns. **b** Part of tumor showing papillary pattern. HE; **a** × 100, **b** × 200

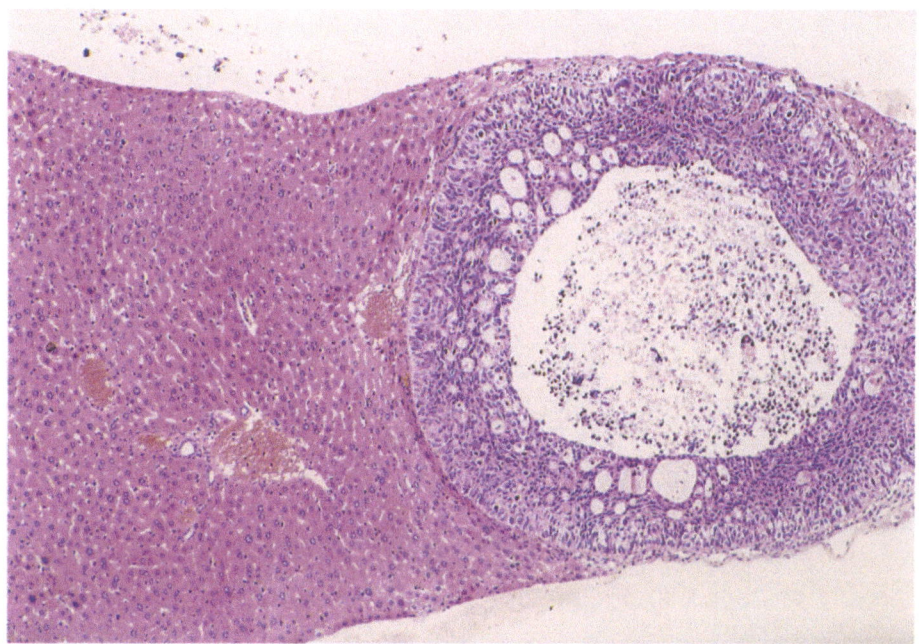

Fig. 14.27. Transplanted tumor (KMCH-1 cells) in the liver of a nude mouse showing cystic change. HE, × 100

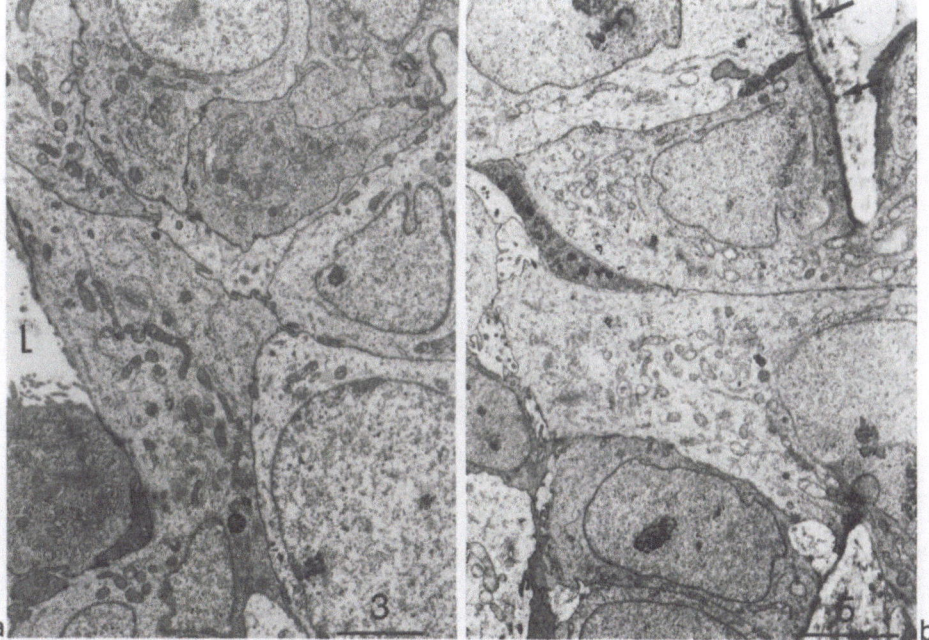

Fig. 14.28. Ultrastructure of transplanted tumor (KMCH-1 cells) in a nude mouse. **a** Tumor cells showing a glandular structure (*L*). The cytoplasmic organelles are poorly developed. **b** Basement-membrane-like structure (*arrows*)

Fig. 8.25. ...

Chapter 15
Metastatic Liver Cancers

It is a well-known fact that hematogenous metastasis frequently involves the liver as welll as the lungs. The occurrence of metastatic carcinoma in the liver is far more frequent than primary carcinona. The ratio of secondary over primary carcinoma has been reported to range from 7 : 1 to 20 : 1.

HCC occurs in men far more frequently than in women in the ratio of 5–7 : 1. Metastatic liver cancer shows a slight tendency to affect men more frequently than women, but the ratio for secondary carcinoma in the liver is 1.5 : 1. This ratio possibly reflects that of 1.7 : 1 for carcinomas in general.

The rate of metastasis to the liver has been reported to be 37.6% by Mori et al. (240), 44% by Arima (241), 49.4% by Abrams et al. (242), and 36.0% by Willis (243). All these rates do not greatly differ from our own estimate of 46.5%. These metastatic cancers arise mainly in the gastrointestinal tract, biliary tract, and lungs.

It has been reported that a cirrhotic liver is infrequently involved in metastatic processes [244–247]. In our series, 80% of HCCs were associated with liver cirrhosis, while liver cirrhosis was found only in 6.4% of livers bearing metastatic cancers.

Macroscopic Findings

Metastatic liver cancer frequently involves both the right and left lobes. Many metastatic liver cancers are seen as multiple nodules of varing size. Unlike HCC, metastases to the liver rarely form a major tumor surrounded by foci caused by infiltration or intrahepatic metastasis through the portal vein. Metastatic cancer nodules are frequently observed as a central depression (umbilication) on the surface of the tumor when the center of the lesion necroses.

The cut surface of the metastatic nodules presents relatively homogenous solid appearance and is gray-white to white. The gross features of the primary tumor are found in the metastatic tumors. Metastasis of choriocarcinoma or angiosarcoma produces hemorrhagic tumors. In the case of a malignant melanoma, the metastatic tumors are black. Metastasis of cystadenocarcinoma produces a multicystic tumor, containing serous or mucinous material. Thus, it is relatively easy to determine the primary tumor by the characteristic gross features of the metastatic foci in some tumors. The metastatic foci are relatively clearly demarcated from the noncancerous tissue and may grow by compressing the surrounding tissue or by infiltration, but without forming the fibrous capsule characteristic of HCC. In HCC, the tumors are frequently divided by fibrous septa and the separate sections show independent morphological features (Figs. 15.1, 2). In general, however, metastatic tumors have no fibrous septa and are monomorphic (Fig. 15.3).

Histological Findings

The histological features of metastatic tumors in the liver are similar to those seen in the tumor at the site of origin. When a metastatic tumor is large, the tumor tissue may frequently undergo necrosis in the center of the lesion and the necrosis becomes replaced by fibrous connective tissue or shows a cystic change. Occasionally, hyalinization is noticeable.

The growth pattern at the tumor-nontumor boundary is mostly sinusoidal, whereby the metastasized tumor cells proliferate along the sinusoids (Fig. 15.4). A replacing growth pattern characteristic of HCC is extremely rare. When the metastasis is well-differentiated, the tumor grows expansively by compressing the normal tissues, leading to a concentration of reticulin fibers and the formation of a capsule-like fibrous band. Infiltration of free cancer cells into the sinusoids around the metastatic tumor sometimes occurs. A tumor thrombus of the portal vein is occasionally observed.

Angioarchitecture

The angioarchitecture of metastatic tumors usually reflects that in the original tumor. In general, metastatic liver cancer is more hypovascular than HCC [24]. Like HCC, however, most metastatic liver cancers receive blood from the artery [248, 249] (Fig. 15.3b). According to Lin et al. [250], postmortem angiography by injecting contrast medium through the hepatic artery and the portal vein revealed evidence of a blood supply to small metastatic foci from the portal vein via the sinusoids and branches of the portal vein. This agrees well with the histological findings that a metastatic liver tumor grows by infiltration into the sinusoids.

The typical angioarchitecture in one case each of HCC and metastatic liver cancer is presented below.

HCC (mixed infiltrative and expansive, single nodular). The cut surface discloses an encapsulated tumor, up to 10 cm in diameter, surrounded by small metastatic foci. The tumor mass is divided into several sections by thin fibrous septa, each section revealing different gross features (Fig. 15.1a). Soft X-ray findings show both hypovascular and hypervascular sections (Fig. 15.1b).

Metastatic carcinoma (lung cancer, poorly differentiated adenocarcinoma). A gray-white solid tumor mass, up to 10 × 10 cm, is seen in the right hepatic lobe, with several small metastatic foci in both lobes (Fig. 15.3a). Soft X-ray findings show a hypervascular tumor (Fig. 15.3b).

Morphological Changes of Metastatic Liver Cancer with Anticancer Therapy

Metastatic liver cancers have been treated by various methods such as surgical excision and chemotherapy. Repeated anticancer therapy, such as transarterial embolization and the intra-arterial injection of anticancer agents, may frequently modify the morphological features of the tumor, occasionally leading to a morphological similarity, both macroscopically and microscopically, to sclerosing-type HCC due to advanced sclerotic changes of the tumor (Figs. 15.5–12).

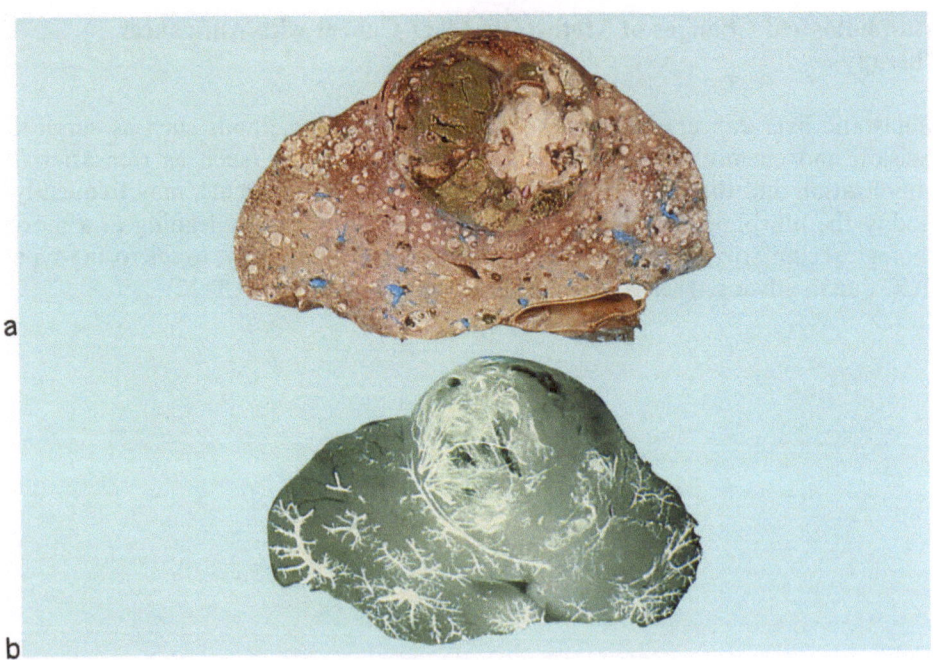

Fig. 15.1. Resected HCC, mixed infiltrative and expansive type. **a** Numerous tiny intrahepatic metastatic nodules are seen around encapsulated main tumor. **b** Angioarchitecture of main tumor is different in each part separated by septa

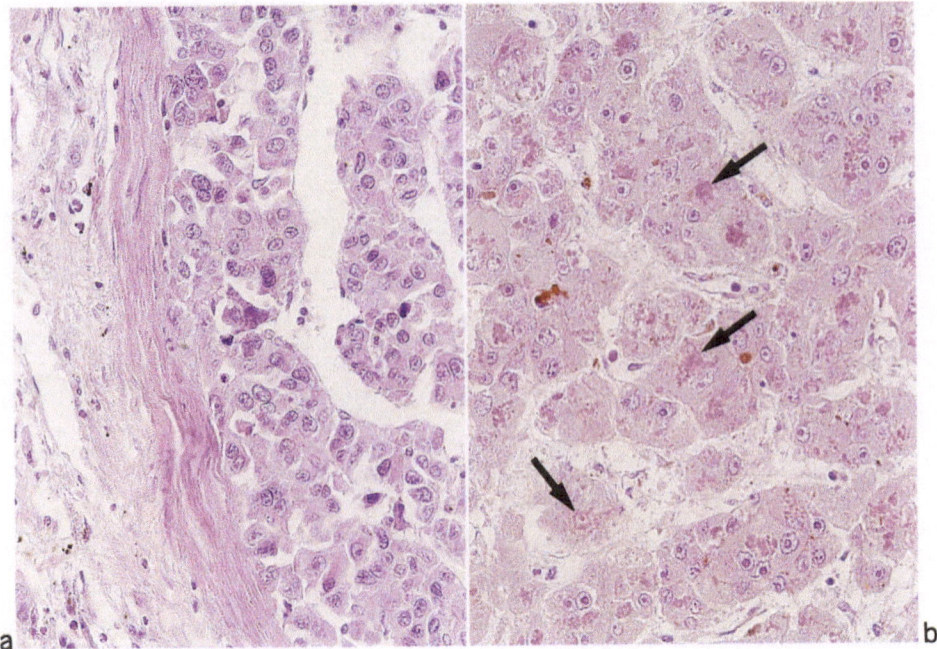

Fig. 15.2. Same case. **a** Fibrous capsule at the boundary. **b** Mallory bodies (*arrows*) in HCC cells. HE; **a, b** × 200

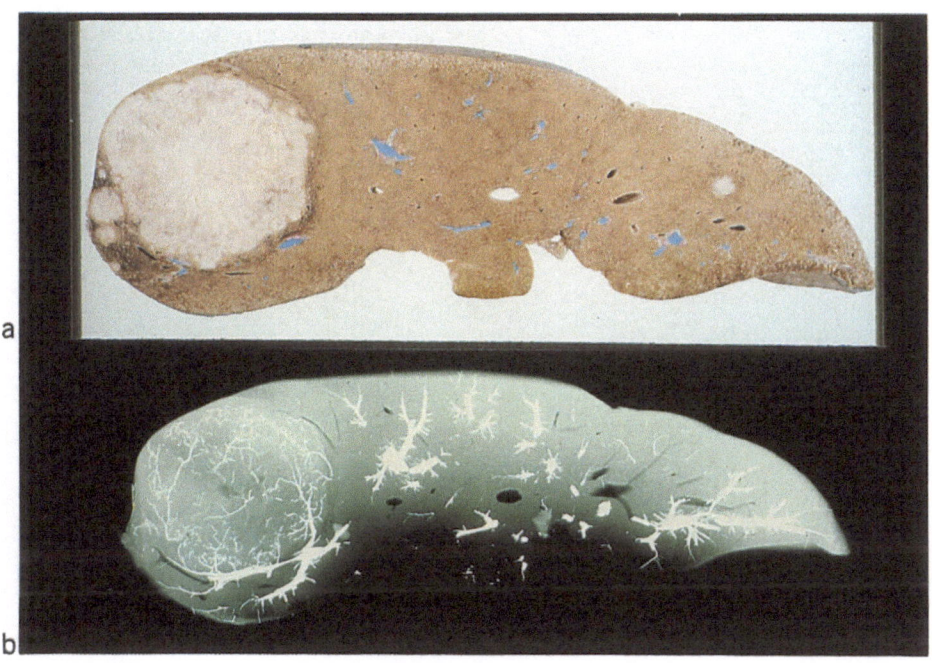

Fig. 15.3. Metastasis of lung cancer. **a** Metastatic tumor is not encapsulated and there are no septa in the tumor. **b** Angioarchitecture of the tumor is uniform

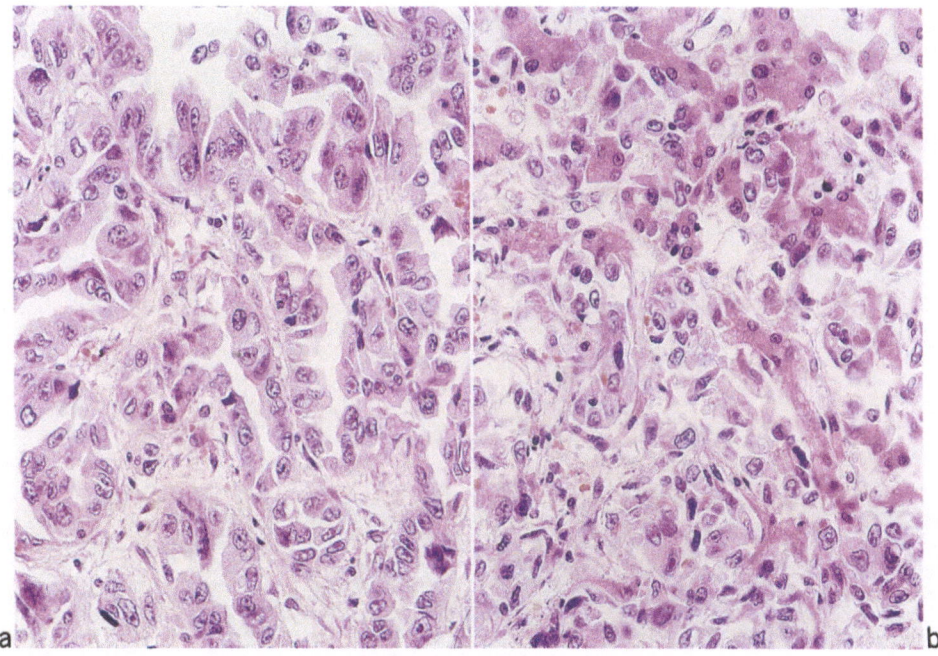

Fig. 15.4. Same case. **a** Metastatic lung cancer showing a papillary pattern. **b** Cancer cells grow in the sinusoids and atrophied hepatocytes are retained among cancer cells. HE; **a, b** × 200

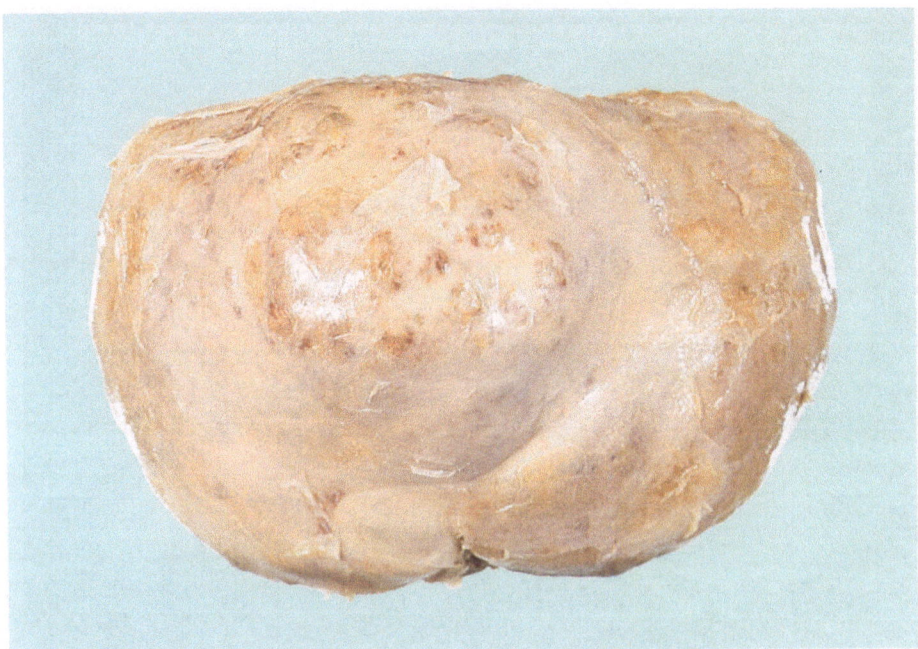

Fig. 15.5. HCC treated by repeated intra-arterial injection of anticancer drugs

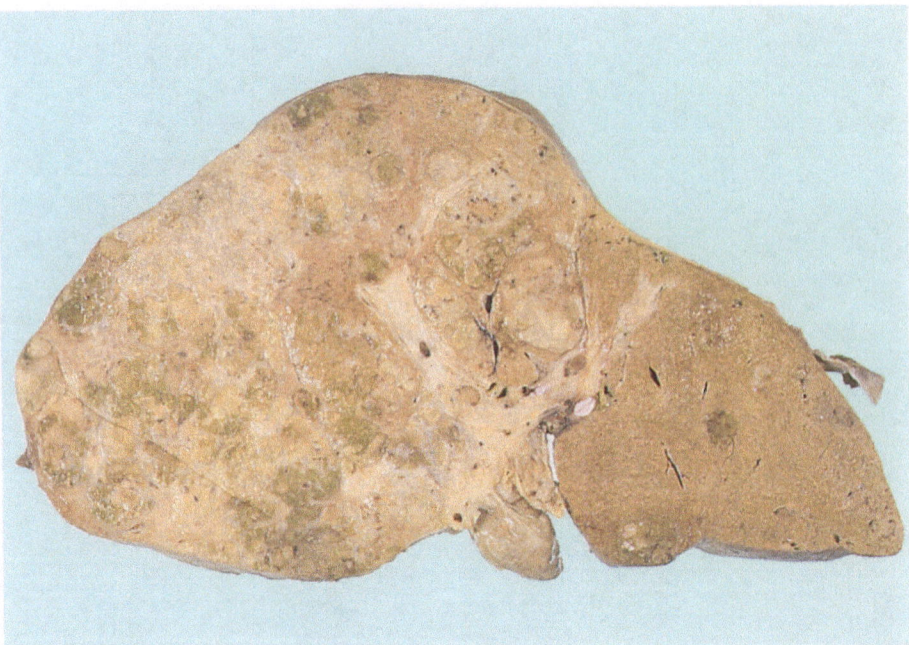

Fig. 15.6. Same case. HCC is diffusely located in the right hepatic lobe and tumor thrombus of the portal trunks is replaced by dense fibrous connective tissue

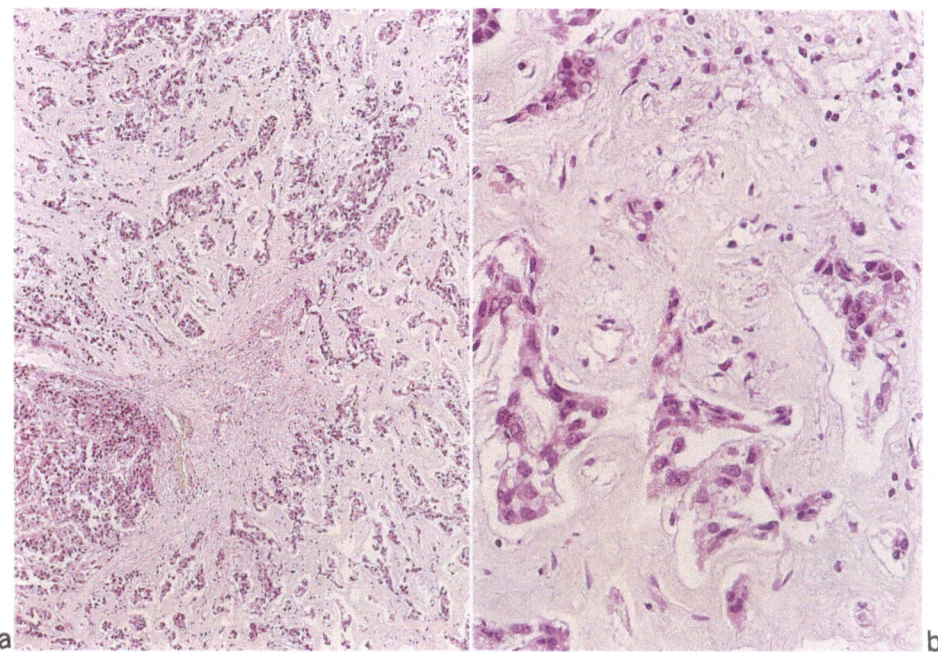

Fig. 15.7. Same case. **a, b** Marked fibrosis in HCC tissue. HE; **a** × 20, **b** × 200

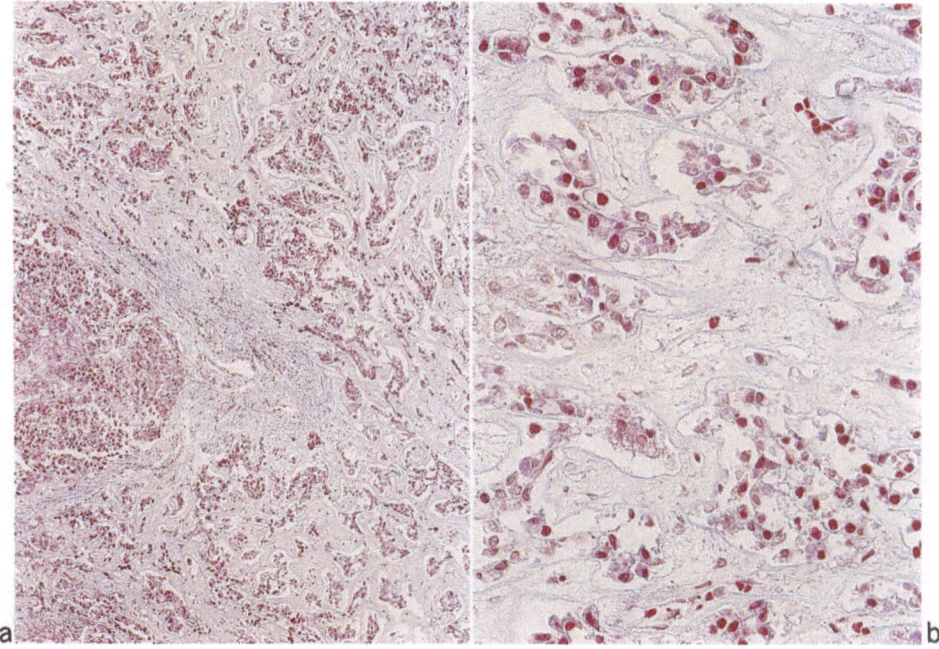

Fig. 15.8. Same case. **a, b** Azan-Mallory. **a** × 20, **b** × 200

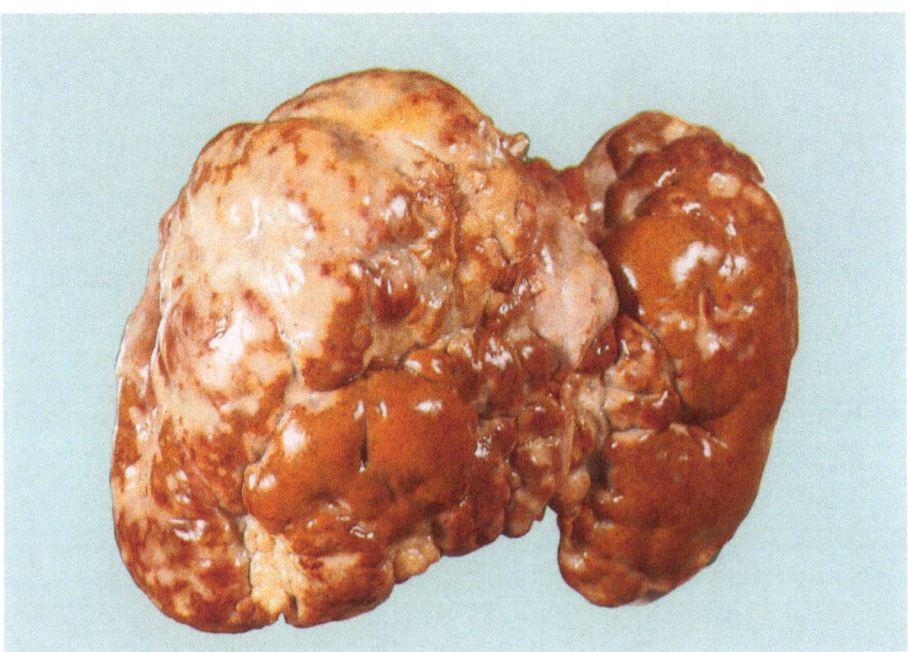

Fig. 15.9. Metastatic breast cancer in the liver treated by repeated intra-arterial injections of anti-cancer drugs. Irregular scarring is dominant

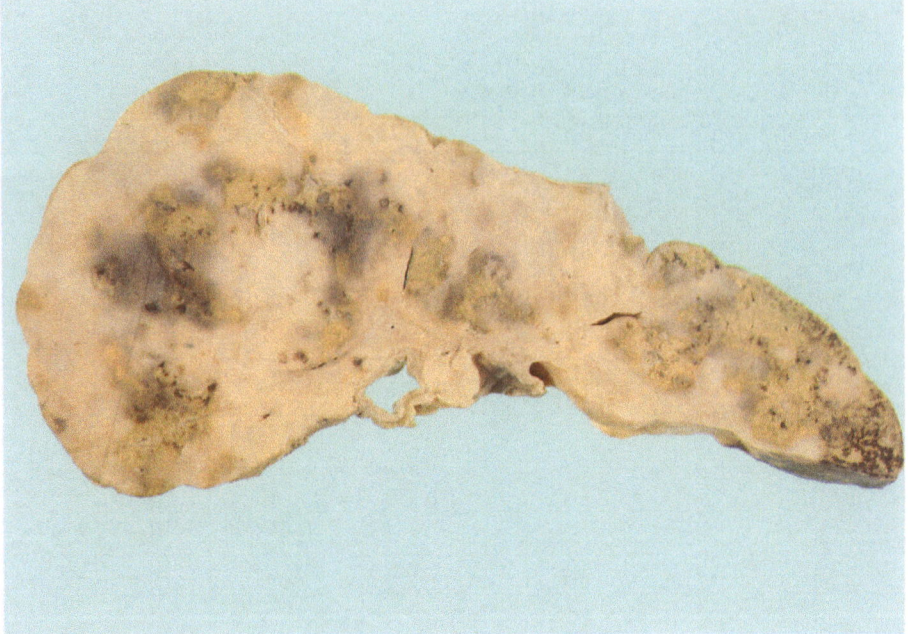

Fig. 15.10. Same case. Metastatic cancer shows scar-like appearance

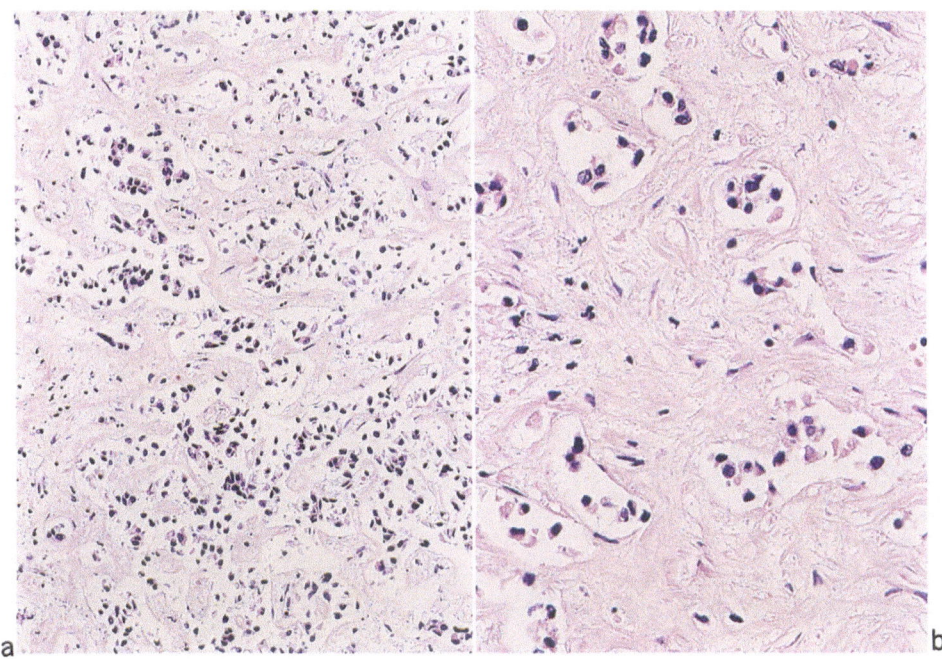

Fig. 15.11. Same case. **a, b** Cancer nests are highly atrophied due to dense fibrosis. HE; **a** × 50, **b** × 200

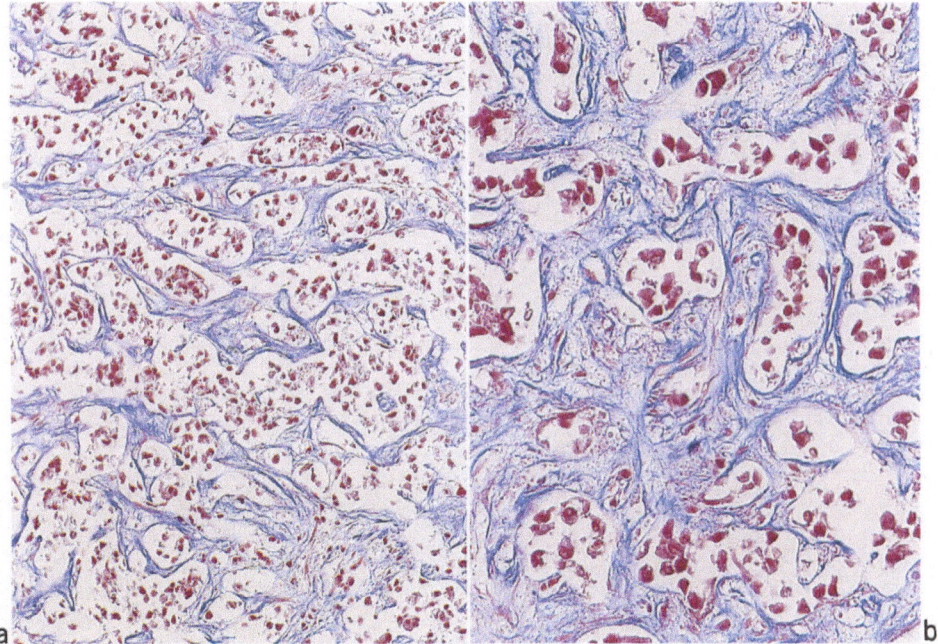

Fig. 15.12. Same case. **a, b** Azan-Mallory. **a** × 50, **b** × 200

References

1. Berman C (1951) Primary carcinoma of the liver. H.K. Lewis, London
2. Morgagni JB (1954) The seats and causes of diseases (Cited in [9])
3. Virchow R (1862) Krankheiten Geschwulste. Hirschwald, Berlin
4. Hansemann D (1890) Über den primären Krebs der Leber. Berl Klin Wochenschr 27: 353–356
5. Hanot V, Gilbert A (1888) Etudes sur les maladies du foie. Asselin and Houzeau, Paris (Cited in [9])
6. Eggel H (1910) Über das primäre Carcinom der Leber. Beitr z path Anat z allg Path 30: 506–604
7. Yamagiwa K (1911) Primary parenchymatous carcinoma of the liver (hepatoma). Gann 5: 225–282
8. Goldzieher M, Bokay Z (1911) Der primäre Leber Krebs. Virchows Arch [A] 203: 75–131
9. Edmondson HA, Steiner PE (1954) Primary carcinoma of the liver. A study of 100 cases among 48 900 necropsies. Cancer 7: 462–503
10. Edmondson HA (1958) Tumors of the liver and intrahepatic bile ducts. Section III, Fascile 25. Armed Forces Institute of Pathology, Washington DC
11. Miyaji T (1977) A close association of hepatocellular carcinoma with cirrhotic changes among 275 857 pathological autopsy cases in Japan during 16 years from 1958 to 1973. Kurume Med J 24: Suppl 63–79
12. Kew MC, Geddes EW (1982) Hepatocellular carcinoma in rural southern African blacks. Medicine 61: 98–108
13. Okuda K, Peters RL, Simson IW (1984) Gross anatomic features of hepatocellular carcinoma from three disparate geographic areas, proposal of new classification. Cancer 54: 2165–2173
14. Craig JR, Peters RL, Edmondson HA, et al. (1980) Fibrolamellar carcinoma of the liver; a tumor of adolescents and young adults with distinctive clinico-pathologic features. Cancer 46: 372–379
15. Pedersen KO (1944) Fetuin, a new globulin isolated from serum. Nature 154: 575
16. Abelev GI, Perova SD, Khramkova NI, et al. (1963) Production of embryonal α-globulin by trasplantable mouse hepatoma. Transplantation I: 174–180
17. Tatarinov JS (1964) New data on the embryospecific antigen components of human blood serum. Vopr Med Khim 10: 584–588
18. Nishi S (1970) Isolation and characterization of a human fetal α-globulin from the sera of fetuses and a hepatoma patient. Cancer Res 30: 2507–2513
19. Vogel CL, Anthony PP, Mody N, et al. (1970) Hepatitis-associated antigen in Ugandan patients with hepatocellular carcinoma. Lancet ii: 621–624
20. Prince AM, Szmuness W, Michon J, et al. (1975) A case control study of the association between primary liver cancer and hepatitis B infection in Senegal. Int J Cancer 16: 376–383
21. Lee YS (1979) Hepatic cirrhosis in Singapore: differences between the Chinese and Indian ethnic groups. Trop Geogr Med 31: 329–338
22. Yap EH, Ong YW, Simons MJ, et al. (1972) Australia antigen in Singapore: II. Differential frequency in Chinese Malays and Indians. Vox Sang 22: 371–375
23. Nishikawa K (1978) Hepatocellular carcinoma and hepatitis B virus. In: Hepatitis virus. Japan Medical Research Foundation, Tokyo University Press, Tokyo, pp 247–255
24. Sherlock S, Fox RA, Niazi SP, et al. (1970) Chronic liver disease and primary liver-cell carcinoma with hepatitis-associated (Australia) antigen in serum. Lancet i: 1243–1247

25. Tong MJ, San SC, Schaffer BT, et al. (1971) Hepatitis-associated antigen and hepatocellular carcinoma in Taiwan. Ann Intern Med 75: 687–691

26. Ohbayashi A, Okochi K, Mayumi M (1971) Familial clustering of asymptomatic carriers of Australia antigen and patients with chronic liver disease or primary liver cancer. Gastroenterology 62: 618–623

27. Alexander JJ, Bay Em, Gedds EW, et al. (1976) Establishment of a continuously growing cell line from primary carcinoma of the liver. S Afr Med J 18: 2124–2128

28. Macnab GM, Alexander JJ, Lecatsos G, et al. (1976) Hepatitis B surface antigen produced by a human hepatoma cell line. Br J Cancer 34: 509–515

29. Huh N, Utakoji T (1981) Production of HBs-antigen by two new human hepatoma cell lines and its enhancement by dexamethasone. Gann 72: 178–179

30. Chakraborty PR, Ruiz-Opazo N, Shouval D, et al. (1980) Identification of integrated hepatitis B virus DNA and expression of viral RNA in an HBs-Ag producing human hepatocellular cell line. Nature 286: 531–533

31. Shafritz D, Shouval D, Sherman HI, et al. (1981) Integration of hepatitis B virus DNA into the genome of liver cells in chronic liver disease and hepatocellular carcinoma. N Engl J Med 305: 1067–1073

32. Brechot C, Pourcel C, Hadchouel M, et al. (1982) State of hepatitis B virus DNA in liver disease. Hepatology 2: 27 S-34 S

33. Chen DS, Hoyer BH, Nelson J, et al. (1982) Detection and properties of hepatitis B viral DNA in liver tissues from patients with hepatocellular carcinoma. Hepatology 2: 42 S-46 S

34. Hino O, Kitagawa T, Koike K, et al. (1984) Detection of hepatitis B virus DNA in hepatocellular carcinoma in Japan. Hepatology 4: 90–95

35. Steiner PE (1960) Cancer of the liver and cirrhosis in Transsaharan Africa and the United States of America. Cancer 13: 1085–1166

36. Nakashima T, Sakamoto K (1977) A study of hepatocellular carcinoma among Japanese from the point of view of morphodevelopmental pathology. Gross anatomical types classified in its relation to capsule formation. Kurume Med J 24 Suppl: 43–62

37. Okuda K, Musha H, Nakajima Y, et al. (1977) Clinicopathological features of encapsulated hepatocellular carcinoma. A study of 26 cases. Cancer 40: 1240–1954

38. Nakashima T, Okuda K, Kojiro M, et al. (1983) Pathology of hepatocellular carcinoma in Japan. 232 consecutive cases autopsied in ten years. Cancer 51: 863–877

39. Okabe M (1979) Patho-morphological studies on hepatocellular carcinoma: A study on a mechanism of capsule formation and septum formation of tumor nodules. Acta Hepatol Jpn 20: 144–156

40. Mori W (1956) Studies of metastasis of hepatoma. Its relationship to liver cirrhosis. Tr Soc Pathol Jpn 45: 224–236

41. Miyagi T, Yuko J, Oda T, et al. (1960) Pathomorphological studies on hepatocellular carcinoma in Japan in recent ten years. Acta Hepatol Jpn 1: 17–36

42. Ikari T (1982) Pathomorphological study on hepatocellular carcinoma: A clinicopathological study of minute hepatocellular carcinoma. J Kurume Med Assoc 45: 302–314

43. Sakamoto K (1976) Pathomorphological study on hepatocellular carcinoma: A study of minute hepatoma. J Kurume Med Assoc 13: 18–33

44. Okuda K, Nakashima T, Obata H, et al. (1977) Clinicopathological studies of minute hepatocellular carcinoma. Gastroenterology 73: 109–115

45. Yoshida T, Okasaki N, Yoshino M, et al. (1982) Minute hepatocellular carcinoma without appreciable change in size for seven years. A case report. Cancer 49: 1491–1495

46. Liver Cancer Study Group of Japan (1983) The general rules for the clinical and pathological study of primary liver cancer. Kanehara, Tokyo.

47. Roux (1897) Un cas de cancer primitif du foie avec pericholicystite calculeuse, perforation intestinale. Hemostase hepatique. Rev med de la Suisse Rome 17: 114–119. (Cited in [9])

48. Goldberg SJ, Wallerstein H (1934) Primary massive liver-cell carcinoma. Rev Gastroenterol 1: 305–313. (Cited in [9])

49. Kato Y, Kurosaki Y, Kobayashi K (1971) A case of hepatocellular carcinoma with large ball-shaped tumor thrombus in the right atrium. Naika 28: 349–353

50. Arakawa M, Kage M, Isomura T, et al. (1982) Pathomorphological studies on hepatocellular carcinoma (HCC): Seven cases of HCC with an extrahepatic tumor growth —"pedunculated hepatoma". Acta Hepatol Jpn 23: 942–948

51. Isomura T, Arakawa M, Wada T, et al. (1979) Hepatocellular carcinoma with sarcoma-like

transformation: A case report. Acta Hepatol Jpn 20: 70–75

52. Teruya K, Kamino T, Wasa T, et al. (1968) A case of hepatoma with an interesting X-ray finding. Geka Chiryo 18: 715–719
53. Horie Y, Kato S, Yoshida H, et al. (1983) Pedunculated hepatocellular carcinoma: Report of three cases and review of literature. Cancer 51: 746–751
54. Ninomiya F, Kawahara T, Yamaguchi G, et al. (1980) A case of pedunculated hepatoma. Acta Hepatol Jpn 21: 1581–1586
55. Kakizoe S, Kojiro M, Nakashima T Pathomorphological study of hepatocellular carcinoma with sarcomatous change. Cancer. (in press)
56. Horiuchi N, Kitamura T, Tateishi R (1973) Hepatoma originated in the retroperitoneal space. Oncology 27: 235–243
57. Miyoshi M, Iwasa N, Fujii H, et al. (1977) A case of pedunculated hepatoma with spontaneous rupture. Acta Hepatol Jpn 18: 765–772
58. Cullen TS (1925) Accessory lobes of the liver. Arch Surg 11: 718–764
59. Broders AC (1920) Squamous-cell epithelioma of the lip, a study of five hundred thirty seven cases. JAMA 74: 656–664.
60. Gibson JB (1978) Histological typing of tumours of the liver, biliary tract and pancreas. International Histological Classification of Tumours, 20. World Health Organization, Geneva
61. Sakurai M, Okamura J, Kuroda C (1984) Transcatheter chemoembolization effective in treating hepatocellular carcinoma. A histologic study. Cancer 54: 387–392
62. Stocker JT, Ishak KG (1978) Undifferentiated (embryonal) sarcoma of the liver. Report of 31 cases. Cancer 42: 336–348
63. Chang WWL, Morgan WS (1983) Primary sarcoma of the liver in the adult. Cancer 51: 1510–1517
64. Jaffe RI (1924) Sarcoma of the liver following cirrhosis. Arch Intern Med 33: 330–342
65. Nagamine Y, Sasaki K, Kaku K, et al. (1978) Hepatic sarcoma associated with hepatoma. Acta Pathol Jpn 28: 645–651
66. Peters RL (1976) Pathology of hepatocellular carcinoma. In: Okuda K, Peters RL (eds) Hepatocellular carcinoma. Wiley, New York, p 107
67. Munoz PA, Rao MS, Reddy JK (1980) Osteoclastoma-like giant cell tumor of the liver. Cancer 46: 771–779
68. Kuwano H, Sonoda T, Hashimot H, et al. (1984) Hepatocellular carcinoma with osteoclast-like giant cells. Cancer 54: 837–842
69. Buchanan TF, Huvos AG (1984) Clear cell carcinoma of the liver. A clinicopathologic study of 13 patients. Am J Clin Pathol 61: 529–539
70. Wu PC, Lai KC, Lok ASF, et al. (1983) Clear cell carcinoma of the liver. An ultrastructural study. Cancer 52: 504–507
71. Sasaki K, Okuda S, Takahashi M, et al. (1981) Hepatic clear cell carcinoma associated with hypoglycemia and hypercholesterolemia. Cancer 47: 820–822
72. Ross JS, Kurian S (1985) Clear cell hepatocellular carcinoma. Sudden death from severe hypoglycemia. Gastroenterology 80: 188–194
73. Mcfadzean AJS, Yeung RTT (1969) Further observations on hypoglycemia in hepatocellular carcinoma. Am J Med 47: 220–235
74. Mallory FB (1911) Cirrhosis of the liver. Five different types of lesions from which it may arise. Bull John Hopkins Hosp 22: 69–75
75. Monroe S, French SW, Zamoboni L (1973) Mallory bodies in a case of primary biliary cirrhosis, an ultrastructural and morphogenetic study. Am J Pathol 59: 254–262
76. Popper H (1968) Comments-103, Wilson's disease. In: Bergman D (ed) Birth defects original articles series, vol. 4, no. 2. The National Foundation-March of Dimes, New York, pp
77. Gerber MA, Denk H, Popper H, et al. (1973) Hepatocellular hyalin in cholestasis and cirrhosis; its diagnostic significance. Gastroenterology 64: 89–98
78. Roy S, Ramalingaswami V, Nayak NC (1971) An ultrastructural study of the liver in Indian childhood cirrhosis with particular reference to the structure of cytoplasmic hyalin. Gut 12: 693–701
79. Michel RP, Limacher JJ, Kimoff RJ (1982) Mallory bodies in scar adenocarcinoma of the lung. Hum Pathol 24: 81–85
80. Kuhn C III, Kuo TT (1973) Cytoplasmic hyalin in asbestosis. Arch Pathol 85: 25–32
81. Norkin SA, Campagna-Pinto D (1968) Cytoplasmic hyaline inclusions in hepatoma. Arch Pathol 86: 25–32

82. Enginger FM, Winshow DJ (1962) Liposarcoma—a study of 103 cases. Virchow Arch [A] 335: 367–388

83. Popper H, Schaffner F (1962) Progress in liver disease. New York, pathology of Kaposi's sarcoma. Un Cintra Cancer 28: 413–428

84. Palmer PE, Wolfer HJ (1976) Alpha-1-antitrypsin deposition in primary hepatic carcinomas. Arch Pathol Lab Med 100: 232–236

85. Pariente EA, Degott C, Martin JP, et al. (1981) Hepatocytic PAS-positive diastase-resistant inclusions in the absence of alpha-1-antitrypsin dificiency: High prevalence in alcoholic cirrhosis. Am J Clin Pathol 76: 299–302

86. Nakanuma Y, Ohta G (1985) Is Mallory body formation a preneoplastic change? A study of 181 cases of liver bearing hepatocellular carcinoma and 82 cases cirrhosis. Cancer 55: 2400–2404

87. Tomimatsu H (1983) Electron microscopic study of Mallory body in hepatocellular carcinoma. Acta Hepatol Jpn 24: 513–520

88. Keeley AF, Iseri OA, Gottlieb LS (1972) Ultrastructure of hyaline cytoplasmic inclusion in a human hepatoma: Relationship to Mallory's alcoholic hyalin. Gastroenterology 62: 280–293

89. Enat R, Buschmann RJ, Chomet B (1973) Ultrastructure of cytoplasmic hyaline inclusions in a case of human hepatocarcinoma. Gastroenterology 65: 802–810

90. Stromeyer FW, Ishak KG, Gerber MA (1980) Ground-glass cells in hepatocellular carcinoma. Am J Clin Pathol 74: 254–258

91. Gregorie HB, Othersen HB, Moore M (1962) The significance of sarcoid-like reaction in association with malignant neoplasm. Am J Surg 104: 577–586

92. Neville E, Piyasena KHG, James DG (1975) Granulomas of the liver. Postgrad Med J 51: 361–365

93. Tomimatsu H, Kojiro M, Nakashima T (1982) Epithelioid granulomas associated with hepatocellular carcinoma. Arch Pathol Lab Med 106: 538

94. Tanikawa K (1979) Ultrastructural aspects of the liver and its disorders, 2nd edn. Igakushoin, Tokyo, pp 338–348

95. Isomura T, Nakashima T (1980) Ultrastructure of human hepatocellular carcinoma. Acta Pathol Jpn 30: 713–726

96. Schaffner F, Popper H (1963) Capillarization of hepatic sinusoid in man. Gastroenterology 44: 239–242

97. Anthony PP (1973) Primary carcinoma of the liver; a study of 282 cases in Uganda Africans. J Pathol 1101: 37–48

98. Cameron HM (1976) Liver cell carcinoma. In: Cameron DA, Linsel GP Warwick (eds) Elsevier, Oxford, pp 21–26

99. Yokoo H, Minick OJ, Batti F, et al. (1972) Morphologic variants of alcoholic hyalin. Am J Pathol 69: 24–40

100. Shirai F (1982) Pathological study on hepatocellular carcinoma. A study of growth pattern. Acta Hepatol Jpn 23: 1034–1042

101. Nakashima T (1985) Metastasis of hepatocellular carcinoma. J Jpn Med Ass 93: 169–172

102. Takemoto N (1982) Pathomorphological study of hepatocellular carcinoma. Ultrastructure of tumor-nontumor boundary. Acta Hepatol Jpn 23: 1–9

103. Sugihara S, Kojiro M, Nakashima T (1985) Ultrastructural study of hepatocellular carcinoma with replacing growth pattern. Acta Pathol Jpn 35: 549–559

104. Bierman HR, Byron RL, Kelley KH, et al. (1951) Studies of blood supply of tumors in man. Vascular pattern of the liver by hepatic arteriography in vivo. J Natl Cancer Inst 12: 107–131

105. Seldinger SI (1958) Catheter replacement of the needle in percutaneous arteriography; a new technique. Acta Radiol [Diagn] 39: 368–376

106. Ödman P (1958) Percutaneous selective angiography of celiac artery. Acta Radiol [Suppl] 159

107. Boijsen E, Abrams HL (1965) Roentgenologic diagnosis of primary carcinoma of the liver. Acta Radiol [Diagn] 3: 257–277

108. Yu C (1967) Primary carcinoma of the liver (hepatoma). Its diagnosis by selective celiac arteriography. Am J Roentenol 99: 142–149

109. Kido C, Sasaki T, Kaneko M (1971) Angiography of primary liver cancer. Am J Roentgenol Rad Ther Nuclear Med 113: 70–81

110. Okuda K, Mucha H, Yoshida T, et al. (1975) Demonstration of growing casts of hepatocellular carcinoma in the portal vein by celiac angiography: The thread and streaks sign. Radiology 117: 303–309

111. Okuda K, Obata H, Jinnouchi S, et al. (1977) Angiographic assessment of gross anatomy of hepatocellular carcinoma: Comparison of celiac angiograms and liver pathology in 100 cases. Radiology 123: 21–29
112. Okuda K, Jinnouchi S, Nagasaki Y, et al. (1977) Angiographic demonstration of growth of hepatocellular carcinoma in the hepatic vein and inferior vena vaca. Radiology 124: 33–36
113. Takashima T, Matsui O (1980) Infusion hepatic angiography in the detection of small hepatocellular carcinoma. Radiology 136: 321–325
114. Yamada R, Nakatsuka H, Nakamura K, et al. (1981) Transcatheter arterial embolization therapy for hepatoma: Assessment in blood chemistry. Jpn J Gastroenterol 78: 214–221
115. Sato M, Yamada R (1982) Conservertive therapy for hepatoma—transcatheter arterial embolization therapy (TEA). Kan Tan Sui 5: 1169–1175
116. Kanno T, Kadona J, Maruge T, et al. (1982) A comparison of transcatheter arterial embolization with intraarterial one-shot injection of anticancer drugs for patients with hepatocellular carcinoma. Acta Hepatol Jpn 23: 622–628
117. Nakashima T (1975) Vascular changes and hemodynamics in hepatocellular carcinoma. In: Okuda K, Peters RL (eds) Hepatocellular carcinoma. Wiley, New York, pp 169–203
118. Kuratomi S (1976) A histopathological study of hepatocellular carcinoma: Pathology of advanced hepatocellular carcinoma and intravascular tumor thrombosis in relation to vascular structure and alterations. Acta Hepatol Jpn 17: 517–527
119. Motoyama F (1982) Pathomorphological studies on hepatocellular carcinoma: A study of angioarchitecture of tumor thrombus of the portal vein. J Kurume Med Assoc 45: 1085–1095
120. Nakashima T, Kojiro M (1983) Pathology of hepatocellular carcinoma. Jpn J Surg 84: 939–942
121. Jimi A (1983) Pathomorphological study on hepatocellular carcinoma: A study of tumor thrombus of the portal vein. Acta Hepatol Jpn 24: 641–647
122. Nakashima T, Kojiro M, Sugihara S, et al. (1984) Tumor thrombus of portal and hepatic veins in hepatocellular carcinoma. J Kurume Med Assoc 47: 454–467
123. Kakizoe S, Kojiro M, Sugihara S, et al. (1985) Pathomorphological studies on hepatocellular carcinoma: A study of histologic features of tumor thrombus in the portal vein. J Kurume Med Assoc 48: 662–668
124. Kitagawa T, Sugioka G, Takazawa Y, et al. (1963) An autopsy case of liver cirrhosis with acute Budd-Chiari syndrome due to complicating liver carcinoma. Naika 12: 1178–1182
125. Takeuchi J. Taketa A, Hasumura Y, et al. (1971) Budd-Chiari syndrome associated with obstruction of the inferior vena cava. Am J Med 51: 11–20
126. Kanayama R, Hirose S, Sawae G, et al. (1969) A case of hepatocellular carcinoma died of acute heart failure due to ball-shaped tumor thrombus in the right atrium. Clin All-Round 18: 825–829
127. Simpson WM (1924) Tumor-thrombosis of the inferior vena cava with four additional cases of neoplastic invasion. Ann Clin Med 3: 29–68
128. Gustafson EG (1937) An analysis of 62 cases of primary carcinoma of the liver based on 24 400 necropsies at Bellevue Hospital. Ann Int Med 11: 889–900
129. Gregory R (1939) Primary carcinoma of the liver. Tumor thrombosis of the inferior vena cava and right auricle. Arch Int Med 64: 566–578
130. MacDonald RA (1957) Primary carcinoma of the liver. Arch Int Med 99: 266–279
131. Kika G (1927) Statistical study of 110 cases of primary liver cancer in Pathology Department of Tokyo University and a study of collateral circulation in hepatoma. Gann 23: 341–37
132. Kikuchi H, Hashimato M, Katagiri H, et al. (1965) Primary liver carcinoma and Budd-Chiari syndrome. Acta Pathol Jpn 6: 337–342
133. Shikara T (1969) Pathology of Budd-Chiari syndrome. Acta Hepatol Jpn 10: 181–184
134. Kojiro M, Nakahara H, Sugihara S, et al. (1984) Hepatocellular carcinoma with intra-atrial tumor growth. A clinicopathologic study of 18 autopsy cases. Arch Pathol Lab Med 108: 989–992
135. Nakamura T, Nakamura S, Aikawa T, et al. (1968) Obstruction of the inferior vena cava in the hepatic portion and the hepatic veins. Angiology 19: 479–498
136. Araki U, Miyazaki T (1974) Primary liver carcinoma. Clinical and statistical studies of Japanese liver carcinoma. Jpn J Clin Med 32: 2231–2262
137. Takada A, Kaneyama R, et al. (1969) Budd-Chiari syndrome. Main study of secondary Budd-Chiari syndrome. Saishin lgaku 24: 1055
138. Hahne OH, Climie ARH (1962) Right atrial thrombi with ball-valve action. Am J Med 32: 942–946

139. Kumagaya Y (1979) Pathomorphological study on hepatocellular carcinoma: A study of intrabile duct tumor growth. Acta Hepatol Jpn 20: 157–163
140. Kojiro M, Kawabata K, Kawano Y, et al. (1982) Hepatocellular carcinoma presenting as intrabile duct tumor growth. A clinicopathologic study of 24 cases. Cancer 49: 2144–2147
141. Gray W, Futterman S (1977) Obstructive jaundice secondary to hepatoma, case report and literature review. Am J Gastroenterol 67: 80–83
142. Mallory TB (1947) Hepatoma with invasion of cystic duct and metastasis to 3rd lumber vertebra. N Engl J Med 2137: 673–678
143. Lin TY (1972) Tumor of the liver. Part 1: Primary malignant tumors. In: Bockus HL, Berk JE, Haubrich WS, Kalser M, Roth LA, Vilardell F (eds) Gastroenterology, 3rd edn. Sanders, Philadelphia, p 522
144. Okuda K, Nakashima T (1967) Primary carcinoma of the liver. In: Berk JE, Haubrich WS, Kalserm, Roth LA, Schaffner F (eds) Bockus Gastroenterology, 4th edn. Sanders, Philadelphia, p 3315
145. Sandblom P (1948) Hemorrhage into the biliary tract following trauma. Traumatic hemobilia. Surgery 24: 581–586
146. Herxheimer G (1930) Lebergewächse. In: Henke F, Lubarsch O (eds) Handbuch der Speziellen pathologischen Anatomie und Histologie V/1, p 797
147. Wilber DL, Wood DA, Wilett FM (1944) Primary carcinoma of the liver. Ann Int Med 20: 453–485
148. Hoyne RM, Kernohan JW (1947) Primary carcinoma of the liver. A study of 31 cases. Arch Int Med 79: 532–554
149. Paget S (1928) The distribution of secondary growth in cancer of the breast. Lancet i: 571–573
150. Hort IB, Fidler IJ (1980) Role of organ selectivity in the determination of metastatic patterns of B 16 melanoma. Cancer Res 40: 2281–2287
151. Berman C (1941) The pathology of primary carcinoma of the liver in the Bantu races of South Africa. S Afr J Med Sci 6: 11–26
152. Meyer PG (1954) Das primäre Lebercarcinom in Basel 1937–1952. Zschr Krebsforsch 60: 115–138
153. Mathhews WF, Abell MR (1954) Primary carcinoma of liver. Univ Michigan M Bull 25: 313–332
154. Tsakraklides V, Templetion AC, Estensen R, et al. (1975) Hepatocellular carcinoma. A clinical and pathological study of 33 cases. Minn Med 58: 450–453
155. Tull JC (1932) Primary carcinoma of the liver: a study of one hundred and thirty-four cases. J Pathol Bact 35: 557–562
156. Okuda K (1976) Clinical aspect of hepatocellular carcinoma. Analysis of 134 cases. In: Okuda K, Peters RL (eds) Hepatocellular carcinoma. Wiley, New York, p 384
157. Strong GE, Pitts HH, Mephee JG (1949) Primary carcinoma of the liver—25 years study. Ann Int Med 30: 791–798
158. Smith KG (1933) Primary carcinoma of the liver. A clinicopathologic study. J Lab Clin Med 18: 915–925
159. Goveia G, Bahn S (1978) Asymptomatic hepatocellular carcinoma metastasis to the mandible. Oral Surg 45: 424–430
160. Ishizu H, Yasumuro Y, Fujit S, et al. (1951) A clinicopathological study on bone metastases in the autopsied cases with hepatocellular carcinoma. Acta Hepatol Jpn 17: 47–53
161. Haratake J, Nakamura Y, Ota G, et al. (1978) An autopsy case of hepatocellular carcinoma presenting main clinical signs of complete spinal transection. Jpn J Gastroenterol 75: 552–556
162. Matsuzaki O, Murata K, Yano S, et al. (1976) Two autopsy cases of metastatic liver tumor to the stomach. Jpn J Gastroenterol 73: 1314
163. Saijo N, Kure Y, Akazawa S, et al. (1978) An autopsy case of hepatoma with metastasis showing a feature of Borrman type I in the stomach. Jpn J Clin Cancer 24: 786–789
164. Shibata T, Nakano T, Kitamura K, et al. (1981) A case of a metastatic hepatocellular carcinoma to the stomach via the blood stream. Jpn J Gastroenterol 78: 1998–2002
165. Kawano Y, Sugihara S, Tomimatsu H, et al. (1982) Metastasis to the stomach, brain and heart in hepatocellular carcinoma. Jpn J Clin Cancer 28: 1157–1162
166. Kimura M, Niwa H, Hirayama Y, et al. (1981) A case of metastatic liver tumor to duodenum. Gastroenterol Endosc 23: 989–995
167. Wada I, Hani H, Hirayama Y (1983) Metastasis of hepatocellular carcinoma to the duodenum: An autopsy case with triple primary carcinoma on heterotaxia (situs inversus transversus

viscerum totalis) Jpn J Gastroenterol 80: 228–231
168. Hanfling SM (1960) Metastatic cancer to the heart. Review of the literature and report of 127 cases. Circulation 22: 474–483
169. Liber AF, Brown CR (1939) Primary liver cell carcinoma with splenic metastases. Am J Cancer 35: 521–527
170. Al-Sarraf M, Kithier K, Vaithericius VK (1974) Primary liver cancer. A review of the clinical features, blood groups, serum enzymes, therapy, and survival of 65 cases. Cancer 33: 574–582
171. Kawabata K (1980) Pathomorphological studies on hepatocellular carcinoma: A study of the lymphnode with marked metastasis of hepatocellular carcinoma. Acta Hepatol Jpn 21: 203–215.
172. Ko S (1978) Lymphatic system of the liver. J Jpn Coll Angiol 18: 233–238
173. Sotsuna M (1968) Lymphatic system in Japanese. Kanehara Shuppan, Tokyo, pp 165–169
174. Sugawara K, Wada T, Yoshioka M (1984) Lymph nodes in hepatocellular carcinoma. In: Hattori N (ed) Viral hepatitis to hepatocellular carcinoma. Gan to Kagakuryoho-sha, Tokyo, p 579
175. Saitsu H, Okuda K, Yoshida K, et al. (1986) Confirmation of the presence of lymph channels in hepatoma nodes for use in the treatment of hepatocellular carcinoma. Acta Hepatol Jpn 27: 1296–1302
176. Orsos F (1930) Zur Struktur und Histogenese der primären Leberkrebs. Beitr z path Anat u z allg Path 84: 33–105 (Cited in [9])
177. Green JM (1939) Primary carcinoma of the liver. A ten year collection review. Surg Gynecol Obstet 69: 231
178. MacSween RNM (1974) A clinico-pathological review of 100 primary malignant tumours of the liver. J Clin Pathol 27: 669–682
179. Inde DC, Sherlock P, Winower SJ, et al. (1974) Clinical manifestations of hepatoma: a review of 6 years experience at a cancer hospital. Am J Med 56: 83–91
180. Shikata T (1976) Primary liver carcinoma and liver cirrhosis. In: Okuda K, Peters RL (eds) Hepatocellular carcinoma. Wiley, New York, p 53
181. Jim WSJ (1980) Hepatoma in Taiwan: a pathological study. Trans Gastroenterol Aoc Roc 9: 3–5
182. Lin DY, Liaq YF, Chu CM (1984) Hepatocellular carcinoma in noncirrhotic patients. A laparoscopic study of 92 cases in Taiwan. Cancer 54: 1466–1468
183. Gall EA (1960) Posthepatitic, postnecrotic and nutritional cirrhosis. A pathologic analysis. Am J Pathol 36: 241
184. Miyake J (1960) Pathology of the liver. Main study of the liver cirrhosis. Tr Soc Pathol Jpn 49: 589–632
185. Nishioka K (1973) Report of WHO associated workshop of hepatitis B antigen. World Health Organization, Geneva
186. Mori W (1967) Cirrhosis and primary cancer of the liver. Comparative study in Tokyo and Cincinnati. Cancer 20: 627–631
187. Karasawa T, Kushida T, Shikata T, et al. (1980) Morphologic spectrum of liver disease among chronic alcoholics. A comparison between Tokyo, Japan and Cincinnati, USA. Acta Pathol Jpn 30: 505–514
188. Nonomura A, Hayashi M, Takayanagi N, et al. (1986) Correlation of morphologic subtypes of liver cirrhosis with excess alcohol intake, HBV infection, age at death, and hepatocellular carcinoma: A study of 234 autopsy cases in Japan. Acta Pathol Jpn 36: 631–640
189. Simson IW (1982) Membranous obstruction of the inferior vena cava and hepatocellular carcinoma in South Africans. Gastroenterology 82: 171–178
190. Rosenthal SR (1932) Hemochromatosis and primary carcinoma of liver; report of case with review of literature and discussion of pathogenesis. Arch Pathol 13: 88–105
191. Berk JE, Lieber MM (1941) Primary carcinoma of the liver in hemochromatosis. Am J Med Sci 202: 708–714
192. Warren SS, Drake WK (1951) Primary carcinoma of the liver in hemochromatosis. Am J Pathol 27: 573–591
193. Nakashima T, Okuda K, Kojiro M, et al. (1975) Primary liver cancer coincident with schistosomiasis japonica. A study of 24 necropsies. Cancer 36: 1483–1489
194. Warvi WH (1944) Primary neoplasm of the liver. Arch Pathol 37: 367–382
195. Prates MD (1957) On etiology of primary cancer of liver in natives of Mozambique. Int J Cancer 13: 662–668

196. Iuchi M, Hayakawa, Kitani K, et al. (1973) Primary liver tumor in chronic schistosomiasis japonica. Acta Hepatol Jpn 14: 249–252
197. Gibson JE (1971) Parasites, liver disease and liver cancer. International Agency for Research on Cancer, Lyon, pp 42–52
198. Hou PC (1985) Relationship between primary carcinoma of the liver and infestation with *Clonorchis sinensis*. J Pathol Bact 72: 239–246
199. Liang PC, Tung C (1959) Morphologic study and etiology of primary liver carcinoma and its incidence in China. Chin Med J 79: 336–347
200. MacMahon E, Murphy AS, Bates MI (1947) Endothelial cell sarcoma of the liver following Thorotrast injection. Am J Pathol 23: 585–613
201. Mori T, Kato Y, Shimamine T, et al. (1979) Statistical analysis of Japanese Thorotrast-administered autopsy cases. Environ Res 18: 231–244
202. Wegner K, Welch H, Kampmann H (1976) Investigations in human thorotrastosis. Virchow Arch A (Pathol Anat) 371: 131–143
203. Umezu T (1984) Pathomorphological study on Thorotrast-induced hepatic angiosarcoma. J Kurume Med Assoc 47: 62–73
204. Kojiro M, Nakashima T, Ito Y, et al. (1985) Thorium dioxide-related angiosarcoma of the liver. Pathomorphologic study of 29 autopsy cases. Arch Pathol Lab Med 109: 853–857
205. Kojiro M, Nakashima T, Ito Y, et al. (1986) Pathomorphological study on Thorotrast-induced hepatic malignancies. In: The radiobiology of radium and thorotrast. Urban and Schwarzenberg, Munich, pp 119–122
206. Hirayama Y (1975) Problems in epidemiology of Au antigen. J Jpn Med Assoc 73: 171–181
207. Alpert E, Isselbacher KJ (1971) Hepatitis-associated antigen and hepatoma in the U.S. Lancet ii: 1087
208. Kew M, Geddes EW (1982) Hepatocellular carcinoma in rural southern African blacks. Medicine 61: 98–108
209. Sung JC, Chen DS (1976) Hepatitis B surface antigen and antibody in liver disease in Taiwan. In: Proceedings Fifth Asian Pacific Congress of Gastroenterology. Abst, Singapore, pp 265–269
210. Beasley RP, Stevens CE (1974) Epidemiology of hepatitis B infection in Taiwan. In: Proceedings International Symposium on Hepatitis in Taipei. Abst, Singapore pp 1–10
211. Sakurai M, Miyaji T (1977) Orcein staining of hepatitis B surface antigen in paraffin section of liver on autopsy cases. Acta Hepatogastroenterol 24: 334–449
212. Bartok I, Remenar E, Toth J (1976) Demonstration of hepatitis B surface antigen by orcein staining in paraffin sections of cirrhotic liver. Virchows Arch [A] 369: 23–248
213. Cohen C, Berson SO, Geddes EW (1978) Hepatitis B antigen in black patients with hepatocellular carcinoma. Correlation between orcein stained liver sections and serology. Cancer 41: 245–249
214. Hsu HC, Jin WSJ, Tsai MJ (1983) Hepatitis B surface antigen and hepatocellular carcinoma in Taiwan, with special reference to types and localization of HBs Ag in the tumor cells. Cancer 52: 1825–1832
215. Nakashima T, Kojiro M, Kawano Y, et al. (1982) Histological growth pattern of hepatocellular carcinoma. Relationship to orcein (hepatitis B surface-antigen) positive cells in cancer tissue. Hum Pathol 13: 563–568
216. Anthony PP, Vogal CH, Barker LF (1973) Liver cell dysplasia; a premalignant condition. J Clin Pathol 26: 217–223
217. Sakurai M (1978) Liver cell dysplasia and hepatitis B surface and core antigens in cirrhosis and hepatocellular carcinoma of autopsy cases. Acta Pathol Jpn 28: 705–719
218. Cohen C, Berson SD, Geddes EW (1977) Liver cell dysplasia. Association with hepatocellular carcinoma, cirrhosis and hepatitis B antigen carrier status. Cancer 44: 1671–1676
219. Okita K, Kodama T, Harada T, et al. (1977) Early lesions and development of primary hepatocellular carcinoma in man—association with hepatitis B viral infection. Gastroenterol Jpn 12: 51–57
220. Kojiro M (1986) Liver cell dysplasia. Digestive Med 4: 6–11
221. The Japanese Pathological Society (1968–1974) Annual of the pathological autopsy cases in Japan, pp 10–17
222. Nakamura K, Aizawa K (1972) A study of multiple cancer from the point of view of combination: Analysis of 1121 cases of multiple cancer. Jpn J Clin Cancer 18: 662–666
223. Kimoto T, Ugaki M (1982) Hepatocellular carcinoma combined with hepatic mesenchymal cell

tumor and sarcoma. Acta Pathol Jpn 32: 1131–1141

224. Hatanaka S, Sawada S, Higawa O (1983) An autopsy case of hepatocellular carcinoma complicated with rhabdomyo-sarcoma considered from the liver. Jpn J Clin Med 42: 895–900

225. Matsu K (1985) Pathological study on hepatocellular carcinoma. A study of histological changes after transcatheter arterial embolization therapy. Acta Hepatol Jpn 26: 1207–1216

226. He L, Isselbacher KJ, Wands JR, et al. (1984) Establishment and characterization of a new human hepatocellular carcinoma cell line. In Vitro 20: 439–504

227. Chen JM, Chu TH, Yen HJ, et al. (1978) The establishment and some characteristics of a human liver carcinoma cell line (BEF-7402) in vitro. Acta Biol Exp Sin 11: 37–50

228. Doi L, Nanba M, Sato J (1975) Establishement and some biological characteristics of human hepatoma cell lines. Gann 66: 385–392

229. Witcultt JM (1975) Establishment of permanent hepatoma cell line from autopsy materials from a case of hepatocellular carcinoma. Proc Mine Med Off Assoc 55: 18

230. Yano H, Kojiro M, Nakashima T (1986) A new human hepatocellular carcinoma cell line (KYN-1) with a transformation to adenocarcinoma. In Vitro (in press)

231. Kuwahara T (1980) Heterotransplantation of human hepatoma in nude mice: Establishment of the serially transplantable hepatoma. Acta Hepatol Jpn 21: 303–315

232. Sasaki F (1983) Establishment of alpha-fetoprotein producing human hepatoma cell line and characteristics. Acta Hepatol Jpn 24: 1274–1281

233. Murakami T (1984) Establishment and characterization of human hepatoma cell line (KIM-1) Acta Hepatol Jpn 25: 532–539

234. Lundholm K, Karlbeg I, Sherstem T (1980) Albumin and hepatic protein synthesis in patients with early cancer. Cancer 46: 71–76

235. Kojiro M, Kawano Y, Isomura T, et al. (1981) Distribution of albumin- and/or α-fetoprotein positive cells in hepatocellular carcinoma. Lab Invest 44: 221–226

236. Motoyama T, Watanabe H (1983) Carcinoembryonic antigen production in vitro and in nude mice. Gann 74: 679–686

237. Murakami T, Kojiro M, Nakahima T, et al. (submitted) Establishment of cell line of combined hepatocellular and cholangiocarcinoma (KMCH-1 cell)

238. Allen RA, Lisa JR (1949) Combined liver cell and bile duct carcinoma. Am J Pathol 25: 647–655

239. Goodman ZO, Ishak KG, Langloss JM, et al. (1985) Combined hepatocellular-cholangiocarcinoma. A histological and immunohistochemical study. Cancer 55: 124–135

240. Mori W, Adachi Y, Okabe H, et al. (1963) Analysis of seven hundred and fifty-five autopsy cases of malignant tumors. Statistical study of metastasis. Jpn J Clin Cancer 9: 351–374

241. Arima M (1966) Clinical aspects of primary and secondary carcinomas of the liver. Acta Hepatol Jpn 7: 224–247

242. Abrams HL, Spiro R, Goldstein N (1950) Metastases in carcinoma. Analysis of 1000 autopsied cases. Cancer 3: 74–85

243. Willis RA (1973) The spread of tumors in the human body. Secondary tumors of the liver, 3rd edn. Butterworth, London, pp 175–183

244. Lisa JR, Solomon C, Gordon EJ (1942) Secondary carcinoma in cirrhosis of the liver. Am J Pathol 18: 137–140

245. Lieber MM (1975) The rare occurrence of metastatic carcinoma in the cirrhotic liver. Am J Med Sci 23: 145–152

246. Inayatullah M, De Peyster FA, Capps RB (1963) Metastatic malignancy in cirrhotic liver. Experimental observation and review of literature. Gastroenterology 44: 485

247. Furui S (1982) Computed tomography (CT) and angiography. Diag Therp 70: 1669–1683

248. Honjo I, Matumura H (1965) Vascular distribution of hepatic tumors. Experimental study. Rev Int Hepatol 15: 681–690

249. Ackerman NB, Lien WM, Kondi ES, et al. (1969) The blood supply of experimental liver metastasis: I. The distribution of hepatic artery and portal vein to "small" and "large" tumor. Surgery 66: 1067–1072

250. Lin G, Lunderquist A, Hagerstrand I, et al. (1984) Postmortem examination of the blood supply and vascular pattern of small liver metastasis in man. Surgery 96: 517–526

Subject Index